HEMATOLOGY

A Pathophysiological Approach

Second Edition

HEMATOLOGY
A PATHOPHYSIOLOGICAL APPROACH

Second Edition

Bernard M. Babior, M.D., Ph.D.

Member and Head, Division of Biochemistry
Member, Division of Hematology/Oncology
Department of Molecular and Experimental Medicine
Research Institute of Scripps Clinic
Scripps Clinic and Research Foundation
La Jolla, California

Thomas P. Stossel, M.D.

Chief, Hematology–Oncology Unit
Massachusetts General Hospital
American Cancer Society Professor of Medicine
Harvard Medical School
Boston, Massachusetts

CHURCHILL LIVINGSTONE
New York, Edinburgh, London, Melbourne

Library of Congress Cataloging-in-Publication Data

Babior, Bernard M., date
    Hematology: a pathophysiological approach/Bernard M. Babior, Thomas P. Stossel, —2nd ed.
      p. cm.
    Includes bibliographies and index.
    ISBN 0-443-08608-7
    1. Hematology.   I. Stossel, Thomas P.   II. Title.
    [DNLM: 1. Hematologic Diseases—physiopathology.   WH 100 B114h]
  RB145.B23   1990
  DNLM/DLC
  for Library of Congress   89-17274
                                                   CIP

Second Edition © **Churchill Livingstone Inc. 1990**
First Edition © **Churchill Livingstone Inc. 1984**

Distributed in the United Kingdom by Churchill Livingstone, Robert Stevenson House, 1–3 Baxter's Place, Leith Walk, Edinburgh EH1 3AF, and by associated companies, branches, and representatives throughout the world.

Accurate indications, adverse reactions, and dosage schedules for drugs are provided in this book, but it is possible that they may change. The reader is urged to review the package information data of the manufacturers of the medications mentioned.

The Publishers have made every effort to trace the copyright holders for borrowed material. If they have inadvertently overlooked any, they will be pleased to make the necessary arrangements at the first opportunity.

Acquisitions Editor: *Beth Kaufman Barry*
Copy Editor: *Ann Ruzycka*
Production Designer: *Angela Cirnigliaro*
Production Supervisor: *Jocelyn Eckstein*

Printed in the United States of America

First published in 1990

Preface

Hematology, the study of the blood, is in our not unbiased view the most beautifully rational and therefore the most intellectually satisfying of all the disciplines of medicine. Hematology achieved this status because blood can be studied in the laboratory more easily than any other human tissue. Through a simple venipuncture, the physician–scientist can obtain the material needed to understand how normal blood works, and what goes wrong when the blood is diseased. Because of the availability of this human tissue, more has been learned about disease mechanisms in hematology than in perhaps any other area of medicine. Through this knowledge of mechanisms, logic and order has been brought to the bewilderingly complex field of hematology, and the modern approach to the patient with a disease of the blood has been developed.

Our plan in writing the first edition of this introduction to hematology was to make this inherent connection between mechanisms and diseases as clear as possible. To achieve this goal, we found it necessary to organize the book in a way that differed from the way many hematology books are put together. These innovations were well received and have been retained. The major approaches in our book are the following:

1. We discuss normal function side by side with diseases pertinent to that function. High-affinity hemoglobins, for example, are treated in one of the first chapters in the red cell section—the chapter on the binding of oxygen to hemoglobin—not in a later chapter on mutant hemoglobins. By a similar token, discussion of the mechanisms of destruction of senescent red cells is not presented in a preliminary chapter on red cell turnover, but is deferred to the chapter on extravascular hemolysis, which is one of the later chapters in the red cell section. This close association between the normal and abnormal is maintained throughout the book, serving as an ongoing "clinical correlation" that emphasizes the way in which the principles of normal function are applied to hematological diseases. In this integrated approach, we have done our best to see that these principles are introduced in a logical order, so that by the time the discussion has reached diseases with a complicated pathophysiology (e.g., sickle cell anemia or disseminated intravascular coagulation), most of the relevant principles will have been explained.

2. We employ a classification of hematological diseases that emphasizes pathophysiological mechanisms. This modified classification places a number of diseases into categories somewhat different from those traditionally used. The most extensive modifications are the introduction of a category called stem cell diseases, in which are included several disorders affecting all three blood cell lines that were heretofore squeezed uncomfortably into categories designed for conditions involving only one cell line (e.g., aplastic ane-

mia, paroxysmal nocturnal hemoglobinuria, and essential thrombocythemia), and the addition of a category called immune-mediated blood cell destruction, into which are placed all diseases caused by the immunological destruction of blood cells, regardless of the cell line affected. Other modifications include the distribution of the mutant hemoglobins into functional categories more explicitly than usual, and division of the acute thrombocytopenias between immune cytopenias and disseminated intravascular coagulation/thrombotic thrombocytopenic purpura. Those familiar with the traditional classifications of hematological disorders will probably recognize other modifications as well, mostly minor.

Why change the classification at all? Because a classification scheme is only a mental crutch—a way of arranging a group of things so they can be thought about more easily—and should be altered when a new mode of classification would seem to serve this purpose better than the old. As mentioned above, our aim in this book is to present hematology through correlations between mechanisms and manifestations of disease. We believe the new classification aids in the fulfillment of this particular aim.

3. We have discussed fully certain rare diseases that shed light on pathophysiological principles in a particularly straightforward way. One example of this is our treatment of the α-thalassemias, a group of conditions that provide a striking example of the clinical ramifications of molecular genetics, though they are of relatively minor clinical importance outside the Orient.

By the time most students get around to the initial study of the blood they will already have received instruction in biochemistry, immunology, and physiology. This background was not taken completely for granted in our explanations of principles. Rather, we have attempted to provide further information concerning aspects of hematology about which the readers may already have been instructed in another context (for example, the morphology of blood cells, and the structure of hemoglobin and of immunoglobulins). This material is presented both to jog the memories of informed readers and to show them how their previously acquired knowledge can be applied to the medical discipline of hematology. Repetition is the mother of learning.

True to its history, the science of hematology has moved rapidly, and we have tried to incorporate important new advances into this edition. Of particular note are discoveries in molecular genetics that have radically improved our understanding of hematologic malignancies and have led to the cloning and expression of recombinant hematopoietic growth factors and blood coagulation proteins, not to mention better comprehension of their structure and function. In addition, we responded to criticisms of the first edition by replacing drawings of cells with photomicrographs. We hope that the text will continue to serve as both a useful introduction to clinical hematology for medical students and as a source of review for residents and practicing physicians in related disciplines.

Finally, and most importantly, we again thank our families, Shirley, Greg, and Jill Babior, and Anne, Scott, and Sage Stossel, for their cheerful forbearance as we abandoned them for nights, weekends, and holidays of writing and revising and for the support we needed to see this book through to its realization.

Bernard M. Babior, M.D., Ph.D.
Thomas P. Stossel, M.D.

Contents

The Hot Temperate Red Humor: An Overview of the Blood

The discipline of hematology encompasses the circulating blood and the function of blood cells throughout the body. Robert Burton, in 1628, characterized the blood as a "hot, temperate, red humor whose office is to nourish the whole body to give it strength and color being dispersed by the veins through every part of it." That elegantly simple and apt description of the blood can now be embellished by our deep understanding of the biology of this most excellent humor.

The mass of the circulating blood comprises 5 to 7 percent of our body weight. The blood is a suspension of cells, called the *formed elements*, in *plasma*, a solution of protein and salts. The blood and the circulatory system, the conduit of sluices, gates, and alleyways through which the blood courses, were required for the evolution of complex higher organisms. In these organisms the blood provides for nutrition, oxygenation, the cleansing of wastes, and the defense of body tissues against ever present assault by microbes.

THE COMPONENTS OF THE BLOOD

The principal component of the blood *plasma*, which comprises over half the total blood volume, is water. Our bodies are 70 per-

cent water, our cells all function in a watery environment, and the blood is responsible for bringing adequate hydration to all our tissues. The blood fluid also contains dissolved ions that are crucial for cell functions. These ions are principally sodium, potassium, chloride, hydrogen, magnesium, and calcium. As will be discussed in Chapter 4, the plasma also transports iron, which is vital for crucial tissue enzymes but is particularly important for the structure and function of red blood cells.

The proteins of the blood plasma can be broadly divided into three classes: *carrier proteins, immunoproteins,* and *coagulation proteins.*

The carrier function of plasma proteins is threefold. First, the plasma proteins can bind molecules in the plasma, thereby diminishing the nonspecific diffusion of these molecules into the tissues or their nonspecific interaction with blood and tissue cells. Second, complexes of carrier proteins and molecules bound to them may be recognized by particular cells with a high degree of specificity. In this way molecules such as iron can be directly targeted to cells that require them, as discussed in Chapter 4. Finally, plasma proteins can diminish the toxic effects of certain molecules in the plasma by binding to them and by carrying these neutralized toxins to specific sites, where they can be eliminated. Examples of these three carrier functions are evident for the plasma proteins described in the following paragraph.

The chief plasma protein is *albumin*. Comprising two-thirds of the mass of plasma protein, albumin is the major source of the osmotic pressure of the plasma. In this sense albumin can be said to be a carrier of water, and when the serum albumin level declines, the tissues of the body become edematous. Albumin is also a carrier of many compounds, examples of which are bilirubin and other bile pigments (described in Ch. 5), and of free fatty acids. Albumin does not bind all such molecules with very high avidity, but because of the high albumin concentration, the proportion of these molecules that remain uncomplexed in the plasma is small. Another class of carrier proteins are the *lipoproteins*, which transport cholesterol, triglyceride, and phospholipid between tissues. Two plasma proteins are particularly important for the transport of nutrients needed by the blood. One of these proteins is *transferrin*, an iron-binding protein described in Chapter 4, which carries iron to developing red blood cells. The second carrier is a class of proteins called *transcobalamins*, proteins that transport cobalamins, vital cofactors for DNA synthesis in blood cells and other tissues. The cobalamins are described in Chapter 6.

Another set of carrier proteins complex to substances that may not ordinarily be present in the plasma but appear following injury or tissue destruction. *Haptoglobin* is a protein that binds hemoglobin if this principal red blood cell constituent appears in the plasma because of red blood cell destruction (Ch. 9). A protein with a similar function is *hemopexin*, which binds to free heme released from denatured hemoglobin (Ch. 9). Two proteins, *alpha-1-antiprotease* and *alpha-2-macroglobulin*, bind and neutralize proteolytic enzymes released from destroyed tissues and phagocytic leukocytes (Ch. 18). The protease–antiprotease complexes are avidly cleared from the circulation by mononuclear phagocytes (Ch. 18). These antiproteases also function in the

tissues. Injury and inflammation frequently increase the permeability of blood vessels, allowing plasma constituents to leak into the injured area. The antiproteases participate in the neutralization of proteolytic enzymes activated by the injury and inflammatory processes (Ch. 18). Another "anti-inflammatory" plasma protein is a copper-binding protein called *ceruloplasmin*. Ceruloplasmin participates in the detoxification of oxygen-free radicals that are released during inflammation by phagocytic cells (Ch. 18). In addition, ceruloplasmin is required to prevent the accumulation of copper in tissues, where it can have toxic effects. A congenital disorder in which ceruloplasmin is absent, *Wilson's disease*, is associated with extensive tissue damage, including red blood cell destruction.

Aside from nutrition, defense is the major function of the blood. Both cells and humors participate in this defense. The blood humors active in defense against invading microorganisms are the immunoproteins, the *immunoglobulins*, and the *complement proteins*. These proteins are described in Chapter 16.

One of the tasks of the blood is to maintain the integrity of its conduit, the vascular system. As in defense against infection, cells and humors cooperate in this endeavor. The humoral arm of this defense is the *coagulation system*, a series of plasma proteins that interact to produce gelatinous plugs for sealing breaks and leaks in the vasculature. As described in Chapter 13, a variety of conditions activate the coagulation protein. The solidification of plasma as a result of this activation is due to the formation of a network of strands composed of the protein *fibrin*. Between the strands of fibrin are water, salts, and the majority of plasma proteins. By centrifugation of the clot, these compounds can be squeezed out; collectively they are called the *serum*. One of the stimuli for blood coagulation is contact of the plasma with foreign surfaces such as glass or plastic. Therefore, any attempt to remove blood from the vascular system results in activation of the clotting system unless coagulation is inhibited in some way. For a number of diagnostic procedures involving blood and for blood transfusion (Ch. 30) it is inconvenient to have clotting occur. Therefore blood is often *anticoagulated*. The coagulation system is very dependent on the presence of ionized calcium (Ch. 13), so that if calcium is lowered by means of a suitable chelating agent coagulation is inhibited. Blood can be drawn into a container containing a sufficient quantity of sodium citrate or else ethylenediaminetetraacetic acid (commonly called EDTA) to complex all the free calcium and will not clot. A system of proteins complementary to the coagulation proteins inhibits the coagulation system. It prevents the whole circulation from clotting up at once, if exposed locally to one of the many coagulation activators, and it also breaks down formed clots when they are no longer needed. This system is called the *fibrinolytic system*. The components and interactions of the coagulation and fibrinolytic systems are described in Chapters 13 and 16.

THE FORMED ELEMENTS

The bulk of the formed elements, about one-half the blood volume, is composed of *red blood cells (erythrocytes)*. The function of these anucleate biconcave discs is to carry oxygen to the tissues and to return to the lungs carrying carbon dioxide. The red blood cells function totally within the vasculature. Chapters 2 through 12 describe the structure, function, and disorders of these *erythroid* cells.

The normal function of *white blood cells (leukocytes)* is to defend the organism against infection. In contrast to the red blood cells, the vasculature is merely a highway for white blood cells, which function mainly in the tissues. The white blood cells are divided into two main categories: the *phagocytes*, cells capable of engulfing particulate matter, and the *lymphocytes*. Both phagocytes and lymphocytes are nucleated ameboid cells capable of

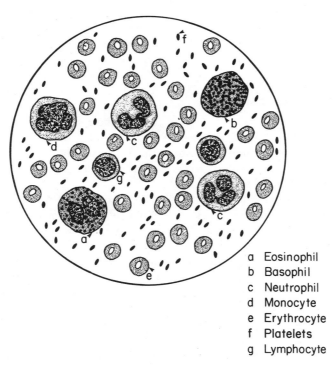

a Eosinophil
b Basophil
c Neutrophil
d Monocyte
e Erythrocyte
f   Platelets
g Lymphocyte

Fig. 1-1. Blood smear.

locomotion within the tissues. Chapters 18 through 26 describe the structure, function, and disorders of white blood cells.

The *platelet*s are disc-shaped anucleate fragments released from a giant cell called the *megakaryocyte*. Platelets, the structure, function, and disorders of which are described in Chapter 14, work with the coagulation proteins to defend the vasculature in case of tears or leaks.

The formed elements of the blood are easily visualized by means of the *blood smear* (Fig. 1-1). A drop of blood is obtained by pricking the finger or else taken from a tube of anti-coagulated blood, smeared out on a class slide or coverslip, and allowed to dry. The dried smear is then stained with *Wright's stain*. This stain is a mixture of dyes dissolved in methanol. During initial exposure of the smear to the dye, the cells are fixed by the methanol and the cell nuclei and certain cell components stain blue. After a few moments, water buffered to an alkaline pH is added, which causes the red blood cells and parts of other cells to stain red. The coloration of cell components described in this text all refer to Wright's-stained cells.

THE LIFE HISTORY OF THE FORMED ELEMENTS

Of the many body cells, blood cells are among those with the highest rate of self-renewal or *turnover*. Each blood cell type has a somewhat different reason for requiring this high rate of turnover. In the course of their meanderings through the circulation, the erythrocytes are subjected to mechanical and oxidant stresses that lead to their destruction. Furthermore, evolution has had to allow for the replacement of red blood cells in case of bleeding following injuries. Phagocytes function continuously in tissues invaded by microorganisms. This invasion is an unending process, particularly in the gastrointestinal tract, oral cavity, and skin, which are zoological gardens teeming in microbial species. In dealing with these microbes, phagocytes are destroyed, and there is, therefore, a continuous demand for their replacement. Lymphocytes perform complex immunological functions that require that discrete lymphocyte populations amplify themselves on demand (Chs. 24 and 25). Finally, platelets are consumed during the process of coagulation and must be replenished. Even in the absence of overt injury, the coagulation system functions at a low level to maintain the integrity of the vascular system.

Except for an early portion of fetal life, the *bone marrow* is the site of production of most blood cells. The ultimate source of blood cells is the *pluripotent hematopoietic stem cell*.

This cell, more about which is discussed in Chapter 28, is present in very small numbers, replicates itself, and differentiates into *committed* stem cells destined to differentiate into erythroid, phagocytic, megakaryocytic, and lymphoid cells (Fig. 1-2). Only cells differentiated beyond the stem cell stage can be recognized by their morphological appearance as belonging to one of these lineages. Early in their differentiation these cells are capable of cell division and are therefore defined as the *mitotic compartment* of blood cells. The more mature forms of differentiation and the fully differentiated erythroid and phagocytic cells, which are incapable of mitosis, are called the *postmitotic compartment*. Although, as described in Chapter 28, there is evidence that stem cells may circulate in the blood, it is primarily the completely mature blood cells that leave the bone marrow and can be observed in the peripheral blood.

Figures 1-2 and 1-3 illustrate that the lymphoid cells are in many respects exceptions to statements that have been made above. First, lymphoid cells, unlike erythroid phagocytic and megakaryocytic forms, do not necessarily follow a unidirectional development from mitotic stem cells to end cells. Rather, lymphoid cells can oscillate between mitotic forms and dormant "memory" cells capable of recruitment into a mitotic pool on demand. Second, lymphoid cells percolate back and forth between various compartments, the bone mar-

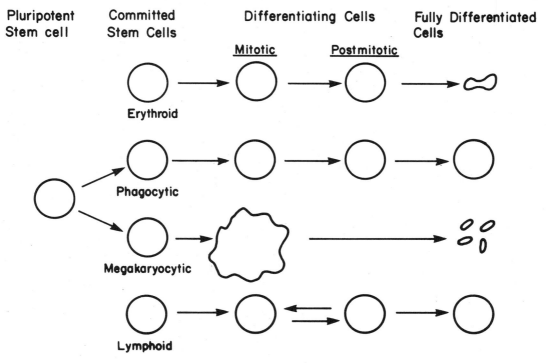

Fig. 1-2. Hematopoiesis.

row, the blood and lymphatic circulations, and the tissues. In contrast, erythrocytes and platelets released from the marrow live out their life spans in the blood. Phagocytes enter the tissues and do not return to the blood.

In the bone marrow, blood cells develop in *sinuses* lined with endothelial cells and fibroblasts. The endothelium, fibroblasts, and abundant fat cells constitute what is termed the *stroma* of the bone marrow. The bone marrow is a rich, seemingly random mixture of blood cells of all types in all stages of maturation. A sample of bone marrow stained with standard histological dyes reveals a beautiful variety of cell shapes, colors, and sizes. Easiest to identify are occasional megakaryocytes, distinctive for their large size and multilobed nuclei. Most of the other cells visible are developing phagocytes, principally polymorphonuclear leukocytes, and developing erythrocytes. The phagocytes outnumber the erythrocytes by a ratio of about 3:1. Mature cells leave the marrow by creating gaps in the endothelial lining of the si-

nuses and enter capillaries in continuity with the circulation. The bone marrow with its remarkable diversity of cellular forms resembles a tropical coral reef.

In a child the entire bone marrow contains growing blood cells (*hematopoietic tissue*). However, of the total mass of bone marrow in an adult, only a fraction contains substantial amounts of hematopoietic tissue, although the absolute amount of this tissue is the same in adults and children. The locations of this *red marrow*, as it is called from its appearance, are illustrated in Fig. 1-4. The rest of the marrow contains principally fat and is therefore called *yellow marrow*.

Examination of a bone marrow sample is an important procedure in hematology because it affords a view, albeit relatively qualitative, of blood cell production. It is quite simple and not too painful to put a suitable needle into the bone marrow (Fig. 1-5) and obtain a small quantity of marrow tissue. Figure 1-4 shows that there is considerable red marrow in the

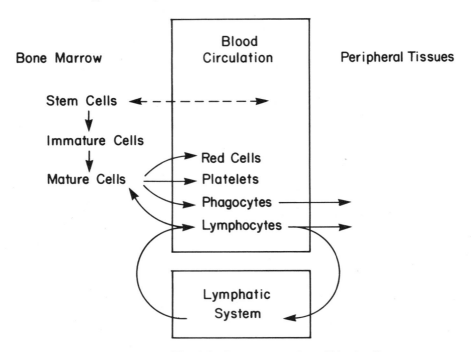

Fig. 1-3. Compartmentation of blood cells.

pelvis. For this reason the posterior superior iliac spine is a site frequently selected for bone marrow sampling. Another location often used is the sternum. The two techniques employed for sampling are the *aspirate* and the *biopsy*. Aspiration through the needle into a syringe disrupts the bone marrow structure but obtains cells in a relatively dispersed form suitable for staining and examination with Wright's or Wright–Giemsa stains. The details of cellular structure are well visualized by this approach, and a general impression of the relative numbers of different cell types in the sample can be obtained. The aspirated marrow sample can also be innoculated into appropriate media for determining whether certain infectious organisms, such as typhoid bacilli, mycobacteria, or fungi, are present. The overall architecture of the bone marrow, however, is not readily appreciated by this approach. Furthermore "sticky" elements, such as tumor cells or fibrotic lesions, cannot be aspirated; and if the

bone marrow contains no hematopoietic tissue, as in aplastic anemia (Ch. 28), the attempt to aspirate will yield a "dry tap." The biopsy, in which a core of marrow is acquired, overcomes some of the limitations of the aspirate and complements it. The biopsied tissue must be decalcified, fixed, and stained with histological dyes, such as hematoxylin and eosin, before visualization. These treatments render the morphology of individual cells considerably less distinct than the stained cells of aspirates. However, it is possible to discern the principal types of bone marrow cells in the fixed specimen. Most importantly, the biopsy sample reveals the architecture of the bone marrow. The presence of clumps of tumor cells, fibrosis, or aplasia is readily appreciated. The decalcification process takes many hours, thereby delaying the opportunity to observe the sample. By placing the biopsy sample on a glass slide before placing the sample in fixative solution, it is sometimes possible to obtain a "replica" of the marrow on the slide that can be observed immediately after staining. This procedure is called a *touch preparation*.

THE REGULATION OF BLOOD CELL RENEWAL

As mentioned above, the high turnover of blood cells is in part geared to the capacity to respond to stress, for example, blood loss (erythrocytes and platelets) and infection (white blood cells). The events leading to the increased demands for blood cells usually occur at sites distant from the bone marrow, the organ of blood cell production. Accordingly, feedback mechanisms involving circulating humors exist to signal the distant bone marrow to increase its output on demand.

The primary signal regulating red blood cell production (*erythropoiesis*) is the tissue oxygen tension (Fig. 1-6). A fall in tissue oxygenation, resulting from anemia or pulmonary insufficiency, is followed by an increase in red blood cell production (Chapter 3). The link between tissue oxygen tension and bone marrow red blood cell production is the glycoprotein hormone *erythropoietin*, which is produced by the kidney. Erythropoietin circulates in the blood and is also excreted into the urine. When tissue oxygenation decreases, the activity of erythropoietin in the plasma and urine rises. The action of erythropoietin is to accelerate the commitment of pluripotent stem cells into erythroid development and to enhance the rate of division and maturation of red cell progenitors. Erythropoietin activity can be demonstrated experimentally by injecting urine or plasma into mice that have been transfused with red blood cells so as to have supernormal oxygen-carrying capacity. Using techniques described in Chapter 4 for assessing red blood cell production, it can be shown that these transfused mice have virtually shut down red blood cell formation in their bone marrow. If urine or plasma containing erythropoietin is

Fig. 1-4. Location of hematopoiesis in the adult bone marrow.

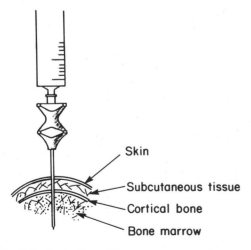

Skin

Subcutaneous tissue

Cortical bone

Bone marrow

Fig. 1-5. Aspiration of bone marrow.

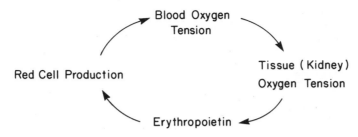

Fig. 1-6. Regulation of erythropoiesis.

injected into these mice, however, their red blood cell production rises significantly.

It is quite clear that oxygen is the "thermostat" for red blood cell production and that erythropoietin is the signal between the thermostat and the bone marrow. The factors regulating phagocyte, lymphocyte, and platelet production are much less well understood at this time, but evidence is rapidly accumulating that growth factors also have an important role (Table 1-1). These factors were initially recognized as glycoproteins in the blood and urine that promoted the growth and differentiation of blood cells in tissue cultures. These hematopoietic hormones caused committed stem cells in samples of bone marrow or blood to develop into colonies of mature phagocytic cells and were therefore named *colony-stimulating factors* (CSFs). CSFs act on stem cells to enter the cell renewal cycle from a dormant state and to differentiate into their mature phenotypes, and they also may enhance some of the mature cell functions. Other agents have been discovered as components in tissue culture media that induced lymphocytes to divide and grow. The CSFs and lymphocyte growth factors are either highly specific for particular cell types (e.g., promoting the development of granulocyte *versus* monocyte and macrophage colonies) or else overlapping in activity (promote the development of granulocyte *and* monocyte colonies). The emergence of molecular cloning techniques has facilitated the identification and characterization of these growth factors, which are also known as *interleukins*. White blood cell growth factors are produced by a number of tissues, including fibroblasts and macrophages. Stimulation of the latter cells in inflammatory states may induce the secretion of CSFs and interleukins.

Table 1-1. Hematopoietic Growth Factors and Related Factors

Factor	Target Cell(s)	Actions
Erythropoietin	Erythroblasts	Promote erythroid growth and differentiation
CSF-G	Phagocyte stem cells	Promote differentiation into neutrophils
CSF-GM	Phagocyte stem cells	Promote differentiation into neutrophils and monocytes/macrophages. Also has some activity for other lineages
CSF-M	Phagocye stem cells	Promote differentiation into monocytes and macrophages
Interleukin 1 (IL1, endogenous pyrogen)	Multiple	Induces fibroblasts to synthesize CSF-GM and CSF-G
Interleukin 2 (IL2)	T lymphocytes	T-cell growth factor Activates natural killer cells (see Ch. 19)
Interleukin 3 (IL3)	Multipotent stem cells	Promote growth of all blood cell lines
Interleukin 4 (IL4)	B lymphocytes Mast cells	B-cell growth factor Mast cell growth factor
Interleukin 5 (IL5)	B lymphocytes Eosinophil precursors	B-cell growth factor Eosinophil growth factor
Interleukin 6 (IL6, interferon 2)	B lymphocytes Multipotent stem cells	B-cell growth factor Potentiates IL3
Interferon	Phagocytes	Induces a variety of antimicrobial functions

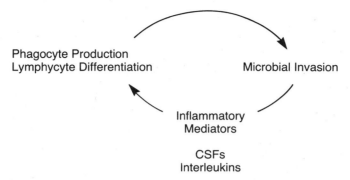

Fig. 1-7. Regulation of white blood cell production.

As is discussed in Chapter 18, the interaction between microorganisms and tissue results in the elaboration of a number of *mediators* of inflammation, some of which include the immunoproteins discussed above and in Chapter 17. These mediators also have the capacity to increase the production of phagocytic leukocytes and call forth these cells into the blood and into the tissues where they are needed (Fig. 1-7). Chapter 20 discusses how lymphoid cells are recruited by exposure to foreign substances to differentiate and acquire the capacity to produce immunoglobulins and then undertake other immunological functions. It also discusses how this recruitment is amplified following repeated exposures to the offending agents. Finally, anemia and bleeding bring about an increase in the number of circulating platelets. Whether this action is in part mediated by erythropoietin or is totally the respon-

sibility of some as yet unidentified humor, called *thrombopoietin*, is not known (Fig. 1-8). It is unclear whether the putative platelet growth regulator acts positively like CSFs and erythropoietin to stimulate platelet production or is rather released by platelets and inhibits megakaryocytes in a suppressive feedback loop.

THE SCOPE OF HEMATOLOGY

The foregoing discussion has provided an overview of and set the stage for the detailed description of the structure and functions of the blood in the remainder of this text. We close this introductory chapter by considering for whom this information can be useful.

In one guise, hematology is a subspecialty of internal medicine. Practitioners of this form of hematology are specialists in dealing with diseases of the blood. They diagnose and treat anemias, coagulation disorders, and malignant neoplasms of blood cells. The treatment of malignancies of the blood, discussed in Chapters 19, 22–28, and 31, is very similar to the treatment of a variety of solid tumors. Conversely, the therapy of solid tumors often has profound effects on the blood. For these reasons, the disciplines of hematology and oncology have always been closely related and in recent years have become even more closely linked. Another close relationship exists between hematology and immunology. Abnor-

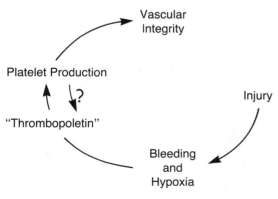

Fig. 1-8. Regulation of platelet production.

malities of the numbers and functions of white blood cells often cause a patient to become abnormally susceptible to infection, a state defined as *immunodeficiency*. On the other hand, perversion of the immune system so that it destroys normal blood cells, a state defined as *autoimmunity*, is frequently encountered in medical practice.

Another aspect of hematology is *blood transfusion therapy*. Replacement of whole blood and blood components is a major medical enterprise, occurring during surgery and following injury. Not only are blood components infused into patients, but, increasingly, abnormal proteins are removed from patients with various diseases. All the procedures described in Chapter 30 are performed in transfusion services that are present in all but the smallest hospitals. Furthermore, in the United States there is a regional network of blood transfusion centers organized by the American National Red Cross. This very active dimension of hematology has enormous medical and economic ramifications.

Finally, nearly every physician is, in a sense, a "hematologist." Because of its access to all tissues of the body, the blood is often one of the first sources of information that indicate changes in the state of health and the development of specific diseases. Changes in the number or appearance of formed elements and in the levels of plasma components are extremely useful to all clinicians. It is not surprising, then, that diagnostic hematology laboratories are consulted by nearly all clinicians and that the total impact of the work of these laboratories on the cost of health care is considerable.

In closing this chapter, we want to emphasize the utility of examination of the blood smear to all physicians. Examination of a Wright's-stained specimen of blood under the microscope may be the first clue to a dangerous depression in the number of circulating platelets and alerts the clinician to the possibility of bleeding. A large number of "bluish" red blood cells on the smear indicates the presence

of *reticulocytes*, young red blood cells, which increase in number when bleeding is occurring. The smear can indicate the presence of elevated numbers of circulating phagocytes and changes in the appearance of these cells, which suggests existence of bacterial infection. In some instances, together with other information, the presence of a specific infection may be suggested. For example, parasitic microorganisms, such as the plasmodia of malaria, may be directly observed. The aggregation of red blood cells on the smear might suggest alterations in the levels of plasma proteins (Ch. 17). Peculiarities in the shapes of the red blood cells can mean the presence of vascular injury, liver disease, or overwhelming infection. We emphasize that the examples given here are not diseases limited to the province of the "hematologist" but are conditions that any physician is likely to encounter. The blood is truly a window into our state of health, and the peripheral blood smear affords a practical and simple glance into that window.

SUGGESTED READINGS

Colman, R.W., Hirsh, J., Marder, V.J., & Salzman, E.W., Eds. (1987) Hemostasis and Thrombosis: Basic Principles and Clinical Practice. 2nd ed. J.B. Lippincott, Philadelphia.

Dexter, T.M., Spooncer, E. (1987) Growth and differentiation in the hemopoietic system. Ann. Rev. Cell Biol. *3*:423.

Nathan, D.G. & Oski, F.A., Eds. (1987) Hematology of Infancy and Childhood. 2nd ed. W.B. Saunders, Philadelphia.

Sachs, L. (1987) The molecular control of blood cell development. Science *238*:1374.

Stomatoyannopoulos, G., Nienhuis, A.W., Leader, P., & Majerus, P.W. (1987) The Molecular Basis of Blood Diseases. W.B. Saunders, Philadelphia.

Westerman, M.P., Ed. (1981) The bone marrow: structure, function and pathology. Semin. Hematol. *18*:177–300.

Zucker-Franklin, D., Greaves, M.F., Grossi, C.E., & Marmont, A.M. (1988) Atlas of Blood Cells. 2nd Ed. Lea & Febiger, Philadelphia.

SECTION I

Red Blood Cells and Their Diseases

In order to survive, the tissues of the body must receive a steady supply of oxygen from the atmosphere. It is one of the functions of the blood to provide this supply of oxygen. This function is performed by the red cells, which take up oxygen as the blood flows through the lungs and release it when the blood reaches the tissues.

For maximum delivery of oxygen, the blood must contain the right proportion of red cells to total volume. Too low a proportion decreases the amount of oxygen that can be carried by the blood; too high a proportion thickens the blood, impeding its flow through the tissues. It is not surprising, then, that the pro-

portion of red cells in the blood is closely regulated and stays within rather narrow limits under normal circumstances.

Red blood cell disorders typically present as abnormalities in the proportion of red cells to total blood volume. Most common by far are those in which this proportion is low. These are the *anemias*. The anemias include many different red cell disorders, some of which are quite prevalent. In fact, most of the hematological conditions seen in daily practice are anemias of one kind or another. Other disorders show an abnormally high proportion of red cells, but these are seen much less frequently than the anemias.

Red Blood Cell Diseases: Red Cell Production, Red Cell Indices, and the Reticulocyte Count

Red cells are the oxygen-carrying elements of the blood. They are highly flexible biconcave discs filled with hemoglobin (Fig. 2-1). Flexibility is necessary to permit them to pass through the very narrow vessels they must negotiate as they pick up oxygen from the lungs and deliver it to tissues. Hemoglobin is the protein that actually carries the oxygen.

RED CELL PRODUCTION

Like all the cells of the blood, red cells arise from bone marrow stem cells that start out with the capacity to become any cell in the blood or lymphatic system but ultimately commit themselves to a single line—in this case, the red cell line. The daughters of these now-committed stem cells differentiate into red cells by passing through a series of stages identifiable under the microscope as successively more mature red cell precursors. Eventually they mature fully and are released into the bloodstream as young erythrocytes. After circulating for a period of time, the erythrocytes are removed from the bloodstream and destroyed.

The earliest red cell precursors, though not recognizable under a microscope, can be detected by marrow culture, a technique in which bone marrow cells are grown in soft agar containing suitable nutrients and hormones. Two types of red cell precursors have been identified by this technique: the CFU-E (colony-forming unit, erythrocyte), a single cell that gives rise to a tight cluster of hemoglobinized cells as it proliferates and differentiates; and the BFU-E (burst-forming unit, erythrocyte), an earlier cell whose descendents, after wandering a short distance, mature into closely spaced CFU-Es that eventually appear as a group of hemoglobinized cell clusters—a so-called "burst" (Fig. 2-2). The CFU-E is thought to be the immediate precursor of the pronormoblast, the earliest erythrocyte precursor that can be identified under the microscope.

As they differentiate further into erythrocytes, the red cell precursors undergo three major changes: (1) they accumulate hemoglobin; (2) they lose their protein-synthesizing apparatus (including all their RNA) and their mitochondria; and (3) their nuclei contract as the chromatin condenses into a functionless mass, and are finally extruded. These changes are responsible for the changes in the appear-

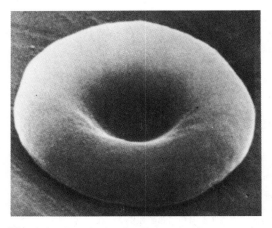

Fig. 2-1. A normal red cell, seen under a scanning electron microscope. (From Wintrobe, M.M. et al. (1974) Clinical Hematology. 7th ed. Lea & Febiger, Philadelphia, with permission.)

ance of the red cell precursors as they pass through the various stages of differentiation (Fig. 2-3). The earliest detectable stage is the pronormoblast, a large cell consisting mostly of a large, purplish nucleus with finely divided chromatin and a couple of dark-staining nucleoli, wrapped in a rim of cytoplasm that is colored a deep rich blue because it contains a very large amount of blue-staining RNA but hardly any pink-staining hemoglobin. Next the red cell precursor becomes a basophilic normoblast, then a polychromatophilic normoblast, and finally an orthochromatic normoblast. As it shrinks in size, its nucleus condenses and contracts, and its cytoplasm turns from blue to pink as RNA is replaced by hemoglobin. Last comes the extrusion of the nucleus—by now nothing more than a small,

Fig. 2-2. Detection of early red cell precursors in bone marrow cultures (**Left**) A cluster of hemoglobinized cells generated by a CFU-E (colony-forming unit, erythrocyte). (**Right**) A closely spaced group of such clusters produced by a BFU-E (burst-forming unit, erythrocyte). (From Zucker-Franklin, D., Greaves, M.F., Grossi, C.E., & Marmont, A.M. (1988) Atlas of Blood Cells. 2nd Ed. Edi Ermes, s.r.l., Milan, with permission.)

Fig. 2-3. (A–E) Stages of maturation of a red cell precursor. (**B, C** from Wintrobe, M.M. et al. (1974) Clinical Hematology. 7th ed. Lea & Febiger, Philadelphia, with permission; **A, D, E** from Lessin, L.S. & Bessis, M. (1972) Morphology of the erythron. In Williams, W.J. et al. (eds.) Hematology. 1st ed. McGraw-Hill, New York, with permission.)

dark, round, structureless mass—and the release of the red cell into the bloodstream. The newly released red cells still contain a few mitochondria and a little RNA, but these disappear within a day or two to produce the fully mature red cell.

Of the four precursor stages—pronormoblast, basophilic normoblast, polychromatophilic normoblast, and orthochromatic normoblast—the first three consist of cells that are able to divide. These cells are said to be in the mitotic compartment (Fig. 2-4). Division and maturation occur at the same time, so a single normoblast will generate several basophilic normoblasts, each of which will produce several polychromatophilic normoblasts, and so forth. The result is that the percentage of red cell precursors in the marrow is much greater for the later stages than for the earlier stages.

It takes about 3 to 5 days for a pronormoblast to become a red cell. Once in the bloodstream, this cell will live for about 4 months. It will then die of old age, and its remains will be degraded for reuse.

The production of red cells is normally controlled fairly tightly, with the fraction of the blood volume occupied by the red cells (this fraction is known as the *hematocrit*) being maintained in the vicinity of 40 to 45 percent. It is probably not a coincidence that 40 to 45

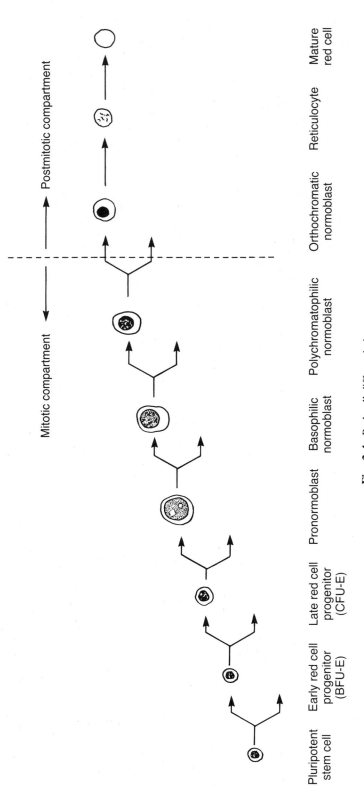

Fig. 2-4. Red cell differentiation.

percent also happens to be the hematocrit range that affords the best delivery of oxygen to the tissues. This optimum range is dictated by two properties of the blood that affect oxygen delivery: its hemoglobin content, which determines how much oxygen the blood can carry, and its viscosity, which influences how rapidly the oxygen-laden blood can flow through the tissues. The hemoglobin content, which is equivalent to the oxygen-carrying capacity of the blood, increases linearly with the rising hematocrit. The viscosity also increases with a rising hematocrit, but in a more complex way, the change being rather small as the hematocrit increases to about 50 percent, but very large as it exceeds this value (Fig. 2-5). Over the flat portion of the viscosity curve, oxygen delivery to the tissues goes up smoothly as the hematocrit rises, because the oxygen-carrying capacity of the blood increases while

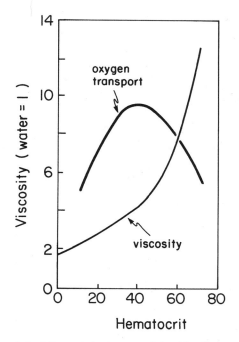

Fig. 2-5. Effect of the hematocrit on blood viscosity and oxygen transport. (Redrawn from Erslev, A.J. & Gabuzda, T.G. (1975) Pathophysiology of Blood. W.B. Saunders, Philadelphia, with permission.)

the blood viscosity stays nearly the same. But in the region of the steep portion, oxygen delivery actually falls as the hematocrit rises, because the increase in the oxygen-carrying capacity of the blood is more than offset by the impedance to tissue blood flow caused by the rapidly increasing blood viscosity. The relationship between these factors is such that oxygen delivery to the tissues is maximum at a hematocrit of 40 to 45 percent.

Red cell production is controlled by several growth factors. The earliest stem cells, those that have not yet committed themselves to a particular line, are regulated by *interleukin 3* and *GM-CSF*, two growth factors that are made in the marrow and act locally (see Ch. 1). Once committed, however, the red cell precursors fall under the control of a glycoprotein hormone called *erythropoietin*. This hormone is manufactured mainly by the kidney, although a small amount is also made by the liver. Its production by the kidney is inversely related to the renal oxygen tension; it is increased when the renal oxygen tension is low and depressed when the renal oxygen tension is high. The hormone is carried by the circulation to the bone marrow, where it augments red cell production by increasing the number of stem cells committed to the red cell line and by shortening the time required for these committed stem cells to mature into reticulocytes (Fig. 2-6).

Erythropoietin is the main factor responsible for the compensatory increase in red cell production that occurs when there is a drop in the oxygen content of the blood, as occurs, for example, in anemia, at high altitudes, and in pulmonary diseases that impede the passage of oxygen from the lungs to the red cells. The drop in blood oxygen content leads to a decrease in the renal oxygen tension, which in turn causes erythropoietin production to rise. As a result, the bone marrow is stimulated, thereby increasing red cell production. The marrow has the capacity to increase red cell production by a factor of seven to eight when maximally stimulated.

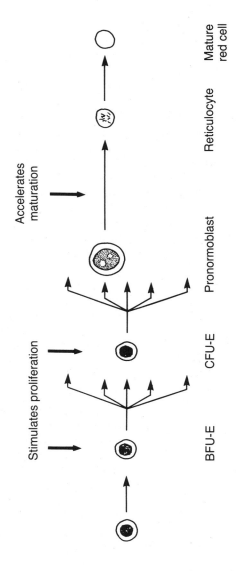

Fig. 2-6. The action of erythropoietin.

Stimulates proliferation

Accelerates maturation

BFU-E

CFU-E

Pronormoblast

Reticulocyte

Mature red cell

RED BLOOD CELL DISEASES: THE RETICULOCYTE COUNT AND THE RED CELL INDICES

Diseases of red cells are by far the most common of the hematological disorders. Almost without exception, these diseases cause a quantitative alteration in the blood hemoglobin level—usually a reduction (anemia), less often an increase (erythrocytosis). An abnormal blood hemoglobin value is the sign that points to the existence of a red blood cell disorder.

Once the presence of a red blood cell disorder has been established, its nature must be determined. This is accomplished by analyzing the clinical and laboratory features accompanying the abnormality in blood hemoglobin in the affected patient. Most of these features are discussed in the chapters that deal with the specific disorders. Two, however, are of very general utility in the evaluation of red blood cell diseases, so it is appropriate to present them here, before discussing each of the specific disorders. These features are the *reticulocyte count* and the *red cell indices* (Wintrobe indices).

The Reticulocyte Count

The RNA of the protein-synthesizing apparatus is degraded as the red cell precursor reaches maturity. Degradation is well under way at the time the cell leaves the marrow, but it does not reach completion until the cell has been in the circulation for a day or two. Newly released red cells therefore contain RNA that is not found in older cells. Because of this RNA, these new cells can be identified morphologically. On a routine smear, which is ordinarily prepared with a hematoxylin-containing stain called Wright's stain, the tinting of the residual RNA by the hematoxylin gives the new cells a distinct bluish cast. Cells with this bluish cast are known as *polychromatophilic cells*. If instead of Wright's stain the smear is prepared with brilliant cresyl blue, the

Fig. 2-7. Reticulocytes. Their dark-staining precipitates distinguish them easily from the homogeneously stained older cells. (From Lessin, L.S. & Bessis, M. (1972) Morphology of the erythron. In Williams, W.J. et al. (eds.) Hematology. 1st ed. McGraw-Hill, New York, with permission.)

RNA precipitates as a deep-blue-staining reticulum of strands and clumps. Cells containing these precipitates are known as reticulocytes (Fig. 2-7). Polychromatophilic cells and reticulocytes are two morphological aspects of the same cell population—that is, red cells that have been released from the marrow 1 to 2 days earlier. These normally constitute about 1 percent of all red cells in the blood.

Reticulocytes are important in the clinical evaluation of the anemias because they provide crucial information on the rate of red cell production. Anemias can be divided into two broad classes: those caused by increased red cell loss from the blood, and those associated with decreased red cell production by the marrow. When an anemia results from increased red cell loss, the marrow compensates by increasing red cell production. New cells are released from the marrow in greater than normal numbers, so the reticulocyte count increases. Conversely, when an anemia is caused by a decrease in red cell production, the release of new cells falls below normal and the reticulocyte count decreases.

Red Cell Indices

Among the features that distinguish one type of anemia from another are the average size and hemoglobin content of the affected red cells. These properties of the red cell are generally expressed in terms of the three red cell (or Wintrobe) indices:

Mean cell volume (MCV), expressed in femtoliters (fl)

Mean cell hemoglobin (MCH), expressed in picograms (pg) per red cell

Mean cell hemoglobin concentration (MCHC), the approximate percentage of the red cell mass that is made up of hemoglobin

Only two of these indices are independent, however; the third can be calculated from the formula

$$MCHC = 100 \times (MCH/MCV)$$

The way in which these indices are determined depends on the method used for quantitating red cells in the blood. Traditionally, red cells were quantitated by hand, using simple equipment. The measurements obtained are the hematocrit, or packed cell volume; the blood hemoglobin; and the red cell count. The hematocrit is the percentage of the total blood volume occupied by the red cells; it is measured by separating the red cells from the plasma by centrifugation and measuring the appropriate volumes. The definitions of blood hemoglobin (g/100 ml blood) and red cell count (cells/μl blood) are self-evident. Red cell indices are calculated from these values according to the formulas:

$$MCV = \frac{hematocrit}{red\ count} \qquad MCHC = \frac{hemoglobin}{hematocrit}$$

Normal 85–100 fl   Normal 32–34 percent

Automated counters are now used for the quantitation of red cells. These instruments measure the MCV directly. In addition, they measure the blood hemoglobin and red cell count. Automated counters can also give the hematocrit value, either by direct measurement or by calculating it by multiplying the MCV by the red count (with an appropriate correction for the units in which these figures are expressed). Indices are calculated directly by the instrument.

The red cell indices are important because they form the basis for an extremely valuable classification of the anemias by pathophysiological category. In the most useful version of this classification, the various anemias are grouped by red cell size into three categories: microcytic (small cell), normocytic (normal size), and macrocytic (large cell). Accordingly, though all three Wintrobe indices are routinely obtained in anemic patients, the only index really needed to classify an anemia is the MCV. The classification of anemias by MCV is given in Table 2-1.

Often, anemias are described in terms of the amount of hemoglobin in the red cells as assessed under the microscope. Cells that look deficient in hemoglobin are termed "hypochromic"; those with normal amounts of hemoglobin are designated "normochromic"; and those with excess hemoglobin are termed "hyperchromic." In practical terms, though, the apparent quantity of hemoglobin in a red cell viewed through a microscope is determined by the size of the cell. Accordingly, microcytic anemias are hypochromic, normocytic anemias are normochromic, and macrocytic anemias are hyperchromic. It is common practice to use

Table 2-1. Classification of the Anemias by Mean Cell Volume (MCV)[a]

Microcytic (MCV low)		Macrocytic (MCV high)		Normocytic (MCV normal)
Disorder	Chapter	Disorder	Chapter	
Iron deficiency anemia	4	Megaloblastic anemia	6	Most other anemias
Thalassemia	10	Hemolytic anemia	8,9	
Sickle cell anemia and related disorders	11	Anemia of liver disease	8	
Sideroblastic anemia	5	Anemia of hypothyroidism	7	

[a] Although this classification scheme is highly useful as a general guide to the diagnosis of anemia, it must be borne in mind that exceptions to these rules do occur.

adjectives describing both cell size and hemo-globin content when classifying an anemia—for example, iron deficiency anemia is gener-ally referred to as a hypochromic microcytic anemia—but little seems to be gained by this dual terminology.

Between the reticulocyte count and the red cell indices, it is usually possible to place an anemia into one of a small number of fairly narrowly defined pathophysiological catego-ries. These pathophysiological categories are the point of departure for the discussions of anemias and other red blood cell disorders pre-sented in the succeeding chapters.

SUGGESTED READINGS

Adamson, J.W. (1986) Evidence for multiple levels of regulation in hematopoiesis. Prog. Clin. Biol. Res. *215*:21–32.

Eaves, C.J. & Eaves, A.C. (1984) Factors and hemopoiesis: Pandora's box revisited. Prog. Clin. Biol. Res. *148*:83–92.

Kurtz, A. (1987) Erythropoietin: structure, func-tion, origin. Adv. Nephrol. *16*:371–378.

Schuster, S.J., Caro, J. & Erslev, A.J. (1987) Erythropoietin: current concepts and future pros-pects. Hematol. Pathol. *1*:193–201.

Spivak, J.L. (1986) The mechanism of action of erythropoietin. Int. J. Cell Cloning *4*:139–166.

Stanley, E.R. & Jubinsky, P.T. (1984) Factors af-fecting the growth and differentiation of hae-mopoietic cells in culture. Clin. Haematol. *13*:329–348.

Hemoglobin and Oxygen Transport: Disorders of Oxygen Binding

Hemoglobin is the oxygen-transporting protein of the red cell. It comprises about 30 percent by weight of the erythrocyte, a concentration high enough that 1 ml of oxygen-saturated packed red cells holds the equivalent of about 0.5 ml of oxygen gas. The hemoglobin picks up oxygen as the red cell passes through the lungs, unloading it when the red cell reaches the capillaries of the tissues. The oxygen-binding properties of hemoglobin are such that it can unload its oxygen even at the relatively high oxygen tensions that prevail in most tissues.

Hemoglobin is actually a family of molecules whose members differ slightly in primary structure. In the context of oxygen binding, however, the most important hemoglobin by far is hemoglobin A, which constitutes more than 95 percent of all the hemoglobin in the normal adult red cell. The following discussion deals with the properties of hemoglobin A. The oxygen-binding properties of other normal hemoglobins differ only in detail from those of hemoglobin A. Clinically important features of oxygen binding by the minor hemoglobins are discussed in connection with diseases of hemoglobin biosynthesis in Chapter 10.

STRUCTURE OF HEMOGLOBIN

The hemoglobin molecule is a tetrameric protein of molecular weight (MW) 65,000. It consists of two types of peptide chains: the α- and β-globin chains. These assemble to form a tetrahedral molecule containing two chains of each kind ($\alpha_2\beta_2$) (Fig. 3-1). The molecule is held together mainly by interactions between dissimilar chains. Because the chains interact less firmly with one of their dissimilar neighbors than they do with the other, the hemoglobin molecule contains a natural plane of cleavage, which will be seen to be important in the regulation of oxygen affinity, and along which the molecule can split into $\alpha\beta$ dimers when it is sufficiently dilute. The portion of the molecule

$$\alpha + \beta \rightarrow \alpha\beta \, (\text{tight}) \rightarrow \alpha\beta \, \cdots \, \alpha\beta$$

lining this plane of cleavage is known as the $\alpha_1\beta_2$ region.

A globin chain itself, containing approximately 150 amino acids, is arranged in a precisely defined configuration resembling a long, thin sausage tied in an elaborate knot (Fig.

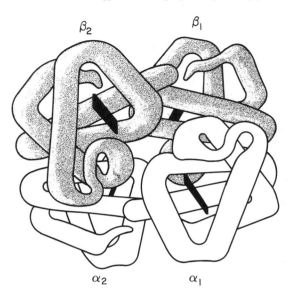

β_2 β_1

α_2 α_1

Fig. 3-1. The hemoglobin tetramer. The molecule consists of two $\alpha\beta$ dimers that combine to form the complete hemoglobin molecule. The region where the two dimers come into contact is known as the $\alpha_1\beta_2$ region. (Modified from Dean, J. & Schechter, A.N. (1978) Sickle-cell anemia: molecular and cellular bases of therapeutic approaches. N. Engl. J. Med. *299*:752–763, with permission.)

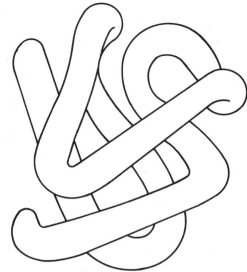

Fig. 3-2. A globin chain: the knotted sausage. (Redrawn from Wintrobe, M.M. et al. (1974) Clinical Hematology. 7th ed. Lea & Febiger, Philadelphia, with permission.)

3-2). Within the knotted chain, regions of particular functional importance can be identified.

The Heme Crevice

Heme is the large, flat, iron-containing disc that actually carries the oxygen molecule. It binds to a specfic region of the globin chain, the heme crevice, by strong but noncovalent forces. Of note are two special histidines in the crevice. Each is directly opposite the iron, one in front and one in back of the ring (Fig. 3-3). The one in back is attached directly to the iron through one of its imidazole nitrogens; the one in front is separated from the iron by a space large enough to accommodate an oxygen molecule. It will be seen that these histidines permit hemoglobin to bind oxygen reversibly.

The $\alpha_1\beta_2$ Region

This region is important because interchain interactions that occur within this region are critical in giving hemoglobin its very remarkable oxygen-binding properties (Fig. 3-4).

The Region of the β-Chain N-Termini

This region contains a pocket lined with positively charged groups consisting of the two terminal amino groups of the β-chains together with positively charged side chains of nearby lysine and arginine residues. This pocket represents a binding site for 2,3-diphospho-glyceric acid (2,3-DPG), a major physiological regulator of the oxygen affinity of hemoglobin. Occupation of this binding site by 2,3-DPG tends to draw together the two $\alpha_1\beta_2$ regions of the hemoglobin tetramer.

Fig. 3-3. The environment of the iron atom in hemoglobin. Oxygen binds to hemoglobin by combining with the iron atoms.

FUNCTION OF HEMOGLOBIN

The function of hemoglobin is to bind oxygen reversibly, delivering it from the lungs, a region of high oxygen tension, to the tissues, a region of much lower oxygen tension. As mentioned earlier, the oxygen-binding site is the iron of the heme group. This iron is in the ferrous (Fe^{2+}) form, and in the normal course of events it takes up and releases oxygen atoms

without undergoing a change in valence. This is a remarkable feature of hemoglobin, because the iron of free heme is very readily oxidized to the ferric (Fe^{3+}) state, and hemoglobin containing Fe^{3+} heme, commonly called *methemoglobin*, is unable to transport oxygen. Stabilization of the iron in the Fe^{2+} state is somehow connected with the special histidine residues at the heme-binding site; disruption of this histidine–iron relationship can result in the rapid oxidation of the hemoglobin iron (see the discussion of hemoglobin M, below).

Oxygen Affinity

The molecule that transports oxygen from the lungs to the tissues is faced with a dilemma. On one hand, it must take up as much oxygen as possible when passing through the lungs. On the other hand, it must unload much of its oxygen at tissue oxygen tensions high enough to support life. Hemoglobin solves this dilemma through its remarkable oxygen-

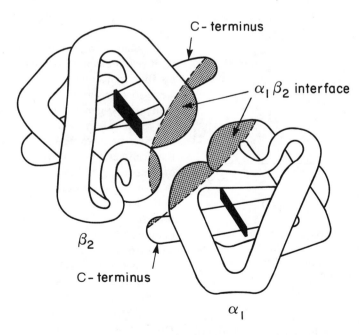

Fig. 3-4. An $\alpha_1\beta_2$ interface. Hemoglobin has two of these.

binding properties. The relationship between the PO_2 and hemoglobin oxygen saturation is sigmoidal (S) shaped (Fig. 3-5), so hemoglobin is able to load up nearly completely in the lungs and yet can release a substantial fraction of its oxygen at the relatively high oxygen levels in the tissues. Specifically, tissues generally take up about 25 percent of the oxygen brought to them by the blood, so that hemoglobin leaving the tissues is about 75 percent saturated. The oxygen saturation curve shows that this corresponds to a tissue PO_2 value of about 40 mm, well within the life-supporting range. Were the relationship between PO_2 and oxygen saturation hyperbolic in shape (i.e., more typical for the binding of a small molecule to a protein), then hemoglobin would be

unable to unload the amount of oxygen required by the tissues until the PO_2 fell to around 2 mm—clearly a metabolic catastrophe that is prevented by the sigmoidality of the hemoglobin oxygen-binding curve.

The characteristics of the saturation curve for this and other hemoglobins are frequently summarized by two numerical parameters. The first is the oxygen tension at 50 percent saturation, known as P_{50}. This is a measure of the inherent oxygen affinity of the hemoglobin; the tighter the oxygen is held, the lower the P_{50}. It is clear from the foregoing discussion that tissue oxygen tensions will correlate roughly with P_{50}, other things being equal.

The second parameter is the Hill coefficient, a number derived from the oxygen-binding curve. This coefficient measures the "S-ness" of the saturation curve. The hemoglobin saturation curve is S-shaped because oxygen binds to hemoglobin in a cooperative fashion. The hemoglobin molecule that is already partly saturated has a higher affinity for oxygen than does a hemoglobin molecule that is completely free of oxygen. Thus the uptake of one oxygen molecule by hemoglobin will facilitate the uptake of the next. It can be shown mathematically that if cooperativity were perfect—that is, if one molecule of hemoglobin were to take up four molecules of oxygen before the next were to take up its first oxygen molecule—then the oxygen saturation curve would obey the relationship: saturation $\approx (PO_2)^4$ (at low and intermediate levels of saturation, where the arithmetic is not affected by the depletion of free oxygen binding sites) (Fig. 3-6). If there were no cooperativity, the oxygen saturation curve would obey the relationship: saturation $\approx (PO_2)$. For intermediate degrees of cooperativity, the power to which PO_2 is raised would take on an intermediate value (i.e., a value between 1 and 4). This exponent thus gives a measure of the degree of cooperativity, which in turn is an index of how effectively hemoglobin can unload oxygen to tissues. The Hill coefficient is an estimate of this exponent. It is determined from the Hill plot, a way of

Fig. 3-5. How the oxygen saturation of whole blood varies with oxygen tension. The sigmoidal shape of the curve is critical for hemoglobin function, permitting hemoglobin to become almost fully oxygen saturated in the lung and yet unload oxygen as required at the relatively high oxygen tensions prevailing in the tissues. (Redrawn from Bunn, H.F., Forget, B.G. & Ranney, H.M. (1977) Human Hemoglobins. W.B. Saunders, Philadelphia, with permission.)

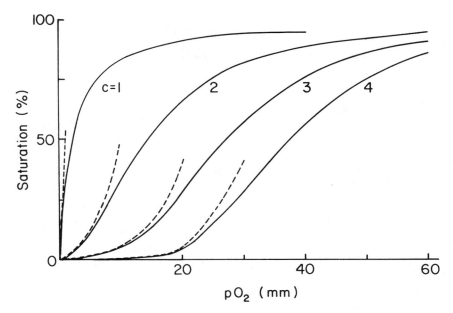

Fig. 3-6. The theoretical oxygen-binding curve of hemoglobin, assuming perfect cooperativity (**right**), intermediate levels of cooperativity, or no cooperativity (**left**). At low levels of saturation, each curve comes very close to the relationship: saturation is approximately equal to $(PO_2)^c$ (*dotted line*). The greater the degree of cooperativity, the greater the value of the exponent c, making this exponent an index of cooperativity. At high levels of saturation, the curves fall away from these relationships because of the progressive depletion of unoccupied binding sites as the hemoglobin takes on its load of oxygen.

plotting saturation against PO_2 that expresses cooperativity in an unusually clear and straightforward manner (Fig. 3-7). The Hill coefficient is simply the slope of the Hill plot at the point where the curve crosses P_{50}. The steeper the slope the greater the Hill coefficient, and the higher the degree of cooperativity in the binding of oxygen of hemoglobin.

The Hill coefficient for hemoglobin A is about 3. Some of the abnormal hemoglobins to be discussed later in this chapter have abnormally low Hill coefficients. This defect in cooperativity adds to the difficulties with oxygen transport in patients burdened with these abnormal hemoglobins.

The molecular basis for cooperativity lies in the fact that hemoglobin exists in two conformations, known as the T and R states, whose oxygen affinities differ from one another (Fig. 3-8). The T (taut) state is characterized by a

relatively low oxygen affinity and a close fit between the two $\alpha_1\beta_2$ regions; the R (relaxed) state has a relatively high oxygen affinity and a wider $\alpha_1\beta_2$ separation than the T state.

In the absence of oxygen, the equilibrium between the two conformers favors the T state. The binding of oxygen to a molecule in the T state induces structural changes that tend to cause the molecule to flip to the R state, whose affinity for oxygen is now higher than it was originally (Fig. 3-9); thus the binding of one oxygen increases the likelihood that a subsequent oxygen atom will bind to the molecule. The greater the number of oxygens bound to a hemoglobin molecule, the more likely it is to be in the R as opposed to the T state. Conversely, a hemoglobin molecule that for one reason or another finds itself in the R state — for example, a molecule in which the $\alpha_1\beta_2$ faces have been permitted to move apart

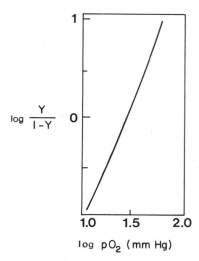

Fig. 3-7. The Hill plot for whole blood. *Y* is the fractional oxygen saturation. By definition, the curve crosses P_{50} at $Y = 0.5$ (i.e., half-saturation). It can be calculated that when $Y = 0.5$, log $[Y/(1 - Y)] = 0$. The slope of the curve at this point is the Hill coefficient. (Redrawn from Bunn, H.F., Forget, B.G. & Ranney, H.M. (1977) Human Hemoglobins, W.B. Saunders, Philadelphia, with permission.)

because of, say, the loss of some protons (see below, The Bohr Effect)—will bind oxygen more tightly than one fixed in the T state. It is important to recognize that the relationship between conformation and oxygen binding is reciprocal. Uptake or release of oxygen by hemoglobin will alter the proportion of T to R, and an alteration in the proportion of T to R will change the oxygen affinity of hemoglobin.

Regulation of Oxygen Affinity

The fitness of hemoglobin as an oxygen-transporting protein is further expressed in the fact that its oxygen affinity is adjustable, varying with its environment. Its alterations in oxygen affinity generally serve to improve the efficiency of oxygen delivery to the tissues. Two mechanisms are responsible for most of the variation in oxygen affinity: the Bohr effect and the effect of 2,3-DPG.

The Bohr Effect

A fall in pH leads to a decrease in the oxygen affinity of hemoglobin (Fig. 3-10). This effect of pH on oxygen affinity is known as the Bohr effect. The Bohr effect facilitates the unloading of oxygen in the tissues. The relatively low pH of actively metabolizing tissues causes a fall in the internal pH of red cells passing through such tissues. The fall in oxygen affinity that results from this drop in pH increases the ease with which oxygen moves from the red cells to the tissues. In the lung, the pH rises, favoring the uptake of oxygen by the red cell.

The Bohr effect occurs because the interaction between the $\alpha_1\beta_2$ faces of the hemoglobin tetramer is strengthened when the molecule takes up protons in response to a fall in pH. The strengthening of this interaction stabilizes the low-affinity (T) conformation of hemoglobin. The fall in oxygen affinity is caused by the stabilization of the T state over the R state as the pH drops.

2,3-DPG

The red cell is unique in containing a glycolytic shunt that permits the accumulation within the cell of large quantities of 2,3-DPG. 2,3-DPG is produced from 1,3-diphosphoglyceric acid, a glycolytic intermediate that normally goes directly to 3-phosphoglyceric acid during the conversion of glucose to lactic acid. The enzyme responsible for the formation of 2,3-DPG is diphosphoglycerate synthetase. The same enzyme can convert 2,3-DPG to 3-phosphoglyceric acid, another glycolytic intermediate. The overall pathway is known as the *Rapoport-Luebering shunt* (Fig. 3-11).

2,3-DPG binds to hemoglobin in the pocket formed by the N-termini of the β-chains (Fig.

Deoxy

Oxy

Fig. 3-8. The two conformations of hemoglobin. In the molecular model, the $\alpha_1\beta_2$ contact areas are enclosed in boxes. The diagram is a highly simplified scheme of the conformational differences between deoxyhemoglobin (*solid lines*) and oxyhemoglobin (*dotted lines*), as seen in the molecular models. The diagram shows how one of the two $\alpha\beta$ dimers rotates with respect to the other on oxygenation of hemoglobin. Besides rotating, the two dimers move closer together by about 1 Å when hemoglobin takes up oxygen. (**Left**: From Muirhead, H. et al. (1967) J. Mol. Biol. *28*:117. © Academic Press Inc. (London) Ltd., with permission. **Right**: Modified from Perutz, M.F. (1979) Regulation of oxygen affinity of hemoglobin. Annu. Rev. Biochem. *48*: 327–386, with permission.)

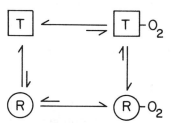

Fig. 3-9. Relationship between hemoglobin conformation and oxygen binding. The preferred conformation of oxyhemoglobin (**right**) is the R conformation, whereas the preferred conformation of deoxyhemoglobin (**left**) is the T conformation. As a result, factors that stabilize the R conformation over the T conformation will favor the binding of oxygen to hemoglobin, whereas factors that preferentially stabilize the T conformation will drive oxygen off the hemoglobin molecule.

3-12). This reduces the affinity of hemoglobin for oxygen by forming a bridge between the two $\alpha_1\beta_2$ faces, stabilizing the T state. The effect of 2,3-DPG on the oxygen affinity of hemoglobin is shown in Figure 3-13. It is probably the most important regulator of the day-to-day oxygen affinity of hemoglobin, providing a baseline setting around which short-term fluctuations in oxygen affinity such as those due to the Bohr effect can take place. Depending on circumstances, the 2,3-DPG concentration will vary so as to promote the normal delivery of oxygen to tissues when the system is stressed. For example, 2,3-DPG levels rise under conditions of hypoxia, promoting more complete unloading of oxygen in tissues to offset the decrease in the amount of ox-

Fig. 3-10. The Bohr effect. How the oxygen affinity of hemoglobin changes with pH. (Redrawn from Wintrobe, M.M. et al. (1974) Clinical Hematology. 7th ed. Lea & Febiger, Philadelphia, with permission.)

Fig. 3-12. The 2,3-disphosphoglycerate pocket is formed by the N-termini of the two β-chains plus some nearby histidines and lysines. (Redrawn from Arnone, A. (1974) *Nature* *249*:34, with permission.)

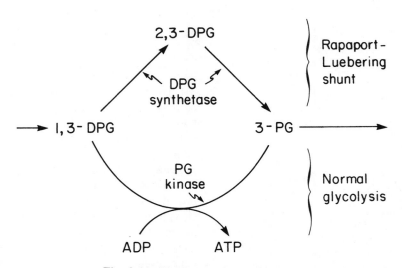

Fig. 3-11. The Rapoport-Luebering shunt.

Fig. 3-13. The effect of 2,3-DPG on the oxygen affinity of hemoglobin. (Redrawn from Benesch, R., Benesch, R.E. (1969) Nature *221*:618, with permission.)

ygen carried by the blood. Similarly, 2,3-DPG levels increase in anemia. Unlike changes in intracellular pH, however, the changes in 2,3-DPG concentration take place over hours to days, a rate consistent with the role of the compound as a sort of thermostat for oxygen affinity.

DISORDERS OF OXYGEN AFFINITY

Certain diseases are characterized by an alteration in the affinity of hemoglobin for oxygen. These diseases fall into two broad classes: those caused by an inherited abnormality of hemoglobin structure, and those caused by abnormalities involving 2,3-DPG.

Hemoglobinopathies

Many hematological disorders result from inherited abnormalities of hemoglobin. Some are caused by defects in the rate of synthesis of structurally normal hemoglobin molecules (i.e., the thalassemias). Most, however, are caused by the production of hemoglobins in

which amino acid substitutions in one of the globin chains result in a molecule with aberrant properties. The precise functional abnormality depends on the nature and location of the amino acid substitution. Some substitutions, for example, lead to a hemoglobin that crystallizes in the red cell; others result in a molecule that is easily denatured under physiological conditions. The substitutions discussed here result in a hemoglobin whose oxygen-binding properties deviate from normal.

High-Affinity Hemoglobins

Most hemoglobins with abnormal oxygen affinity bind oxygen too tightly. Tissue oxygen tensions are therefore lower than normal, leading to the release of erythropoietin, the hormone that stimulates red cell production. Clinical manifestations are largely due to the increase in erythropoiesis that results from the action of this hormone on the bone marrow.

The disease is expressed as one type of familial polycythemia. Its inheritance pattern is autosomal dominant, for reasons that will be discussed below, so that on the average half the family members will be affected by the condition. Hematocrits may range as high as

70, but levels around 60 are more common. Other signs and symptoms are discussed in the chapter on polycythemia (Ch. 12).

Laboratory manifestations in addition to the increased hematocrit and red cell mass include an arterial oxygen saturation exceeding 90 percent and a normal serum uric acid. (Uric acid, a breakdown product of purine metabolism, is often elevated in conditions of accelerated myelopoiesis, some of which also show polycythemia.) The bone marrow examination shows an excessive number of normal red cell precursors. Hemoglobin electrophoresis is sometimes helpful, because in about one-half of affected patients the mobility of the abnormal hemoglobin in an electric field is different from hemoglobin A. The best clues to the disease are listed below.

Clinical Manifestations That Should Raise the Suspicion of High-Affinity Hemoglobin

A family history of erythrocytosis
No splenomegaly
Normal white count, platelet count, and uric acid
Arterial oxygen saturation greater than 90 percent

The diagnosis is made by demonstrating an abnormality in hemoglobin oxygen affinity. This is usually done with intact red cells, although measurements made with hemolysates have the theoretical advantage that effects of oxygen affinity regulators are minimized. The oxygen dissociation curve of red cells from a patient with hemoglobin Bethesda ($\alpha_2\beta_2^{145}$ $^{his\rightarrow tyr}$),* a typical high-affinity hemoglobin,

is compared with that of normal red cells in Figure 3-14 (left). The shift of the curve to the left is very apparent. What is less apparent in this figure, but becomes very evident in the Hill plot (Fig. 3-14 right), is the biphasic nature of the oxygen dissociation curve. This is because the red cells from these patients actually contain both the normal and the high affinity hemoglobins, so the oxygen dissociation curve reflects the combined properties of both hemoglobins. Inspection of the left-hand segments of the Hill plot indicates a P_{50} for hemoglobin Bethesda of about 2.8 mm Hg and a Hill coefficient of about 1.

The fact that clinically significant high-affinity hemoglobin disease occurs when only part of the hemoglobin A is replaced by the abnormal hemoglobin explains why this condition is inherited as an autosomal dominant trait. For part of the hemoglobin A to be replaced by an abnormal hemoglobin, it is only necessary for an individual to inherit a single mutant hemoglobin gene from one parent. The disease is therefore transmitted by a single affected parent: the autosomal dominant mode of transmission.

The diagnosis of high-affinity hemoglobin disease is generally confirmed by family studies, and the workup is terminated there. It is possible to identify the amino acid substitution by purifying the abnormal hemoglobin and examining its structure, but this is almost never done except for research purposes.

To date, more than 40 different high-affinity hemoglobins have been reported. The locations of the altered amino acids in several of these high-affinity variants are shown in Figure 3-15. The alterations cluster in the $\alpha_1\beta_2$ region and the nearby C-terminal ends of the globin chains, just the right locations to disrupt the $R \leftrightarrows T$ transitions that play so important a role in the binding of oxygen to hemoglobin. It is not surprising that alterations affecting these

---

*Amino acid substitutions in mutant hemoglobins are indicated by abbreviations of this sort. This particular abbreviation means that the β-chain of hemoglobin Bethesda contains a tyrosine instead of normal histidine at position

145. In hemoglobin Chesapeake, another high-affinity hemoglobin, leucine replaces arginine at the 92 position of the α-chain. This substitute is abbreviated $\alpha_2^{92arg \rightarrow leu}\beta_2$.

pO_2 (mm Hg)

Fig. 3-14. (Left) The oxygen dissociation curve of a patient with hemoglobin Bethesda, a high-affinity hemoglobin. (*Thick line*) Patient cells. (*Thin line*) Normal cells. The patient's oxygen dissociation curve is not only shifted to the left, but has a peculiar graceless shape. This is because the curve is actually the sum of the oxygen dissociation curves of two hemoglobins, the high-affinity hemoglobin and hemoglobin A, both of which are present in equal amounts in the red cells. **(Right)** The biphasic Hill plot for red cells from the patient with hemoglobin Bethesda. The two hemoglobins in the red cells take up oxygen independently, so that the high-affinity hemoglobin has become largely saturated at a point where the normal hemoglobin has taken up very little oxygen. Each of the two segments can therefore be regarded as a full Hill plot for one of the two hemoglobins. Seen in that way, it becomes clear that one of the two hemoglobins is half-saturated when one-quarter of the total hemoglobin is in the oxy form ($Y/(1 - Y) = 0.25$), and the other is half-saturated at the three-quarter point ($Y/1 - Y) = 0.75$). The P_{50} values can be read off the Hill plots at these points. For the plot shown, these are 2.8 mm (Hb Bethesda) and 26.5 mm (Hb A). (Redrawn from Bunn, H.F., Forget, B.G. & Ranney, H.M. (1977) Human Hemoglobins. W.B. Saunders, Philadelphia, with permission.)

regions give rise to hemoglobins with altered oxygen-binding properties.

Treatment is not necessary in most patients. If problems arise because of high blood viscosity, phlebotomy may be useful to reduce the hematocrit and relieve symptoms.

Low-Affinity Hemoglobins

Patients have been described whose hemoglobins show sharply reduced oxygen affinity. Oxygen binding is ordinarily sufficiently poor that the abnormal hemoglobin is largely in the deoxyhemoglobin form even at normal arterial oxygen partial pressures. Deoxyhemoglobin is

an off-colored hemoglobin that imparts a dusky bluish hue known as cyanosis to the skin and nail beds when it is present in the blood in sufficiently high concentrations (>5 g/dl). Such concentrations are routinely found in patients with low-affinity hemoglobins. These patients therefore present with chronic cyanosis. Cyanosis is also seen in family members, because, like high-affinity hemoglobin disease, and for the same reason, low-affinity hemoglobin disease is transmitted as an autosomal dominant trait. The hematocrit and red cell mass are usually normal, an uncommon feature in diseases associated with chronic cyanosis, in which hematocrits tend to be high.

As with high-affinity hemoglobins, the diag-

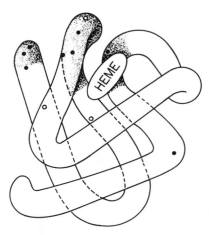

HEME

Fig. 3-15. Locations of the amino acid substitutions in some hemoglobins with abnormal oxygen affinity. The region of the $\alpha_1\beta_2$ interface is stippled. (●) High affinity. (○) Low affinity. (Modified from Wintrobe, M.M. et al. (1974) Clinical Hematology, 7th ed. Lea & Febiger, Philadelphia, with permission.)

nosis of a low-affinity hemoglobin is made by measuring the oxygen dissociation curve. The changes are opposite those seen with high-affinity hemoglobins; the dissociation curve is shifted to the right, not the left, and the P_{50} values from the biphasic Hill plot are high and normal, not low and normal.

Low-affinity hemoglobins are rarer than high-affinity hemoglobins. As with the high-affinity hemoglobins, the amino acid alterations that give rise to low-affinity hemoglobins occur largely in the $\alpha_1\beta_2$ region of the molecule.

This condition does not require treatment.

Alterations in 2,3-DPG Concentration

A number of conditions are characterized by changes in red cell 2,3-DPG levels that lead to alterations in the binding of oxygen to hemoglobin (Table 3-1).

By far the most important factor affecting the level of 2,3-DPG in the red cell is the

Table 3-1. Conditions Causing Abnormalities in Red Cell 2,3-DPG Levels

Increase	Decrease
Alkalosis	Acidosis
Hypoxia	Shock
Anemia	Hypophosphatemia
Hepatic cirrhosis	Bank blood
Uremia	

acid–base status of the patient. 2,3-DPG rises with alkalosis and falls with acidosis, a consequence of the effect of pH on the enzyme responsible for its production and consumption. If the acidosis or alkalosis lasts long enough, the 2,3-DPG eventually reaches a level at which it compensates almost exactly for the Bohr effect caused by the acid–base disturbance, restoring the hemoglobin oxygen affinity to normal. The increases in 2,3-DPG observed in hypoxia and in cirrhosis of the liver appear to be caused by the accompanying respiratory alkalosis; the increase seen in anemia may also be caused by that factor, at least in part. Acidosis is responsible for the fall in 2,3-DPG in patients in shock. The fall in 2,3-DPG levels in bank blood, which is stored in an acid anticoagulant, may also be an example of the effect of acid on red cell 2,3-DPG levels.

Other factors affect red cell 2,3-DPG as well. 2,3-DPG rises and falls with the serum phosphate, accounting for its increase in uremia and its decrease in hypophosphatemia. Inherited deficiencies in glycolytic enzymes are rare causes of abnormal 2,3-DPG levels (e.g., pyruvate kinase deficiency). An inherited deficiency of DPG synthetase caused an isolated drop in 2,3-DPG, with erythrocytosis secondary to the resulting increase in the in vivo oxygen affinity of normal hemoglobin.

METHEMOGLOBINEMIA

When oxyhemoglobin dissociates, the oxygen almost always leaves the same way it arrived—namely, as an oxygen molecule. Every once in a while, though, the oxygen takes an extra electron with it when it goes. The products of this aberrant dissociation reaction are superoxide (O_2^-), which is rapidly destroyed in the red cell, and a form of hemoglobin in which the heme iron has been oxidized by one electron from Fe^{2+} to Fe^{3+}. This form of hemoglobin, known as *methemoglobin*, is unable to take up oxygen. It must therefore be converted back to deoxyhemoglobin if the red cell is to retain its capacity to carry oxygen to the tissues.

The reduction of methemoglobin back to hemoglobin is accomplished in the red cell by a short electron-transport chain that transfers an electron from NADH to the heme iron atom (Fig. 3-16). Reading backward from methemoglobin, the components of the chain are cytochrome b_5, a heme enzyme that passes the electron to methemoglobin, and methemoglobin reductase (more accurately NADPH-cytochrome b_5 reductase), a flavoenzyme that takes the electron from NADH and gives it to the cytochrome. In the normal red cell, the rates of methemoglobin formation and reduction are such that methemoglobin amounts to less than 1 percent of the total hemoglobin in the cell. In certain diseases, this balance is altered, and methemoglobin accumulates in the red cell. This condition is known as *methemoglobinemia*. There are three categories of diseases in which methemoglobinemia occurs:

Hemoglobin M

Hemoglobin M refers to a group of mutant hemoglobins whose iron atoms are fixed in a partly oxidized state. In these hemoglobins, there is a mutant chain (α or β) that has lost its ability to stabilize the heme iron in the reduced

Table 3-2. Hemoglobins M[a]

Hemoglobin	Substitution
M$_{Boston}$	$\alpha 58^{his \to tyr}$
M$_{Hyde\ Park}$	$\beta 92^{his \to tyr}$
M$_{Iwate}$	$\alpha 87^{his \to tyr}$
M$_{Saskatoon}$	$\beta 63^{his \to tyr}$
M$_{Milwaukee}$	$\beta 67^{val \to glu}$

[a] The substitution in M$_{Milwaukee}$ is the only one not involving the special histidines near the heme iron. It is nonetheless a heme crevice substitution, as can be seen by comparing its position with that of M$_{Saskatoon}$.

state because of an amino acid substitution in the vicinity of the metal. This chain remains perpetually in the methemoglobin form, so hemoglobins containing this chain will always be partly oxidized.

There are five known types of hemoglobin M. These are listed in Table 3-2. It is of interest that in four of these five types, one of the two iron-coordinated histidines is replaced by a tyrosine.

How much mutant chain is actually present in hemoglobin M red cells? In the heterozygote, about 25 percent. This can be understood by considering a patient who is heterozygous, for, say hemoglobin M$_{Saskatoon}$, a β-chain mutant. Red cells from this patient will contain equal quantities of α- and β-chains. All the α-chains will be normal, as will one-half the β-chains. The other half of the β-chains will be mutants, because the heterozygote makes the normal and mutant β-chains in roughly equal amounts. Accordingly, this patient's red cells will contain globin chains in the proportion: 2α to $1\beta^A$ to $1\beta^M$.

Methemoglobin levels in patients with hemoglobin M are equivalent to the level of the mutant chain. Red cells in affected heterozygotes therefore contain about 25 percent methemoglobin. This level is high enough to be

Fig. 3-16. The reduction of methemoglobin. This is the normal route of methemoglobin reduction. The electron donor for this pathway is NADH.

clinically significant (for clinical manifestations, see below). Consequently, hemoglobin M is a disease that is seen in the heterozygote —that is, a disease transmitted as an autosomal dominant.

Methemoglobin Reductase Deficiency

This disease results from a deficiency of the NADPH-cytochrome b_5 reductase. Methemoglobinemia occurs because the rate of spontaneous methemoglobin production, slow though it is, is fast enough to outstrip its rate of reduction in these defective cells.

Methemoglobin reductase deficiency is inherited as an autosomal recessive trait. It is not seen in heterozygotes because their reductase levels, though decreased, are high enough to handle the normal methemoglobin load without difficulty. Methemoglobin levels in homozygotes with this disease generally range between 10 and 40 percent. The fact that methemoglobin is reduced at all seems to be due to the presence in the red cell of a group of NADPH-dependent reducing systems whose normal functions have nothing to do with hemoglobin but which can reduce methemoglobin slowly in a pinch.

Ingestion of Oxidizing Agents

Certain oxidizing agents produce methemoglobinemia by entering the red cell and oxidizing the hemoglobin directly. Such agents include inorganic nitrite (NO_2^-), the classic source of which is contaminated well water; organic nitrites, which are used to produce methemoglobinemia in the treatment of cyanide poisoning; and chlorate (ClO_3^-), a constituent of safety match heads.

Clinical Manifestations

The hallmark of methemoglobinemia is *cyanosis*. The bluish cast to the skin, most often caused by deoxyhemoglobin, is also seen when the blood contains sufficient amounts of circulating methemoglobin, the other off-colored hemoglobin. It is generally easy to distinguish between deoxyhemoglobinemia and methemoglobinemia: deoxyhemoglobinemia is almost invariably associated with diminished arterial oxygen tension, whereas the partial pressure of oxygen in methemoglobinic blood is normal (though the oxygen *saturation* of the arterial hemoglobin is reduced, because methemoglobin does not bind oxygen), and the cardiorespiratory diseases that cause arterial hypoxemia are absent. Furthermore, most patients with methemoglobinemia tend to be clinically well, because their modest methemoglobin levels have little practical effect on the oxygen-carrying capacity of their blood; serious problems do not appear until methemoglobin levels reach 40 percent or so.

It is in patients with acquired methemoglobinemia that trouble occurs. When methemoglobin reaches very high levels, oxygen transport by the blood is grossly deranged: The methemoglobin chains are no longer able to carry oxygen, and the normal chains in extensively oxidized hemoglobin molecules (i.e., molecules in which two or three of the four chains are in the methemoglobin form) are fixed in their high-affinity configuration and cannot release their oxygen to the tissues. Any patient whose methemoglobin level exceeds 60 percent is in mortal danger from anoxia. Methemoglobinemia of this degree constitutes a medical emergency that must be dealt with instantly.

The diagnosis of methemoglobinemia should be considered in any patient exhibiting cyanosis. For any patient who is both cyanotic and sick, acquired methemoglobinemia must be considered, because it is a life-threatening illness that can be cured by immediate treatment. Congenital methemoglobinemia should be suspected in a cyanotic patient who is otherwise healthy, especially if the cyanosis was present at birth or appeared in early childhood as expected for congenital diseases. A normal arterial oxygen pressure (not hemoglobin saturation) provides an important clue to methemoglobinemia. An even more important clue is

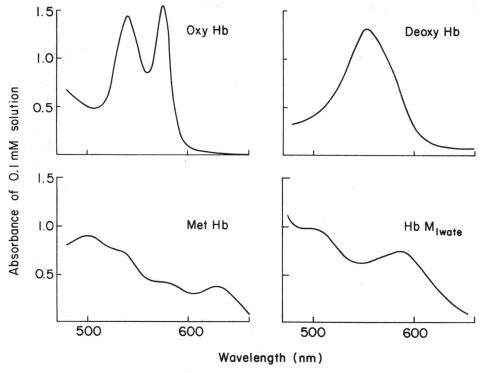

Fig. 3-17. Hemoglobin spectra. Oxyhemoglobin is bright red; the others are dark. The methemoglobins all have the same brownish hue in the test tube, but the spectrum of "normal" methemoglobin is different from that of the M methemoglobins because of the differences in the environment of the heme iron. (Redrawn from Bunn, H.F., Forget, B.G. & Ranney, H.M. (1977) Human Hemoglobins. W.B. Saunders, Philadelphia, with permission.)

the color of drawn blood, which is dark red to brown and does not change on shaking in air. In chronic methemoglobinemia the hematocrit will be elevated, a response to the diminished oxygen-carrying capacity of the blood, but red cell survival does not seem to be compromised by uncomplicated methemoglobinemia (contrast this with the red cell destruction of oxidant hemolysis). The diagnosis is made by demonstrating the presence of methemoglobin in the blood by spectrophotometry (Fig. 3-17) or by electrophoresis. The cause is then established by measuring methemoglobin reductase or by looking for one of the five types of hemoglobin M, or, if acquired, from the history.

Therapy depends on the cause. Acquired methemoglobinemia can be treated by methylene blue, a harmless reducing agent that enters the red cells and passes electrons from an

> ## Clinical Features Associated with Congenital Methemoglobinemia
>
> Cyanosis since infancy
> Good health otherwise
> Normal arterial oxygen saturation
> Off color of drawn blood

NADPH-dependent reductase to methemoglobin (Fig. 3-18). If methemoglobin levels are high enough to cause life-threatening hypoxia, a procedure known as exchange transfusion, in which the patient's blood is replaced with normal blood, may be required. Methemoglobin reductase deficiency is also treated with as-

Fig. 3-18. Methylene blue-mediated reduction of methemoglobin. The electron donor for this pathway is NADPH.

corbate or methylene blue. Treatment is not necessary, however, in mild cases of the disease. No treatment is available for hemoglobin M disease, but none is needed.

SULFHEMOGLOBIN

Sulfhemoglobin is an altered form of hemoglobin that is produced when blood is exposed to powerful oxidizing agents, especially in the presence of sulfides. It is thought to arise when methemoglobin generated by the oxidizing agent undergoes a further reaction with a nearby -SH group (either a cysteine residue or an exogenous sulfhydryl compound). Unlike methemoglobin, sulfhemoglobin cannot be turned back into normal hemoglobin, so the oxygen-carrying capacity of any hemoglobin that has been converted to sulfhemoglobin is irretrievably lost.

Clinically, sulfhemoglobinemia usually results from exposure to an oxidant drug (e.g., dapsone, or an aniline derivative such as phenacetin). Cyanosis is generally the only finding. The diagnosis is made by spectrophotometry, a method that distinguishes sulfhemoglobinemia from other causes of cyanosis. Treatment is usually unnecessary except for withdrawal of the offending agent, but patients with a life-threatening level of sulfhemoglobin may require exchange transfusion.

SUGGESTED READINGS

Adamson, J.W. (1975) Familial polycythemia. Semin. Hematol. *12*:383–396.

Bunn, H.F. & Forget, B.G. (1984) Human Hemoglobins. 2nd ed. W.B. Saunders, Philadelphia.

Bunn, H.F. (1981) Evolution of mammalian hemoglobin function. Blood *58*:189–197.

Golde, D.W., Hocking, W.G., Koeffler, H.P. & Adamson, J.W. (1981) Polycythemia: mechanisms and management. Ann. Intern. Med. *95*:71–87.

Hall, A.H., Kulig, K.W. & Rumack, B.H. (1986) Drug- and chemical-induced methaemoglobinaemia. Clinical features and management. Med. Toxicol. *1*:253–260.

Hanash, S.M. & Rucknagel, D.L. (1980) Clinical implications of recent advances in hemoglobin disorders. Med. Clin. North. Am. *64*:775–800.

Harrison, B.D. & Stokes, T.C. (1982) Secondary polycythaemia: its causes, effects and treatment. Br. J. Dis. Chest *76*:313–340.

Jaffé, E.R. (1981) Methaemoglobinaemia. Clin. Haematol. *10*:99–122.

Jaffé, E.R. (1986) Enzymopenic hereditary methemoglobinemia: a clinical/biochemical classification. Blood Cells *12*:81–90.

Meldon, J.H. (1985) Blood gas transport and 2,3-DPG. Adv. Exp. Med. Biol. *191*:63–73.

Nagel, R.L. & Bookchin, R.M. (1974) Human hemoglobin mutants with abnormal oxygen binding. Semin. Hematol. *11*:423.

Perutz, M.F., Molecular anatomy, physiology, and pathology of hemoglobin, in Stamatoyannopoulos, G., Nienhuis, A.W., Leder, P. & Majerus, P.W., eds., Molecular Basis of Blood Diseases, Saunders, 1987, p. 127.

Rose, Z.B. (1980) The enzymology of 2,3-bisphosphoglycerate. Adv. Enzymol. *51*:211–53.

Sacks, L.M. & Delivoria-Papadopoulos, M. (1984) Hemoglobin-oxygen interactions. Semin. Perinatol. *8*:168–183.

Stephens, A.D. (1977) Polycythaemia and high affinity hemoglobins. Br. J. Haematol. *36*:153–159.

Heme Formation: The Supply of Iron. Iron Deficiency and Iron Excess

Heme is a complex molecule consisting of four pyrrole groups joined by one-carbon bridges into a large ring that contains an iron at its center (Fig. 4-1). It has many roles in biological systems, serving as the oxygen-carrying component of hemoglobin and as an electron carrier for a variety of enzymes that catalyze oxidation-reduction reactions. Because of its central importance in the function of the red cell, abnormalities in heme production are associated with well-defined hematological diseases.

Heme production involves two basic processes: the acquisition of iron and the synthesis of the heme itself. Problems with the former give rise to conditions of iron deficiency or iron overload. These are discussed in this chapter. Problems with the latter present as porphyrias and sideroblastic anemias, which are discussed in the next chapter.

IRON METABOLISM

Every day the normal adult destroys about 15 ml of senescent red cells and produces an equal quantity of new red cells to replace them. For the daily production of new erythrocytes, about 15 mg of iron is required. Almost all this iron is drawn from stores laid down when old red cells are destroyed. The movement of iron back and forth between the red cells and the iron storage pool involves a sequence of steps called the *iron cycle*. A small but critical fraction of red cell iron is obtained from the diet.

Iron Cycle

The iron cycle is illustrated in Figure 4-2. It can be considered arbitrarily to begin with the uptake of iron by transferrin. This is a plasma protein to which almost all the circulating iron is bound. It carries two atoms of ferric (Fe^{3+}) iron, binding them so avidly ($K_{diss} = 10^{-30}$) that the plasma contains virtually no free iron.

The red cell precursors obtain their iron from circulating transferrin. On the surface of these cells are binding sites for transferrin, the so-called transferrin receptors. Precursors as late as reticulocytes possess transferrin receptors, their number declining as the cell matures; fully mature erythrocytes, however, have no transferrin receptors. Iron-loaded transferrin binds to these receptors, which are then carried into the cell along with their cargo by an invagination of the surface membrane that seals and breaks free to form an intracellular vacuole (Fig. 4-3). Fusion of the vacuole

Pyrrole

Heme

Fig. 4-1. Pyrrole and heme. The heme is composed of four pyrroles fused into a large ring. The letters at the periphery of the ring refer to substituents attached to the carbons indicated. The substituents are M, methyl; V, vinyl ($-CH=CH_2$); P, propionyl ($-CH_2CH_2 COOH$). (The structure and biosynthesis of heme are discussed in Ch. 5.)

with a lysosome followed by acidification releases the iron from the internalized iron–transferrin complexes. The liberated iron then makes its way into the cytoplasm, while the vacuole migrates to the cell surface, rejoining the outer membrane and returning the now unloaded transferrin molecules to the plasma. During this passage, the iron is reduced from ferric to ferrous.

In the red cell precursor, the newly acquired iron atom may follow one of two paths. It may become incorporated directly into a molecule of heme, or it may be reoxidized and taken up into a molecule of ferritin. Ferritin, a storage form of iron, consists of a core of ferric hy-

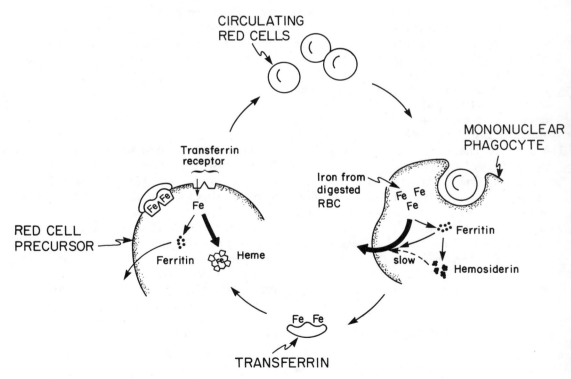

Fig. 4-2. The iron cycle. In the blood, iron circulates in association with transferrin, its carrier protein. It is delivered by transferrin to the red cell precursors, where most of it is incorporated into hemoglobin. These mature and are released as circulating red cells. After 4 months, these cells are removed from the bloodstream by mononuclear phagocytes, which digest them and return their iron to transferrin, either directly or after storing it for a while as ferritin/hemosiderin.

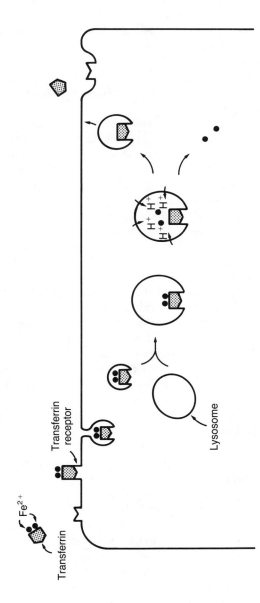

Fig. 4-3. Iron transport into cells. A circulating transferrin molecule loaded with iron binds to a transferrin receptor on the cell surface. The membrane in the region of the loaded receptor invaginates and detaches to form a small vacuole that carries the receptor and its bound cargo into the cytoplasm of the cell. The vacuole fuses with a lysosome to form a combined vacuole whose interior then acidifies, releasing the iron from the transferrin. The iron passes into the cytoplasm, while the vacuole fuses with the plasma membrane, returning the transferrin receptor to the cell surface and liberating the now unloaded transferrin molecule back into the surrounding fluid.

droxide encased in a protein shell composed of 24 identical subunits. The empty shell, known as *apoferritin*, is filled atom by atom with iron, so that ferritin molecules with widely varying core sizes are present in red cell precursors and other storage iron-containing cells.

In normal red cell precursors, the storage iron may be seen as a few tiny grains of Prussian-blue-staining material representing microscopically visible aggregates of ferritin. Cells containing these aggregates are known as *sideroblasts*. They may represent up to 50 percent of all red cell precursors in the normal marrow. Almost all this surplus iron is extruded from the precursors before they leave the marrow, explaining why very few circulating red cells contain ferritin granules. It is important to distinguish these normal marrow sideroblasts from ringed sideroblasts, a type of iron-containing red cell precursor seen only in the sideroblastic anemias.

Mature erythrocytes circulate for about 4 months. They are then taken up by mononuclear phagocytes, primarily in the spleen, and are disposed of by these cells. During the course of destruction of the outdated red cells, the heme is freed from the globin, the ring is opened, and the iron is released into the phagocyte. Most of this iron is delivered immediately to plasma transferrin. However, a portion stays behind in the phagocyte, where it becomes incorporated into ferritin. In a normal person on a normal diet, substantial quantities of ferritin accumulate in the cells of the mononuclear phagocyte system. During the course of time, some of this ferritin undergoes partial degradation, forming heterogeneous aggregates known as *hemosiderin* (Fig. 4-2). The combination of ferritin and hemosiderin in the mononuclear phagocyte system represents the major iron storage pool of the body. It is readily visible on Prussian-blue-stained smears of bone marrow, where it is described as "stainable iron." From this storage pool, iron is released to plasma transferrin as necessary. The transfer of iron from the phagocyte to the circulating transferrin completes the iron cycle.

A recurring theme in the iron cycle and in the mechanism of gastrointestinal iron absorption is the series of changes in oxidation-reduction state that iron undergoes during the course of its movements. These changes make sense if the following rule is kept in mind: Iron is trivalent (ferric) when it is bound, or about to become bound, to a carrier (transferrin or ferritin); otherwise it is divalent (ferrous).

Absorption of Iron

Although the vast majority of the iron is retained in the body as it moves from one compartment to another, a small amount—1 to 2 mg—is lost every day; the iron cycle is not a fully closed loop. Iron is lost from the gastrointestinal tract in the form of blood and sloughed epithelium. Secretions and exfoliated skin also account for a small fraction of the loss. Menstruating women lose iron each month in the menstrual flow, and a pregnancy costs nearly 1 g, as iron is transferred to the newborn and the placenta and is lost with blood at delivery.

These losses are replenished by absorption of iron from diet. Dietary iron is supplied largely as heme, but also as inorganic iron derived from nonheme iron-containing enzymes and storage iron. Both forms of iron can be absorbed throughout the length of the small intestine, but because the first encounter between iron and the gut epithelium takes place in the upper small intestine (duodenum and upper jejunum), most iron absorption takes place there. Heme is absorbed as such, whereas the inorganic iron is reduced to the divalent form (Fe^{2+}) before being absorbed in a reaction facilitated by the low pH of the stomach.

In the intestinal mucosal cell, a complex series of events takes place (Fig. 4-4). The heme is split open just as it is in the mononuclear phagocyte, and its iron is released as Fe^{2+} to join the Fe^{2+} taken up as such by the mucosal cell. This Fe^{2+} then follows one of the two paths. Some is transported out of the mucosal cell to be oxidized in the plasma, then to bind to transferrin and enter the iron cycle.

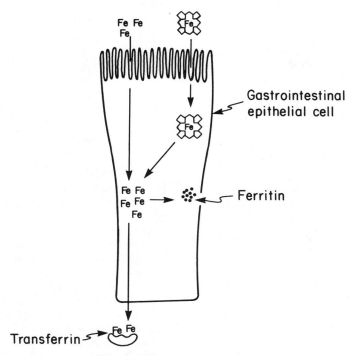

Fig. 4-4. Absorption of iron by the intestinal epithelial cell. Some of the iron taken up by the cell is passed into the bloodstream. The rest is sequestered as ferritin, which is lost when the cell is sloughed into the intestinal lumen.

The rest is oxidized to Fe^{3+} to be incorporated into ferritin, which remains sequestered in the mucosal cell until the cell is shed from the tip of the intestinal villus.

It is at the level of intestinal absorption that the total body iron load is regulated. Under normal circumstances, the amount of iron transported into the blood is a small fraction of the amount ingested, the fraction falling as the ingested load rises (Fig. 4-5). This fraction is such that on the usual diet, iron absorption is equal over time to iron losses, so the total amount of iron in the body remains roughly constant. Under conditions of stress, however, the mucosal cell alters its capacity to absorb iron. Two kinds of stresses elicit this response from the mucosal cell:

Fig. 4-5. Relationship between iron ingestion and iron absorption. (Redrawn from Fairbanks, V.E. & Beutler, E. (1972) Iron metabolism. In Williams, W.J. et al. (eds) Hematology. 1st ed. McGraw-Hill, New York, with permission.)

1. *Alterations in body iron stores.* Iron absorption changes to correct for deviations in iron stores in either direction. When stores are low, iron absorption increases. When stores are overloaded, iron absorption falls, sometimes to very low levels.

2. *Alterations in red cell turnover.* Mucosal cells somehow sense the rate of red cell production and adjust their iron absorption accordingly, regardless of the state of the iron stores. Iron absorption increases sharply in anemias characterized by the destruction of red cells (e.g., immune hemolytic anemias) or their precursors (e.g., thalassemia), disorders in which red cell formation can be increased as much as six- to sevenfold. Conversely, iron absorption falls when red cell formation is depressed. The paradoxical augmentation in iron absorption in the face of greatly increased iron stores can add substantially to the problems faced by iron-overloaded patients with hyperproliferative anemias (discussed below; see Hemochromatosis).

Despite many years of research on the cellular basis for these alterations in iron absorption, their mechanism remains largely obscure. The amount of iron a mucosal cell is capable of transporting into the bloodstream seems to be programmed into the cell at birth, by a mechanism that is not understood (Fig. 4-6). Part of the variability in iron transport appears to depend on the amount of intracellular Fe^{2+} transported into the blood, as opposed to the amount sequestered as ferritin; how the decision is made as to the partitioning of Fe^{2+} between transport and ferritin is not known.

Ferrokinetics

Useful clinical information can be obtained by measuring the movement of iron through its various pools. This is done by administering ^{59}Fe intravenously and measuring the distribution of isotope among these pools as a function of time. These measurements permit determi-

Fig. 4-6. Regulation of intestinal iron absorption. Intestinal epithelial cells live for 2 days, then are sloughed off and replaced. Because of this rapid turnover, it is possible to change the absorptive properties of the entire intestinal epithelium within 48 hours by replacing the current cells with cells possessing new characteristics. This appears to be how iron absorption is regulated. Iron absorption is increased by replacing the epithelial cells with a new crop that takes up more iron from the gut and delivers a greater proportion of this iron to the bloodstream, as opposed to the inert ferritin pool. Absorption is decreased by replacement with cells having the opposite properties.

nation of how rapidly iron is transferred from plasma to tissues, what fraction of this iron is incorporated into the red cells, and how much of the iron is held by the marrow, liver, and spleen, the major storage organs.

The plasma iron turnover (PIT) rate measures the amount of iron moving from plasma to tissue in a day. This value is calculated by multiplying the fractional iron turnover in plasma by the total amount of plasma iron. The fractional iron turnover is equal to the fraction of total plasma iron that moves into the tissues in a given interval of time. The plasma iron concentration does not change in that interval of time because the iron lost into tissues is replaced by an equal quantity of iron from stores and from the diet. The fractional iron turnover, however, can be measured by measuring the rate at which ^{59}Fe is lost from the plasma, as there are no tissue stores of radioactive iron to replenish the supply, permitting the one-directional flux to be measured directly. The procedure is to give ^{59}Fe intravenously, then follow its disappearance from plasma over time. From this disappearance curve, which is exponential for the first few hours and falls on a straight line in a semilog plot, the half-time for disappearance is measured. This half-time is usually expressed in minutes. Dividing this figure into 0.693 (the reciprocal of *e*, the base of the natural logarithms) and multiplying the result by 1440 (the number of minutes in a day) gives the fractional turnover expressed in its most useful form: the fraction of plasma iron turned over per day. When this figure is multiplied by the total plasma iron (plasma iron concentration × plasma volume), the result is the plasma iron transfer rate, the complete formula of which is

$$\text{PIT (mg/day)} = \frac{1{,}440 \times 0.693 \times \text{total plasma iron}}{t_{1/2}}$$

A low plasma iron turnover implies sluggish red cell production, as in certain hypoproliferative anemias; a high plasma iron turnover means more rapid than normal erythropoiesis and is seen especially in conditions associated with the destruction of red cells or their precursors.

The red cell iron utilization rate (RCU) measures the fraction of the iron transferred from plasma to tissues that is actually incorporated into circulating red cells. To make this measurement, a quantity of ^{59}Fe is given intravenously, and the amount of label in the total of the circulating red cells is measured after 14 days. This interval is long enough so that no labeled red cell precursors would be left in the marrow. The amount of label in all the red cells is determined by measuring the radioactivity in 1 ml of packed red cells and multiplying by the red cell mass. Normally the RCU is 80 percent; the remaining 20 percent is accounted for by incorporation of iron into other tissue proteins and by the destruction of iron-labeled red cell precursors in the marrow before release (ineffective erythropoiesis).

The amount of iron in the marrow, liver, and spleen can be measured by scanning after injection of ^{59}Fe. (Marrow iron is measured by scanning the sacrum). Normal values, expressed as the fraction of the value measured shortly after injecting the isotope, are given in Figure 4-7. The early reciprocal changes in blood and marrow iron represent the incorporation of iron into red cell precursors followed by its release into the circulation in the form of new erythrocytes. Liver and spleen iron represent part of the 20 percent that does not get into the red cells. Characteristic changes in these patterns in disease states are discussed in connection with the diseases themselves.

IRON DEFICIENCY

The amount of iron in the normal diet is only slightly greater than the amount necessary to replace the small quantities lost through normal processes. Even a modest increase in these daily iron losses will lead to iron depletion unless measures are taken to increase the amount of iron taken in with the diet. Iron deficiency is therefore an exceedingly common condition, probably the most common of all causes of anemia.

Causes

Increase in iron requirements occur under a variety of circumstances. Any of these may lead eventually to iron deficiency, even on a normal diet.

Physiological Increase in Iron Requirements

The normal adult male requires 1 to 2 mg of iron a day to make up for iron lost from the gastrointestinal tract and through other pro-

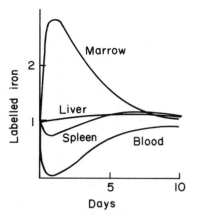

Fig. 4-7. Movement of labeled iron through various tissues during the first 10 days after administration. Characteristic changes in these patterns are seen in patients with shortened red cell survival (hemolytic anemia), destruction of red cell precursors in the marrow (ineffective erythropoiesis), or diminished red cell production (aplastic anemia). (From Finch, C.A. et al. (1970) Ferrokinetics in man. Medicine *49*:17, with permission.)

Causes of Iron Deficiency Anemia

Increased requirements
   Early childhood and adolescence
   Women during the reproductive years
Losses from the GI tract
Losses from urine or sputum (rare)

cesses. In other populations, however, iron requirements are substantially greater (Fig. 4-8). Children require unusually large amounts of iron during the first 5 years and during early adolescence, periods of exceptionally rapid growth. During their reproductive years, women require an additional 1 mg of iron a day to make up for menstrual losses (about 50 ml blood/month), and each pregnancy uses up about 0.7 g of iron, which must be replaced

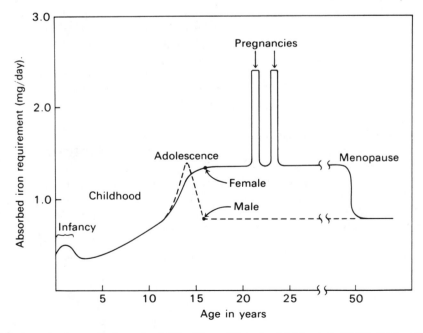

Fig. 4-8. Iron requirements throughout life. (From Wintrobe, M.M. et al. (1974) Clinical Hematology. 7th ed. Lea & Febiger, Philadelphia, with permission.)

through the diet. Iron deficiency in these populations is frequent.

Gastrointestinal Bleeding

Gastrointestinal bleeding is by far the commonest pathological cause of increased iron losses. Any bleeding lesion may lead to iron deficiency, including peptic ulcer, drug- or alcohol-induced gastritis, hookworm, inflammatory bowel disease, or cancer. Cancer of the right side of the colon is notorious for presenting as an isolated iron deficiency anemia in the absence of other signs or symptoms.

Menometrorrhagia

A large number of gynecological conditions can cause abnormally heavy menstrual periods (menorrhagia), nonmenstrual bleeding from the uterus (metrorrhagia), or both. Iron deficiency attributable to excessive vaginal blood loss is the rule in these conditions.

Other Causes

Chronic loss of iron in the urine or sputum is an occasional cause of iron deficiency. Iron deficiency anemia has been produced in hospitalized patients by enthusiastic withdrawal of samples for blood tests.

MANIFESTATIONS

Iron Deficiency Anemia

The major manifestation of iron deficiency is a characteristic anemia. The red cells are small, pale, and irregularly shaped (Fig. 4-9); indices show a hypochromic microcytic anemia. Marrow red cell precursors may also be pale and moth-eaten. Under ultraviolet light the cells fluoresce because of the accumulation of abnormal amounts of iron-free porphyrins

Fig. 4-9. (A,B) Blood smear in iron deficiency anemia. Red cells are small and misshapen. The area of central pallor is disproportionately large because the cells are deficient in hemoglobin. (From Wintrobe, M.M. et al. (1981) Clinical Hematology. 8th ed. Lea & Febiger, Philadelphia, with permission.)

(iron-containing porphyrins do not fluoresce). The white blood cell count is normal, but platelets are often increased, and the spleen and lymph nodes may be slightly enlarged in an occasional patient.

The basis for this clinical picture is the lack of iron to incorporate into heme. With the deficiency of heme, the cells grow poorly, an abnormality perhaps related to the finding that heme deficiency can retard protein synthesis by causing the reversible inactivation of the enzyme responsible for elongating the peptide chain. Nevertheless, porphyrin synthesis continues, with the result that porphyrins containing zinc instead of iron at the center accumulate in the iron-deficient red cells. In iron deficiency anemia, the red cell precursors also seem to undergo an extra division before extruding their nuclei, another factor causing a reduction in the size of the red cell; the reason for this extra division is unknown.

Alterations in the Iron Cycle

Alterations in the iron cycle designed to compensate for the iron-depleted state also take place in iron deficiency and can be de-

Fig. 4-10. Absence of stainable marrow iron in iron deficiency anemia. The "stainable iron" is the hemosiderin in the mononuclear phagocytes, a storage pool drawn on when iron requirements exceed iron intake. Prussian blue stains these hemosiderin granules a deep, intense blue (**A,** *arrows*). Disappearance of this hemosiderin is the first sign of iron deficiency (**B**).

tected by appropriate tests. These alterations are the earliest manifestations of iron deficiency, preceding the development of the anemia.

In iron deficiency, storage iron falls because of the transfer of iron from the storage pool to the red cell precursors. Iron deficiency as the cause of an anemia is indicated by the absence from the marrow of storage iron (detectable as stainable marrow iron (Fig. 4-10)) or by a reduction in the level of serum ferritin (a useful noninvasive index of storage iron).

Iron absorption from the small intestine

increases, as does the serum transferrin, although the amount of iron carried by the transferrin is reduced. The transferrin-bound iron is measured as the serum iron, and the total transferrin as the total iron-binding capacity (TIBC); the serum iron:TIBC ratio in iron deficiency anemia is less than 1:6. The marrow is avid for iron, so ferrokinetic measurements show an increased PIT and an increase in the amount of iron that appears in the marrow at early times.

Other Signs and Symptoms

Patients with iron deficiency anemia sometimes show fatigue and lethargy out of proportion to their degree of anemia (Fig. 4-11). This might be attributable to depletion of iron from iron-requiring enzymes, as has been shown in iron-deficient animals by a correlation between physical endurance and tissue levels of the nonheme iron enzyme glycerol phosphate dehydrogenase. The tongue becomes smooth and sore. Pica, a peculiar desire to eat substances such as ice, laundry starch, and clay, is also seen in iron deficiency anemia. No one knows why. Koilonychia, or spooning of the fingernails, is occasionally seen in severe iron deficiency. Finally, some patients with severe iron deficiency, particularly women, may acquire a web high in the esophagus, with dysphagia; this lesion, which is thought to be premalignant, resolves when the iron deficiency is corrected.

Management

The first principle of management is to discover the reason for the patient's iron deficiency. The diagnosis of iron deficiency anemia is easily made by measuring the serum iron and TIBC; it may be confirmed by measuring iron stores, because a low serum iron, the hallmark of iron deficiency anemia, is also seen in the anemia of chronic disease, but in this condition iron stores are full. The source

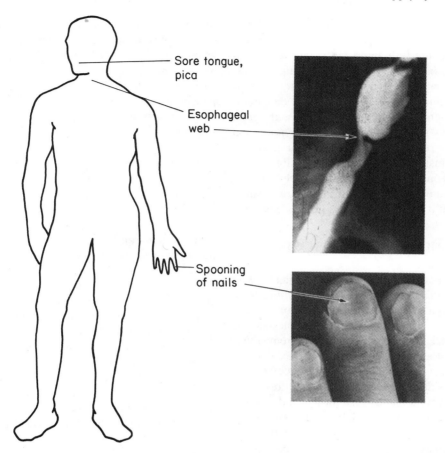

Fig. 4-11. Auxiliary manifestations of iron deficiency. (**Top right:** From Hutton, C.F. (1956) Plummer Vinson syndrome. Br. J. Radiol. *29*:81–85, with permission. **Bottom right:** From Rosenbaum, E. & Leonard, J.W. (1964) Nutritional iron deficiency anemia in an adult male. Ann. Intern. Med. *60*:683, with permission.)

The Diagnosis of Iron Deficiency

Hypochromic microcytic anemia
Low serum iron
High total iron-binding capacity (TIBC)[a]
Low serum ferritin[b]
Absent marrow iron stores[b]

---

[a] In iron deficiency, TIBC may be high, normal or low. High values are very suggestive of iron-deficiency anemia; normal or low values are of no help in making the diagnosis.
[b] The best indicators of iron deficiency.

of iron loss must be established in every patient, paying special attention to occult blood in the stool as a clue to chronic gastrointestinal blood loss. This must be done even in a woman with a history of seven pregnancies and 25 years of heavy menses; she, too, may have a bleeding ulcer.

Iron deficiency is treated by replacement therapy and by correcting the iron-losing condition, if correction is indicated. Iron is usually replaced orally, with therapy continuing well beyond the point where anemia is corrected, in order to replenish depleted stores. The amount of iron that the body can assimilate by this route is small, even in severe iron deficiency, so the response is relatively slow. Generally, a reticulocyte response does not reach a peak until 10 days after treatment is begun, and the anemia is not fully corrected for weeks. Occasionally, parenteral iron therapy is useful; this is ordinarily given by injection into the gluteus, a painful procedure, but it may be administered intravenously slowly and with great care to avoid the sometimes fatal hypotension that may result from anaphylaxis or from too rapid infusion of the iron with resulting acute iron poisoning. Iron stores are rapidly repleted by the parenteral route, but its hazard is sufficient that it should be used as little as possible.

HEMOCHROMATOSIS

It is not uncommon to see patients with modest increases in iron stores resulting from the anemia of chronic disease or from diseases associated with increased erythropoiesis. The occasional patient accumulates a tremendous load of storage iron, depositing the excess iron not only in the mononuclear phagocytes but also outside the phagocytes in locations such as hepatocytes and cardiac muscle cells, where the metal causes potentially fatal tissue damage. Generally speaking, patients with modestly increased stores of iron deposited primarily in the mononuclear phagocytes are said to have *hemosiderosis*; patients with greatly increased iron stores and substantial deposits outside the phagocytes are said to have *hemochromatosis*. The distinction between these two disorders is somewhat arbitrary but is useful because the term "hemochromatosis" implies a dangerous predisposition to iron accumulation that will require therapeutic removal of iron either immediately or at some future time.

Causes of Hemochromatosis

Long-Term Transfusion Therapy

Patients with forms of anemia for which there is no effective specific therapy sometimes require transfusion on a long-term basis to maintain their hematocrits at a level sufficient to prevent secondary complications, such as congestive heart failure or ischemic disease. These patients receive 250 mg of iron with each unit of blood. It is easy to see how such a patient, who may require an average of a unit of blood a week and who can only eliminate iron by the usual physiological mechanisms, can quickly accumulate iron to the point of hemochromatosis.

Increased Iron Absorption

If enough iron accumulates through gastrointestinal absorption, hemochromatosis may develop. In some instances, this condition is thought to result from a combination of hepatic cirrhosis, which leads to augmented iron absorption, together with an abnormally large quantity of iron in the diet. This combination is most frequently seen in alcoholics, especially those who drink red wine, a beverage rich in iron. In other instances, hemochromatosis results from an inherited defect in which the gastrointestinal mucosa is unable for some reason to regulate iron absorption in a normal manner.

Manifestations of Hemochromatosis

Clinical

Cardiac

The accumulation of iron in the heart leads to serious cardiac disease (Fig. 4-12). Both the operation of the myocardial conduction system and the strength of contraction of the muscle itself are compromised. Abnormal cardiac rhythms are therefore frequent, and heart failure with its symptoms of fluid retention and shortness of breath is a common occurrence. Studies in severely affected patients show a heart that is diffusely enlarged, beating rapidly but with little force. The clinical picture is that

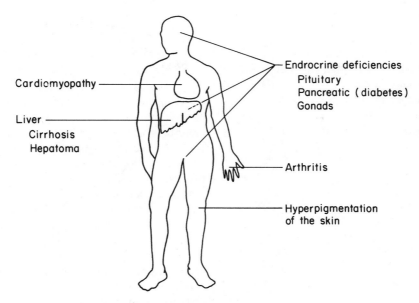

Fig. 4-12. Manifestations of hemochromatosis.

of a generalized cardiomyopathy that develops over the course of months to a few years and is refractory to standard therapy for arrhythmias or heart failure. More than one-half the patients with untreated hemochromatosis die a cardiac death.

Hepatic

The accumulation of iron in the liver leads to cirrhosis and liver failure. Cirrhosis is expressed clinically as an enlargement of the liver and spleen and the development of increased pressure in the portal venous circulation, with dilated veins at the lower end of the esophagus (esophageal varices) that can rupture and bleed, sometimes massively. Liver failure leads to a rise in serum bilirubin with jaundice because of the inability of the affected organ to handle the breakdown products of hemoglobin; a defect in coagulation because of an impairment in the production of certain clotting factors made by the liver; a fall in albumin production, leading to the retention of fluid that, because of increased portal venous pressure, accumulates mainly in the peritoneal

cavity as ascites; and in severe cases stupor or coma because of the failure of the liver to destroy toxins generated by bacteria in the gastrointestinal tract and absorbed into the bloodstream. Hepatoma is a frequent consequence of hemochromatosis of the liver. Most patients with untreated hemochromatosis who do not die from their heart disease will die of liver disease.

Endocrine

The other major clinical manifestations of hemochromatosis involve the endocrine system. Like the cardiac and hepatic disease, the endocrine abnormalities seen in hemochromatosis are thought to result from the destruction of cells by iron deposits. The glands affected are the pancreatic islets, the pituitary, and the adrenals. Islet cell disease leads to diabetes mellitus, a common complication of hemochromatosis. Pituitary disease causes hypogonadism, a problem to which the hepatic disease also makes a contribution. Adrenal insufficiency occurs, but is rare.

Other

Involvement of the skin by hemochromatosis causes increased pigmentation resulting from an increase in dermal melanin, not hemosiderin. The combination of diabetes and increased skin pigmentation has been termed "bronze diabetes." An arthritis typically affects the joints of the hands.

Laboratory

The increased iron stores in hemochromatosis are reflected in the laboratory findings. Serum iron is high while the serum transferrin (measured as the TIBC) is normal, so the ratio of serum iron to TIBC is increased. Serum ferritin, the best noninvasive indicator of iron stores, is higher than normal, as is the stainable marrow iron. Liver biopsy specimens are loaded with iron; this is apparent both under the microscope and by direct measurement, which shows that liver iron may be increased above normal by a factor of 20 or more. Finally, the amount of iron appearing in the urine after administration of the chelating agent desferrioxamine is greatly increased by hemochromatosis.

The Diagnosis of Hemochromatosis

High serum iron
Excessive iron stores
   High serum ferritin
   Increased marrow iron stores
   Increased iron in the liver biopsy[a]
Increased iron mobilization by chelators

---

[a] Quantitation of iron in the liver biopsy is the best way to diagnose hemochromatosis.

Chelation

Chelation is a means by which excess iron (or other metals) can be removed from the body. The term "chelation" refers to the ability of compounds that possess several metal-binding groups to attach to a metal ion by more than one of these groups. Such chelation complexes can be so tight that the metal ion is trapped and for all practical purposes removed from the environment.

Desferrioxamine is a chelating agent that reacts with iron to form a very tight complex (Fig. 4-13). In both its free and iron-bound forms, the agent is relatively nontoxic and is rapidly excreted in the urine, making it useful in the diagnosis and management of iron overload states. Only a very small fraction of the body iron is available for complexation by desferrioxamine at a given time, so that after a single injection of desferrioxamine only a small amount of iron (about 0.01 percent of

Fig. 4-13. Desferrioxamine. The iron-binding element of desferrioxamine is the hydroxamic acid residue

$$\left|\ \overset{\displaystyle O\quad OH}{\underset{\displaystyle (-C-N-)}{\parallel\quad\ |}}\ \right|$$

a group having an unusually high affinity for iron. The desferrioxamine molecule contains three of these groups. They are close enough to each other so that a single iron atom bound to desferrioxamine is held by all three at once. (Modified from Emery, T. (1971) Hydroxamic acids of natural origin, in Meister A. Adv. Enzymol. *35*:125, with permission.)

Fig. 4-14. Removal of iron by chelation. Giving a single injection of desferrioxamine is like draining the chelatable pool once. This pool empties quickly and completely, then refills slowly from the storage pool. Because the chelatable pool contains only a tiny fraction of the iron, draining it once has little effect on total iron stores. Infusing desferrioxamine continuously is equivalent to draining the chelatable pool on a continuous basis. As iron moves from the storage pool into the constantly emptying chelatable pool, it is steadily drained away. Under these conditions, iron stores will slowly but inevitably decline.

total body stores) appears in the urine (Fig. 4-14). This chelatable iron, however, exchanges with the nonchelatable iron in the storage pool (i.e., ferritin and hemosiderin). As a result, when desferrioxamine is given by continuous infusion, substantial amounts of iron can be unloaded over the course of a day, because of the continuous movement of iron from the storage pool through the chelatable pool and into the urine as the desferrioxamine complex. Single injections of desferrioxamine followed by measurements of urine iron are therefore useful in making the diagnosis of hemochromatosis, because the urine iron level after a dose of desferrioxamine is a good measure of iron stores. Treatment with desferrioxamine requires long-term infusions, however, because only in this way can clinically significant reductions in iron stores be achieved.

Management of Hemochromatosis

The management of hemochromatosis involves the removal of the excess iron from the patient. The method used depends on whether or not iron accumulation resulted from long-term transfusion therapy.

Long-Term Transfusion Therapy

Hemochromatosis attributable to long-term transfusion therapy is treated by long-term subcutaneous infusion of desferrioxamine using an infusion pump to deliver the chelating agent. Daily overnight infusions delivered by a portable pump that can be used at home are given initially. When iron stores reach normal levels, treatment may be given less frequently.

Idiopathic Hemochromatosis

Patients with hemochromatosis not caused by transfusion therapy are managed by phlebotomy. The program is similar to the infusion pump program in that the frequency of therapy is high early in the course of the disease and is reduced substantially after normalization of iron stores. It is important to investigate family members of patients with idiopathic hemochromatosis as well, because relatives with asymptomatic increases in iron stores may benefit from treatment to forestall clinical disease. Tissue typing, normally used in marrow transplantation (see Ch. 32), can help identify family members at risk, because there is a very close genetic linkage between the gene for idiopathic hemochromatosis and the tissue type HLA-A3.

Prognosis

In following patients with hemochromatosis, the best measure of iron stores is the ferritin level (Fig. 4-15). Serum iron generally does not fall until late in the course of therapy. Treatment will correct the cardiac disease and

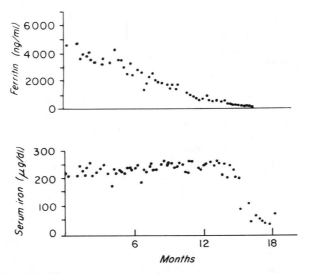

Fig. 4-15. Changes in iron during the treatment of hemochromatosis. Ferritin levels fall steadily. Serum iron remains elevated until iron stores are near normal. (From Milder, M.S. et al. (1980) Idiopathic hemochromatosis, an interim report. Medicine *59*:34–49, with permission.)

hepatic cirrhosis, with a substantial prolongation of life, but diabetes appears to be permanent, and the incidence of hepatoma in patients treated successfully for hemochromatosis remains high.

ANEMIA OF CHRONIC DISEASE

In disorders associated with chronic inflammation, including chronic infections, malignancies, and connective tissue diseases such as rheumatoid arthritis, a characteristic anemia often develops. This anemia results from an impairment in the transfer of storage iron from mononuclear phagocytes back to the hematopoietic tissues. This impairment is thought to result from the effects of certain cytokines that are released in these disorders.

The cytokines are a family of peptides containing, at last count, over two dozen members, including the interleukins, the interferons, and certain hematopoietic growth factors. The cytokines act as mediators in a fantastically tangled network of regulatory interactions involving certain cells of mesodermal origin

(e.g., fibroblasts, endothelial cells, lymphocytes, hematopoietic cells). These cells secrete the cytokines in response to infections and other forms of tissue injury, and at the same time are regulated by these cytokines, both their own and those produced by other cells.

In the anemia of chronic disease, apoferritin synthesis by mononuclear phagocytes is increased in response to a cytokine (possibly interleukin 1, a cytokine that acts on mononuclear phagocytes after being secreted by mononuclear phagocytes that have been activated by an encounter with T lymphocytes that themselves have been activated by the binding of antigen to receptors on their surfaces—a clear, if oversimplified, illustration of the labyrinthine ways of the cytokines, their sources, and their targets). This excess apoferritin directs newly mobilized iron into the storage pool, thereby blocking its release from the mononuclear phagocyte and preventing the red cell precursors from obtaining the iron they need to make hemoglobin (Fig. 4-16). The red cell precursors find themselves in the ancient mariner's predicament, except that what they need and cannot get is iron, not water.

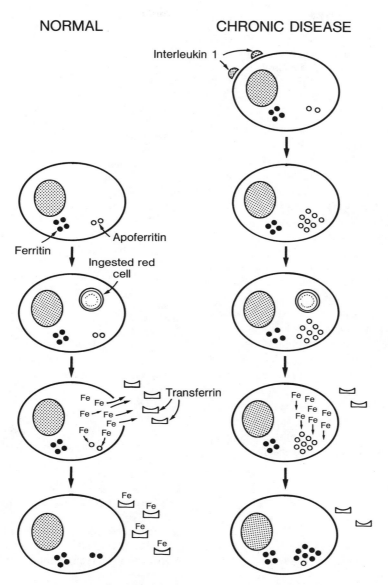

Fig. 4-16. Proposed basis for the anemia of chronic disease. In inflammatory states, a cytokine is released that stimulates the synthesis of apoferritin by mononuclear phagocytes. As a result, some of the iron released into the phagocyte during the breakdown of ingested red cells is not secreted into the plasma, its usual fate, but instead is taken up by the extra apoferritin to form ferritin, the storage form of iron. Iron stores are thereby increased at the expense of the iron supply available for red cell production.

The anemia in this condition develops fairly rapidly (2 to 4 weeks), but remains mild; hematocrits below 30 ml/dl are distinctly unusual. The red cells usually look normal on the smear, but in some cases they may be rather small and pale, perhaps because of their iron-deficient state. Because the anemia is caused by a decrease in red cell production by the marrow, reticulocyte counts are normal to low. The serum iron is low, but the serum iron binding capacity (i.e., transferrin) does not show a compensatory increase as in iron deficiency. Instead, it drops too, and the paradoxical combination of a low serum iron and a low iron binding capacity is the hallmark of the anemia of chronic disease.

There is plenty of iron around, however—in fact, more than normal. It is all locked away in the mononuclear phagocytes as storage iron. The superabundance of storage iron is manifested clinically as an elevation in serum ferritin and a marrow that on staining is loaded with iron, completely the opposite of the iron-free marrow seen in iron deficiency anemia.

As to management, there is little that can be done, and little that needs to be done. Transfusions are not warranted by the degree of anemia seen in the uncomplicated condition and should not be given. Iron therapy is obviously useless. The only effective therapy is the treatment of the underlying condition; alleviate this, and the anemia will cure itself.

SUGGESTED READINGS

Adams, P.C., Halliday, J.W. & Powell, L.W. (1989) Early diagnosis and treatment of hemochromatosis. Adv. Intern. Med. *34*:111–126.

Aisen, P. & Brown, E.B. (1977) The iron-binding function of transferrin in iron metabolism. Semin. Hematol. *14*:31–53.

Bentley, D.P. (1985) Iron metabolism and anaemia in pregnancy. Clin. Haematol. *14*:613–628.

Cook, J.D. & Skikne, B.S. (1987) Intestinal regulation of body iron. Blood Rev. *1*:267–272.

Dallman, P.R. (1986) Biochemical basis for the manifestations of iron deficiency. Annu. Rev. Nutr. *6*:13–40.

Dallman, P.R., Beutler, E. & Finch, C.A. (1978) Effects of iron deficiency exclusive of anaemia. Br. J. Haematol. *40*:149–184.

Finch, C.A. & Cook, J.D. (1984) Iron deficiency. Am. J. Clin. Nutr. *39*:471–477.

Finch, C.A., Deubelbeiss, K., Cook, J.D. et al. (1970) Ferrokinetics in man. Medicine *49*:17.

Finch, C.A. & Huebers, H.A. (1986) Iron metabolism. Clin. Physiol. Biochem. *4*:5–10.

Gordeuk, V.R., Bacon, B.R. & Brittenham, G.M. (1987) Iron overload: causes and consequences. Annu. Rev. Nutr. *7*:485–508.

Jacobs, A. & Worwood, M., eds, Iron in Biochemistry and Medicine, II, Academic Press, London, 1980.

Lee, G.R. (1983) The anemia of chronic disease. Semin. Hematol. *20*:61–80.

Morgan, E.H. & Baker, E. (1988) Role of transferrin receptors and endocytosis in iron uptake by hepatic and erythroid cells. Ann. N.Y. Acad. Sci. *526*:65–82.

Morgan, P.G. & Turner-Warwick, M. (1981) Pulmonary haemosiderosis and pulmonary haemorrhage. Br. J. Dis. Chest *75*:225–242.

Wickramasinghe, S.N. (1988) Nutritional anaemias. Clin. Lab. Haematol. *10*:117–134.

Worwood, M. (1986) Serum ferritin. Clin. Sci. *70*:215–220.

Heme Formation: Biosynthesis of the Tetrapyrrole. Porphyrias and Sideroblastic Anemias

Heme biosynthesis, although complicated at first glance, is actually a very straightforward process involving a logical sequence of biochemical steps. The process can be divided into three stages: (1) the synthesis of the five-carbon building block from which heme is made, (2) the formation of a tetrapyrrole from this building block, and (3) the conversion of this tetrapyrrole into the heme molecule. Disorders of the latter two stages give rise to the porphyrias, a group of diseases in which the relationships between the biochemical and clinical manifestations are unusually well worked out. Disorders of the first stage appear to be responsible for many of the characteristic features of the sideroblastic anemias, but these diseases are not nearly as well understood as the porphyrias.

BIOSYNTHESIS OF HEME

The stages involved in the formation of a heme molecule are (1) the production of δ-aminolevulinic acid (ALA), the building block; (2) the formation of the first tetrapyrrole by

two successive condensation reactions, the first producing a monopyrrole from ALA and the second producing the tetrapyrrole from 4 monopyrroles; and finally (3) the conversion of this tetrapyrrole into heme. This sequence is outlined in Figure 5–1.

The Building Block

ALA is produced by the enzyme ALA synthetase in a reaction in which glycine and succinyl coenzyme A are joined end to end. The reaction requires pyridoxal phosphate, a point of clinical importance (Fig. 5–2).

The First Tetrapyrrole

This is synthesized in two steps. The first is the condensation of two molecules of ALA to form the monopyrrole, porphobilinogen (PBG); this reaction is catalyzed by PBG synthetase (Fig. 5–3). The first tetrapyrrole is then formed by the one-step condensation of four PBGs, catalyzed by an enzyme with the

Fig. 5–1. Three stages of heme biosynthesis.

Fig. 5–2. The production of δ-aminolevulinic acid (ALA) by the condensation of glycine and succinyl coenzyme A (CoA).

uninformative name *PBG deaminase*, so called because it splits an ammonia out of each PBG molecule during the condensation (Fig. 5–4). The product of the two successive condensation reactions is called uroporphyrinogen (UROGEN). The suffix -ogen refers to the fact that the tetrapyrrole is partly reduced, with the one-carbon bridges each containing two hydrogen atoms.

Hanging from the pyrrole ring of each PBG molecule are two carboxylic acid side chains: an acetate (A) and a propionate (P). PBG deaminase acting by itself causes the PBG monomers to condense in a head-to-tail manner, so that the order of the side chains around the tetrapyrrole ring is as follows: A—P—A—P—A—P—A—P—. This compound, known as UROGEN I, is normally made in small amounts, but cannot be further metabolized: it is a dead-end product. The true precursor of heme is UROGEN III, a molecule in which the order of side chains is A—P—A—P—A—P—P—A— (see Fig.5-4). It is produced by the combined action of PBG deaminase and a second enzyme, cosynthetase. It will be seen

that the order of the substituents around the periphery of the tetrapyrrole, seemingly a trivial matter, is actually of clinical significance.

To summarize, PBG is formed by the condensation of two ALA molecules in a reaction catalyzed by PBG synthetase. Four PBG molecules then condense to yield UROGEN. When condensation is catalyzed by PBG deaminase

Fig. 5–3. The first tetrapyrrole. Porphobilinogen (PBG), the first tetrapyrrole, is formed by the condensation of two molecules of ALA. This reaction is catalyzed by PBG synthetase.

Fig. 5–4. Formation of UROGEN III by the condensation of four molecules of PBG. This reaction is catalyzed by two enzymes: PBG deaminase and cosynthetase.

plus cosynthetase, the product is UROGEN III, which can be metabolized further to heme. When condensation is catalyzed by PBG deaminase alone, the product is UROGEN I, a dead-end metabolite.

Heme

Heme is produced by three successive modifications in the tetrapyrrole followed by the insertion of an iron atom to yield the final product (Fig. 5–5). In the first modification, CO_2 molecules are removed from the acetate side chains to produce coproporphyrinogen III (COPROGEN III), containing four methyl groups (M) instead of the four acetates. The order of side chains in COPROGEN III is M—P—M—P—M—P—P—M— The four CO_2 molecules are all removed by a single enzyme, coproporphyrinogen synthetase.

In the next modification, the two nonadjacent propionate side chains are oxidized. Oxidation of these chains is accompanied by the departure of two more CO_2 molecules. The product is protoporphyrinogen IX (PROTOGEN IX), containing vinyl groups (V) instead of propionyl groups in two of the peripheral locations. The order of side chains in PROTOGEN IX is M—V—M—V—M—P—P—M—. The enzyme catalyzing this reaction is coproporphyrinogen oxidase.

The final modification is the oxidation of the ring. Four additional double bonds are created

to produce the fully oxidized porphyrin, protoporphyrin IX (PROTO IX). This reaction is catalyzed by protoprophyrinogen oxidase.

Finally, heme is produced by the enzyme-catalyzed insertion of an iron atom into the center of the porphyrin ring. This reaction is catalyzed by ferrochelatase.

The four steps involved in the conversion of UROGEN III to heme are summarized in Table 5–1.

PORPHYRIAS

The rate of porphyrin synthesis is tightly controlled by the intracellular concentration of free heme, which regulates its own production by acting as a feedback inhibitor of ALA synthetase. When the activity of one of the porphyrin-synthesizing enzymes is decreased, the resulting slowdown in heme synthesis causes the release of this feedback inhibition, with an increased flow of precursors into the porphyrin synthetic pathway. This increase in flow, combined with the restriction in the rate of one of the porphyrin synthetic steps, causes the accumulation of the intermediate whose further metabolism is restricted by the enzymatic defect (Fig. 5–6). All the intermediates in the porphyrin biosynthetic pathway are toxic compounds whose accumulation leads to disease. The diseases produced by these intermediates are the porphyrias.

The porphyrias are a confusing group of conditions, because there is a different form of

UROGEN III   COPROGEN III   PROTOGEN IX

Protoporphyrinogen   Protoporphyrin   Heme

Fig. 5–5. Conversion of UROGEN III to heme. (**Top row**) Side-chain modifications, leading successively from UROGEN III through COPROGEN III to PROTOGEN IX. (**Bottom row**) Last two steps in heme synthesis: the oxidation of protoporphyrinogen to protoporphyrin and the insertion of the iron. For clarity, the nitrogens and most of the hydrogens have been omitted and the side chains have been left off the figures in the bottom row.

porphyria for each enzyme, and these different forms vary in their manifestations depending on the nature of the intermediate that accumulates. There is, however, a series of logical principles that can serve as a guide through this rather bewildering thicket of diseases:

1. A 50 percent reduction in the activity of one of the porphyrin-synthesizing enzymes is often enough to lead to symptomatic porphy-

ria. Inheritance therefore tends to be *autosomal dominant*.

2. PBG causes neurological abnormalities, possibly because PBG or a metabolite can mimic a normal neurotransmitter. Tetrapyrroles, however, act mainly in the skin, where they are deposited and cause a photosensitivity dermatitis whose severity varies depending on which compound accumulates.

3. Porphyria is generally diagnosed by mea-

Table 5-1. The Conversion of UROGEN III to Heme

Step	Reaction	Enzyme
UROGEN → COPROGEN	4 Acetate → 4 methyl	Uroporphyrinogen decarboxylase
COPROGEN → PROTOGEN	2 Propionate → 2 vinyl	Coproporphyrinogen oxidase
PROTOGEN → protoporphyrin	Oxidation of the ring	Protoporphyrinogen oxidase
Protoporphyrin → heme	Insertion of iron	Ferrochelatase

Fig. 5–6. The origin of porphyria. (**Top**) Normal situation. Heme feeds back on the enzyme that makes ALA, controlling ALA production. (**Bottom**) Porphyria attributable to a deficiency of COPROGEN oxidase. Heme production is decreased. This lifts the feedback inhibition of the ALA-forming enzyme, causing ALA production to increase. Intermediates down the line, however, accumulate behind the partial block. These increased quantities of intermediates push heme synthesis back toward normal, but their toxicity also causes the signs and symptoms of porphyria. U, UROGEN; C, COPROGEN; P, PROTOGEN.

suring the excretion of heme precursors in the urine and stool. The distribution of a precursor between the urine and the stool depends on its water solubility, which is related to the number of negatively charged carboxyl groups at its periphery (Fig. 5–5). PBG and UROGEN, which contain two carboxyl groups/pyrrole, are excreted in the urine. COPROGEN, which contains one carboxyl group/pyrrole, is excreted partly in the urine and partly in the stool. Later precursors are excreted entirely in the stool.

Acute Intermittent Porphyria

Acute intermittent porphyria (AIP) is caused by a partial deficiency of PBG deaminase, the tetrapyrrole-forming enzyme. Under normal circumstances, patients with this disease are usually clinically well, and precursors do not accumulate in detectable quantities. When the deficient patient is stressed, however, levels of PBG and ALA build up, provoking one of the recurrent attacks that characterize the disease (Fig. 5–7). The symptoms of the attack are widespread, but they can all be ascribed to abnormalities of the nervous system (Fig. 5–8). Psychosis and convulsions indicate disease of the cerebral cortex. Instability of temperature and blood pressure are caused by brain-stem disease; this may lead to death. Abdominal and pelvic pain that can be so severe as to mimic an acute abdomen are thought to be caused by dysfunction of the autonomic nervous system. Acute peripheral neuropathy, most typically an acute paralysis involving one or more motor nerves, may also be seen, and respiratory paralysis leading to death can occur in this condition.

Several types of stresses can precipitate attacks of AIP. They may occur during the menstrual period, and in fact women are generally more susceptible to attacks of AIP than are men. Infections and acidosis may initiate attacks of AIP. Attacks are characteristically

$$\longrightarrow \text{PRECURSORS} \longrightarrow \text{ALA} \longrightarrow \text{PBG} \overset{\text{deficient}}{\dashrightarrow}_{\text{U}} \longrightarrow$$

Fig. 5–7. Site of the blockade of porphyrin synthesis in acute intermittent porphyria.

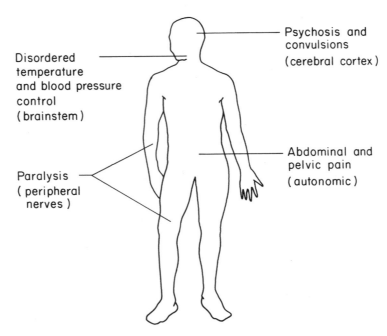

Fig. 5–8. Signs and symptoms of acute intermittent porphyria. These occur as attacks. They are thought to be caused by the neurotoxicity of PBG or its metabolites.

precipitated by certain drugs, of which barbiturates are the most frequent offenders. These AIP-precipitating drugs have in common the capacity to induce the formation of hepatic drug-metabolizing enzymes, including cytochrome P-450, and it is thought that the attack results from the increase in heme formation that is required to provide the cytochrome with its prosthetic group.

Factors Precipitating Attacks of Acute Intermittent Porphyria

Menstrual periods
Infections
Acidosis
Drugs
    Barbiturates
    Birth control pills
    Others

The diagnosis of AIP is made by demonstrating the presence of ALA and PBG in the urine during the course of an attack. These are generally not found in the urine between attacks. Furthermore, tetrapyrroles are not found in either the urine or stool at any time during the course of this disease; their presence should raise doubts about the accuracy of the diagnosis. The diagnosis may also be made by demonstrating reduced levels of PBG deaminase in liver biopsies, but this is mainly a research method and is not widely available.

The management of AIP has been at least partly rationalized on the basis of an understanding of the precipitating factors and the control of the heme biosynthetic pathway. Between attacks the patient should be on a high carbohydrate diet to prevent minor degrees of acidosis that increase susceptibility to an attack; drugs that can precipitate attacks should be scrupulously avoided. An attack is treated with intravenous heme, which terminates the attack by blocking ALA synthetase (Fig. 5–6).

Porphyria Cutanea Tarda

Porphyria cutanea tarda is caused by hepatic cirrhosis from any cause combined with an inherited partial deficiency of UROGEN decarboxylase, the enzyme that converts URO-GEN to COPROGEN (Fig. 5–9). An isolated partial deficiency of the decarboxylase normally causes no disease, because even with a 50 percent reduction in the level of the enzyme, the rate of conversion of UROGEN to COPROGEN is rapid enough to prevent an accumulation of precursors. When the liver is cirrhotic, however, the activity of the hepatic decarboxylase is further reduced, apparently because of inhibition by the iron that invariably builds up in the parenchymal cells of cirrhotic livers. This further reduction in the activity of the decarboxylase is enough to cause an accumulation of precursors and the onset of symptoms.

The precursors that accumulate are tetrapyrroles, as expected from the location of the

$$\longrightarrow \text{ALA} \longrightarrow \text{PBG} \longrightarrow \overset{\text{deficient}}{\text{U}} \cdots\overset{\text{g}}{\longrightarrow} \text{c} \longrightarrow$$

Fig. 5–9. Site of the blockade of prophyrin synthesis in porphyria cutanea tarda.

block in porphyrin synthesis. The tetrapyrroles are UROGEN III and some partially decarboxylated products that arise because of the incomplete decarboxylation of UROGEN by the decarboxylase, a single enzyme that removes all four CO_2 molecules in the course of converting UROGEN to COPROGEN. The accumulation of the tetrapyrroles leads to a dermatitis in sun-exposed portions of the skin that may be very severe, with painful bullae that heal with scarring, irregular increased pigmentation, and hair growth in affected areas (Fig. 5–10).

A clue to the presence of porphyria cutanea tarda is provided by clinical examination of the urine from suspected patients. The heme precursors excreted in the urine of patients with

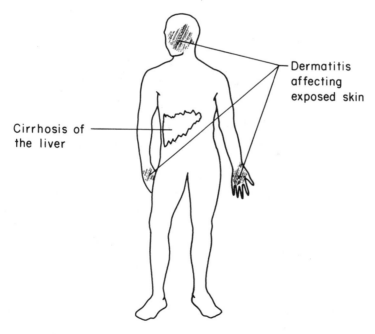

Dermatitis affecting exposed skin

Cirrhosis of the liver

Fig. 5–10. Signs and symptoms of porphyria cutanea tarda. Hepatic cirrhosis is a contributing cause of the disease. The dermatitis is caused by the deposition of porphyrins in the skin, sensitizing it to damage by the sun.

Colorless porphyrinogen   Red porphyrin

Fig. 5–11. Spontaneous oxidation of a porphyrinogen to a porphyrin in voided urine. The side chains and nitrogens are omitted for clarity.

porphyria cutanea tarda are porphyrinogens, which are tetrapyrroles containing a partially reduced ring (see above). Porphyrinogens are colorless, so that freshly voided urine containing these compounds is normal in color. On standing, however, the porphyrinogens in this urine undergo oxidation to the corresponding porphyrins, which are deep red (Fig. 5–11). Urine from patients with porphyria cutanea tarda therefore turns dark with time.

The diagnosis is made by the method used to diagnose all porphyrias: the demonstration of porphyrin precursors in the urine or stool. In porphyria cutanea tarda, precursors are found in both, the relative proportions varying with the number of carboxyl groups, as discussed above. Owing to their susceptibility to oxidation, however, the -ogen precursors are not found as such, but will have been converted to the fully oxidized porphyrins by the time the measurement is made. Thus UROGEN III, a major component of the porphyrin

precursors excreted in porphyria cutanea tarda, is found mostly in the urine, where it is detected as uroporphyrin III. Partially decarboxylated precursors, however, appear in both urine and stool as fully oxidized 5- to 7-carboxyporphyrins. This is summarized in Figure 5–12.

On the basis of pathogenetic mechanisms, a rational approach to the management of porphyria cutanea tarda has been developed. The mainstay of treatment is phlebotomy, which in removing excess iron from the liver relieves the inhibition of the decarboxylase and permits precursors to flow normally into heme. Treating the underlying cirrhosis will also alleviate the porphyria, but this is usually much less successful because of the difficulty in eliminating the cause of the cirrhosis, usually alcohol.

Other Porphyrias

Porphyrias have now been associated with deficiencies of each of the enzymes of the heme synthetic pathway, except for ALA synthetase. The features of these porphyrias are summarized in Table 5–2.

SIDEROBLASTIC ANEMIAS

The sideroblastic anemias are a group of conditions in which the incorporation of iron into heme is impaired. Uptake of iron by the red cell precursors is intact, however, and iron

```
        URINE   │   STOOL
                │
Uroporphyrin    │
  7-carboxyl porphyrin
      6-carboxyl porphyrin
         5-carboxyl porphyrin
                │
```

Fig. 5–12. Porphyrin excretion in porphyria cutanea tarda.

Table 5-2. The Porphyrias

Deficiency	Disease	Products Excreted[a]	Manifestations[b]
PBG deaminase	Acute intermittent porphyria	ALA–PBG[c]	N
UROGEN decarboxylase	Porphyria cutanea tarda	U, decarboxy U	D
Cosynthetase	Erythropoietic porphyria	U I (not U III)	D (very severe)
COPROGEN oxidase	Hereditary coproporphyria	C, ALA–PBG	N, D
PROTOGEN oxidase (?)	Variegate porphyria	C, P, ALA–PBG	N, D
Ferrochelatase	Erythropoietic *proto*porphyria	P	D

[a] Principal compounds: U, uroporphyrin; C, coproporphyrin; P, protoporphyrin. U is found mainly in the urine, C and P mainly in the stool.

[b] Manifestations correlate with the products excreted. N, neurological: attacks like those in acute intermittent porphyria. D, dermatological; solar dermatitis.

[c] ALA and PBG are always excreted together in the hereditary porphyrias.

accumulates in these precursors in a characteristic pattern. The basis for the problem with iron metabolism is not well understood, but there is some evidence that it may be associated with a defect in the formation of ALA, the starting material for heme synthesis. Although this evidence is not abundant, the concept of a defect in ALA formation provides both a rationale for understanding the pathophysiology of sideroblastic anemias and a thread that ties together a number of otherwise unrelated facts about the diseases. They will therefore be discussed within the context of this idea.

Ineffective Erythropoiesis

The sideroblastic anemias, as well as the megaloblastic anemias, thalassemias, and certain hematological malignancies, are characterized by an aberration in red cell formation known as *ineffective erythropoiesis*. This term is used to describe the destruction of red cell precursors in the marrow before they can mature fully to appear in the blood as reticulocytes.

The occurrence of ineffective erythropoiesis has been established by observing the fate of newly synthesized heme over time. Newly made heme can be tagged by administering isotopically labeled glycine to a subject. A portion of the labeled glycine is incorporated into heme, whereas the rest is rapidly metabolized by other routes. The labeled glycine is

thus available only for a short period of time, and only those heme molecules that were synthesized during that short time interval will carry the label.

The tagged heme is then incorporated into proteins—mostly hemoglobin, but also heme-requiring enzymes, of which the most abundant by far is the cytochrome P-450 of the liver. When these proteins are degraded, the heme is converted into bilirubin, which is excreted in the bile. Tagged bilirubin will appear when proteins containing tagged heme molecules are degraded. It is possible, therefore, to determine the lifetime of heme-containing proteins by measuring the interval between the administration of labeled glycine and the appearance of labeled bilirubin in the bile. This method, of course, only indicates that some heme-containing proteins have been degraded; the identity of the degraded protein must be determined by other types of studies.

The fate of newly synthesized heme has been followed in humans using ^{13}C-labeled glycine (Fig. 5–13). Three peaks of labeled bilirubin appear in the bile. The first two are the so-called "early labeled" peaks. They appear 1 to 4 days after the tagged glycine is given and contain about 15 percent of the total excreted label. The first peak has been shown to result from the breakdown of cytochrome P-450; the second is from hemoglobin that has been degraded during the destruction of red cell precursors in the marrow—that is, from ineffective erythropoiesis. The third peak, by far the largest, appears about 4 months after

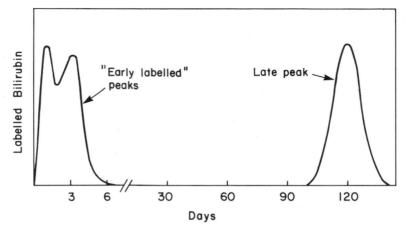

Fig. 5–13. Fate of newly synthesized heme in humans, as measured by the production of labeled bilirubin from heme tagged in vivo with labeled glycine. A small fraction of the new heme is in the liver, where it is incorporated mostly into cytochrome P-450; turnover of this protein accounts for the first of the two "early labeled" peaks. Almost all the rest of the new heme is made in the red cell precursors. About 10 percent of these are destroyed before they leave the marrow, their heme producing the second of the two "early labeled" peaks. The rest develop into red cells, which enter the bloodstream and circulate for about 4 months. They are then destroyed, producing the late peak of labeled bilirubin. (Note the change in scale on the X-axis.)

the labeled glycine is given and is caused by the destruction of the cohort of red cells that had formed in the marrow at the time the tagged heme was available. From the ratio of the second and third peaks, it can be calculated that ineffective erythropoiesis accounts for about 10 percent of total red cell production under normal conditions.

In patients with sideroblastic anemias and the other anemias listed above, the percentage of red cell precursors destroyed in the marrow is much greater than normal. In especially severe cases, ineffective erythropoiesis may amount to 90 percent of total red cell production. This increase in ineffective erythropoiesis could in principle be diagnosed by the tagged heme method. This method, however, is not practical for the routine investigation of anemic patients. At the bedside, ineffective erythropoiesis is generally diagnosed from the results of the bone marrow examination combined with ferrokinetic data. As expected from the very high rate of erythropoiesis necessary to maintain an adequate hematocrit in this con-

dition, the marrow is grossly hypercellular, with almost no fat, and the myeloid:erythroid ratio is shifted far in the direction of the red cell series. The increased marrow iron requirement necessary to meet the demands of erythropoiesis is reflected in ferrokinetic measurements, which show a greatly increased plasma

---

Diagnosis of Ineffective Erythropoiesis

Hypercellular marrow with a disproportionate increase in the red cell series (increased erythroid/myeloid ratio)
Increased plasma iron turnover
Erythrocyte iron turnover < 70 percent of plasma iron turnover
Increased uptake and retention of iron by the marrow[a]

---

[a] See Figure 5–9 for further details.

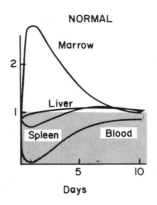

Fig. 5–14. Movement of labeled iron through various tissues during the first 10 days after administration in a patient with ineffective erythropoiesis. Note especially that after 8 to 10 days there is more iron in the marrow and less iron in the blood than is seen in normal circulation. (From Finch, C.A. (1982) Clinical aspects of iron deficiency and excess. Semin. Hematol. *19*: 1–67, with permission.)

iron turnover and an increase in the amount of iron taken up by the marrow. In this respect, the ferrokinetics of ineffective erythropoiesis are the same as those of iron deficiency. They differ, however, in that most of the iron in ineffective erythropoiesis does not end up in the red cells, but remains in the marrow, where the hemoglobin-containing precursors are destroyed. This is most apparent in the fact that the erythrocyte iron turnover, instead of being 80 to 90 percent of the plasma iron turnover, is considerably lower, indicating that a substantial amount of the iron taken up from the plasma did not reach the peripheral blood. Studies of iron distribution show that iron is preferentially retained by the marrow at the expense of the peripheral blood (Fig. 5–14). All the ferrokinetics can be understood in the context of a marrow that is taking up iron avidly to make cells of the erythropoietic series, most of which are destroyed in situ before thay can be released into the bloodstream.

Causes of Sideroblastic Anemia

In understanding the causes of sideroblastic anemia, it is useful to have a rationale to explain its characteristics—especially the iron accumulation, which is its most typical feature. Such a rationale is available, although it must be emphasized that the supporting evidence is at present skimpy and indirect. Nevertheless, this rationale is presented, because it provides a convenient way of thinking about these conditions and pulls together a lot of information about what otherwise appears to be a rather heterogeneous group of diseases.

The sideroblastic anemias can be considered in terms of a blockade in heme synthesis at the level of ALA production (Fig. 5–15). This blockade occurs so early in the heme biosynthetic pathway that monopyrroles and tetrapyrroles are prevented from accumulating. Instead, iron accumulates, perhaps because it is

blockaded

succinyl CoA + glycine ⟶ ALA ⟶ PBG → → → Heme

Fig. 5–15. Sideroblastic anemias may be caused by a blockade in the synthesis of ALA.

Causes of Sideroblastic Anemias

Drugs
    Alcohol
    Antituberculosis drugs
    Lead
    Others
Inherited
Idiopathic (stem cell mutation)

taken up by the red cell precursors at a near normal rate, but cannot be disposed of by the usual route of incorporation into heme.

As to causes, the sideroblastic anemias arise either spontaneously or as the side effect of a drug. Many of these causes can be understood in terms of the rationale presented above.

Drugs

Most drug-related sideroblastic anemias are caused by one of two types of agents: alcohol or certain agents used against tuberculosis. The latter include isoniazid (INH), cycloserine, and pyrazinamide. What these appear to have in common is an antagonism against pyridoxal phosphate, the cofactor necessary for the synthesis of ALA. The antipyridoxal effect of INH has been especially well shown and results from the addition of INH to pyridoxal phosphate to form a compound excreted in the urine. With alcohol, there may be interference with the conversion of the vitamin pyridoxine to the coenzyme pyridoxal phosphate.

Other

Most of the non-drug-related sideroblastic anemias appear to arise through the replacement of the normal hematopoietic stem cells by a line of mutant stem cells that have ac-

quired a defect in heme production, resulting in a sideroblastic state. Such a sideroblastic anemia—actually a form of myelodysplasia (see Ch. 27)—generally develops in late middle age. It can be a premalignant condition, with some patients going on to develop acute myeloblastic leukemia. A small percentage of patients with this condition respond to very large doses of pyridoxine.

Sideroblastic anemia may also be inherited, presenting in childhood. The mode of transmission may be autosomal dominant, autosomal recessive, or X-linked.

Manifestations of Sideroblastic Anemia

Sideroblastic anemia looks at first like a disease caused by a deficiency of precursor cells in the bone marrow (i.e., a hypoproliferative or hypoplastic anemia). It is characterized by a low hematocrit combined with a reticulocyte count that is low for the degree of anemia, a combination suggesting that marrow red cell precursors are lacking. On the peripheral smear, the cells usually look smaller than normal (Fig. 5–16), an appearance borne out by microcytic red cell indices. A significant minority of patients, however, have cells that are larger than normal (macrocytosis), and a few show both microcytes and macrocytes, a so-called dimorphic smear. A characteristic feature of the red cell is basophilic stippling, a finding that results from incomplete degradation of RNA as the red cell matures. Normally, the RNA in the red cell precursor is broken down to its nucleotides when the cell reaches maturity. Residual RNA is found only in the youngest circulating cells (see reticulocytes, Ch. 2), and then only in small amounts. If RNA degradation is impaired, however, red cells containing large amounts of RNA will be present in the circulation. In these cells, the nucleic acid can precipitate as visible deep blue aggregates when the smear is stained with

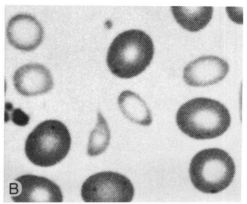

Fig. 5–16. Peripheral smear in sideroblastic anemia. (**A**) Normal smear. (**B**) Sideroblastic anemia. The red cells are irregular in shape (poikilocytosis). Some are small and pale; others appear to be slightly macrocytic. This dual population is characteristic of sideroblastic anemia. Basophilic stippling is seen in an occasional cell. (From Wintrobe, M.M. et al. (1974) Clinical Hematology. 7th ed. Lea & Febiger, Philadelphia, with permission.)

Wright's stain.* Cells containing these aggregates are said to display basophilic stippling. This morphological abnormality is typical of sideroblastic anemia and is seen in several other forms of anemia as well.

The bone marrow examination establishes the diagnosis of sideroblastic anemia. Contrary to what might be expected from the hypoproliferative picture in the periphery, the marrow is packed with red cell precursors. Furthermore, the mononuclear phagocytes of the marrow are loaded with iron in the form of hemosiderin, a consequence of the high rate of local destruction of red cell precursors (i.e., the abnormally high level of ineffective erythropoiesis). Most importantly, it is in the marrow that the diagnostic cell of sideroblastic anemia is found.

The diagnostic cell is a ringed sideroblast. This red cell precursor accumulates large quantities of iron in the mitochondria, a situation

---

*Wright's stain is the stain used for routine blood smears. It can precipitate high concentrations of RNA, but it cannot precipitate the small quantity of RNA in a reticulocyte; for this, cresyl violet is needed.

> ## Anemias in Which Basophilic Stippling May Be Seen
>
> Sideroblastic anemia
> Megaloblastic anemia
> Thalassemia
> Sickle cell anemia

that does not occur in normal erythropoiesis. When an iron-stained marrow sample is examined under the light microscope, the ringed sideroblast appears as a nucleated red cell precursor with a necklace of coarse, iron-containing granules around the nucleus (Fig. 5–17). Electron microscopic examination shows these iron-containing granules to be the mitochondria, which cluster around the nucleus in this cell giving it its characteristic "ringed" appearance.

The accumulation of iron in the mitochondria of these cells may have to do with the fact that the incorporation of iron into heme takes place in mitochondria. The iron is supplied by a mitochondrial iron-transporting system that

Fig. 5–17. Bone marrow in sideroblastic anemia. (**A**) Prussian blue stain. The marrow is packed with red cell precursors. Iron (dark granules) is abundant. The ringed sideroblast (*arrow*) is a red cell precursor with a necklace of prominent iron granules around the nucleus. These granules are iron-filled mitochondria (**B**). (**A**, from Castoldi, G.L. (1981) Erythrocytes. Ch. 3, pp. 33–145. In Zucker-Franklin, D. et al. (eds.) Atlas of Blood Cells: Function and Pathology. Edi. Ermes s.r.l., Milan, with permission. **B**, from Wintrobe, M.M. et al. (1974) Clinical Hematology. 7th ed. Lea & Febiger, Philadelphia, with permission.)

Clinical Iron Measurements in Sideroblastic Anemia

High serum iron
Normal total iron-binding capacity (equivalent to a normal transferrin level)
High transferrin saturation
High serum ferritin

normally seems to maintain a balance between the iron supply and the rate of porphyrin formation, as there is little free iron in the mitochondria of normal red cell precursors. It is conceivable that an impairment in porphyrin synthesis out of proportion to any change in mitochondrial iron transport occurs in sideroblastic anemia. In that event, iron would pile up in the mitochondria, because no porphyrin is available to which it can be transferred.

Other general features of sideroblastic anemia have to do with abnormalities in iron metabolism. Serum iron is high and transferrin saturation is greater than normal, because iron stores are elevated and iron absorption from the small intestine is increased in association with the increase in marrow erythropoietic activity. Serum ferritin is high, another indication of increased iron stores. Ferrokinetics are altered in the characteristic way.

Features may also be seen that are specific for the cause of the sideroblastic anemia. For example, a history of alcoholism or antituberculosis therapy may be obtained. Family studies may provide evidence for an inherited condition. In the spontaneously appearing sideroblastic anemias, other hematopoietic lines may be shown to be involved, indicating a stem cell abnormality (see Ch. 28).

Management of Sideroblastic Anemia

Once the diagnosis is made, the management of sideroblastic anemia is straightforward. If the anemia is iatrogenic, the drug can

be discontinued, unless its use is essential to the patient's welfare. High-dose pyridoxine should always be tried in spontaneously acquired sideroblastic anemia, although the likelihood of success with this form of treatment is not great. In sideroblastic anemias that do not respond to these measures, transfusion may be used, but it must be remembered that hemochromatosis is a serious consideration with long-term transfusion therapy, particularly in anemias with ineffective erythropoiesis in which iron stores are expanded by the nature of the disease itself.

LEAD

Lead is an inhibitor of several of the enzymes of the heme synthetic pathway, affecting PBG synthetase as well as enzymes catalyzing later steps. Perhaps because of its effect on these enzymes, chronic lead poisoning causes a disease exhibiting features of both sideroblastic anemia and porphyria. Porphyria-like features include a motor neuropathy and a characteristic pattern of recurrent abdominal pain with constipation (so-called "lead colic"); coproporphyrin and ALA (but not PBG, an important distinction from the inherited porphyrias) are excreted in the urine. The anemia of lead poisoning is a typical sideroblastic anemia, with microcytosis, basophilic stippling, an elevated serum iron, and ringed sideroblasts in the marrow. Red cell porphyrin is increased, probably reflecting the inhibition of ferrochelatase by the toxic metal.

Other manifestations of chronic lead intoxication include renal failure, hypertension, and gout. Psychosis may also result from chronic lead poisoning; the decline of the Roman empire has been attributed in part to psychosis among the Roman rulers arising from their practice of drinking wine from lead vessels. The "lead line" is a bluish-black deposit seen in the gingival margin; such a line is highly suggestive of intoxication by lead or other heavy metals, but it is seen only in patients with poor dental hygiene. Acute lead poisoning may lead to an acute encephalopathy with greatly increased intracranial pressure, papilledema, and coma.

Lead poisoning typically affects persons exposed to the metal in the course of their work. It used to be particularly common among painters, because of the lead-based pigments at one time present in paints. The paint content has changed, so that lead poisoning in painters is not the problem it once was. Lead-containing paint, however, may still be found on the walls of old houses. This paint represents an insidious source of lead poisoning in children, who flake it from the walls and eat it because of its sweet flavor. In working up any child displaying signs of lead poisoning, this possibility must always be kept in mind.

The diagnosis of lead poisoning is made by the demonstration of elevated lead levels in the blood or urine. The condition is treated by chelation therapy with calcium EDTA and by removal of the patient from the source of poison.

SUGGESTED READINGS

Beris, P., Graf, B.J. & Miescher, P.A. (1983) Primary acquired sideroblastic and primary acquired refractory anemia. Semin. Hematol. *20*:101–113.

Bloomer, J.R. & Bonkovsky, H.L. (1989) The porphyrias. Dis. Mon. *35*:1–54.

Bottomley, S.S. & Muller-Eberhard, U. (1988) Pathophysiology of heme synthesis. Semin. Hematol. *25*:282–302.

Cartwright, G.E. (1975) Sideroblasts, siderocytes, and sideroblastic anemia. N. Engl. J. Med. *292*: 185–193.

Cullen, M.R., Robins, J.M. & Eskenazi, B. (1983) Adult inorganic lead intoxication: presentation of 31 new cases and a review of recent advances in the literature. Medicine *62*:221–247.

Felsher, B.F. & Kushner, J.F. (1977) Hepatic siderosis and porphyria cutanea tarda: Relation of iron excess to the metabolic defect. Semin. Hematol. *14*:243–251.

Lindenbaum, J. & Roman, M.J. (1980) Nutritional anemia in alcoholism. Am. J. Clin. Nutr. *33*: 2727–2735.

Mufti, G.J. & Galton, D.A. (1986) Myelodysplastic syndromes: natural history and features of prognostic importance. Clin. Haematol. *15*:953–971.

Pasanen, A. & Tenhunen, R. (1986) Heme synthesis in sideroblastic anaemias. Scand. J. Haematol. Suppl. *45*:60–65.

Yunis, A.A. & Salem, Z. (1980) Drug-induced mitochondrial damage and sideroblastic change. Clin. Haematol. *9*:607–619.

DNA Replication and Hematopoiesis: Megaloblastic Anemias

In most tissues of the body, cell division is a rare event, taking place only as needed to replace losses resulting from damage or to provide an increase in organ mass in order to handle a functional overload (e.g., the hypertrophy of the remaining kidney that follows unilateral nephrectomy). There are a few tissues, however, in which cell division is a continuous process. These tissues include the hematopoietic system, the gastrointestinal epithelium, the epidermis, and the germinal epithelium of the testis. In all these tissues, normal function involves a continuous loss of cells, so constant production of new cells is necessary to maintain the tissue in a normal state.

The key event of cell division is the synthesis of new DNA. This process occurs only in an occasional cell in slowly dividing tissues, but it is the rule in the hematopoietic system and the other continuously dividing tissues. All these tissues are therefore sensitive to damage by factors that disrupt DNA synthesis, in contrast to slowly dividing tissues, which tend to be resistant to such factors.

In the hematopoietic system, impaired DNA synthesis is expressed clinically as a characteristic disorder of hematopoiesis known as *megaloblastic anemia*. The term *megaloblastic* refers to the abnormally large (megalo-) red

cell precursors (blasts) that populate the marrow in this disorder. Megaloblastic anemia is most often caused by a deficiency of folate or cobalamin, the two vitamins necessary for normal production of deoxyribonucleotides. Drugs that inhibit DNA synthesis may also cause megaloblastic anemia. Occasionally, megaloblastic anemia appears as a manifestation of an acquired stem cell disorder.

MEGALOBLASTIC ANEMIA

Unlike most of the conditions discussed so far, megaloblastic anemia involves all three hematopoietic cell lines—red cells, white cells, and platelets. This is because all three lines are produced continuously by the marrow, and as a result all three lines are affected when a megaloblastic state develops because of a disturbance in DNA synthesis. Accordingly, wide-ranging abnormalities are seen in the peripheral blood of patients with megaloblastic anemia. In addition, a diagnostic cell appears in the marrow—an abnormal red cell precursor known as the megaloblast.

In the peripheral blood, a macrocytic anemia is the rule. By mean cell volume (MCV), the red cells are large; in some cases they are huge, exceeding the normal MCV by 50 percent or more. The blood smear contains many macroovalocytes—the oversized, elliptical, hemoglobin-stuffed red cells characteristic of megaloblastic anemia—but also contains many cells that are smaller than normal. Gross macrocytosis is virtually diagnostic of megaloblastic anemia, but minor degrees (MCV increased by up to 10 percent) occur in some sideroblastic anemias, in the anemias of hypothyroidism and liver disease, and in anemias with large numbers of circulating reticulocytes, which are bigger than mature red cells and will cause an increase in the MCV.

As to the other formed elements, the white blood cell count may be low because of neutropenia, and the platelet count may be reduced as well. "Hypersegmented polys"—neutrophils with more than the normal three to five nuclear lobes—are seen on the smear (Fig. 6–1) in many cases. This abnormality is caused by a defect in nuclear segmentation, and not, as was formerly postulated, by the release of hypermature neutrophils from the marrow.

The anemia in megaloblastic anemia is caused by ineffective erythropoiesis. Accordingly, the marrow is packed with red cell precursors, yet the reticulocyte count is low for the degree of anemia and in many cases is reduced in absolute terms as well. The serum bilirubin is elevated because of the increase in the "early label" peak caused by the degradation of hemoglobin released when red cell precursors are destroyed in the marrow. The serum iron is increased as well. The serum lactate dehydrogenase reaches remarkable heights because of the release of the enzyme from the red cell precursors as well as from leukocyte and megakaryocyte precursors, which are also thought to be destroyed in the marrow (ineffective myelopoiesis and thrombopoiesis).

The hallmark of megaloblastic anemia is the *megaloblast*. This cell, seen in the marrow, is a red cell precursor in which DNA synthesis is retarded (the common feature of megaloblastic anemia), whereas protein and RNA synthesis proceed at a normal rate. The result is a cell in which cytoplasmic differentiation has out-

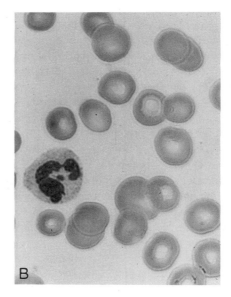

Fig. 6–1. Blood smear in megaloblastic anemia. (**A**) Megaloblastic smear. This field shows several macroovalocytes (*arrows*) as well as a neutrophil with greater than five lobes in its nucleus (a "hypersegmented poly"). The typical variability in red cell size is also evident. (**B**) A normal smear for comparison.

Fig. 6–2. Marrow in megaloblastic anemia. (**A**) Megaloblastic marrow. This marrow is packed with megaloblastic red cell precursors. The megaloblast can be identified by the large cell size and the immature-looking nucleus with its characteristically open chromatin. (**B**) Normal marrow, for comparison.

stripped nuclear maturation, so that the nucleus appears younger than it should for the stage of development of the cell. The nucleus is larger than it ought to be, and its chromatin meshwork is more open. Furthermore, the entire cell is larger than normal, because it undergoes fewer divisions before reaching maturity than does the normal cell. All these features are most readily seen in the final stages of red cell differentiation, but they can be detected at all stages (Fig. 6–2). Greatly enlarged late-stage white cell precursors (giant metamyelocytes and bands) may also be seen in megaloblastic bone marrow.

The foregoing features are common to all megaloblastic anemias. Other clinical manifestations, not common to megaloblastic anemias in general, but seen in only specific types, are described in the sections dealing with the anemias in which they occur.

Clinical Features of Megaloblastic Anemia

Blood cells
  Reticulocytes decreased
  Mean cell volume increased
  Macroovalocytes and hypersegmented
    polymorphonuclear leukocytes on
    smear
Blood chemistries
  Iron increased
  Bilirubin increased
  Lactate dehydrogenase increased
Marrow
  Packed with red cell precursors
  Megaloblasts present

FOLATE AND MEGALOBLASTIC ANEMIA

Folate is required for the synthesis of three of the four bases found in DNA. Deficiency of this vitamin is probably the most common cause of megaloblastic anemia.

Fig. 6–3. Folic acid. The three parts of the molecule are indicated in the figure. For the sake of clarity, some of the hydrogens have been omitted.

Normal Function

Metabolic Role

An understanding of the basis for the megaloblastic anemia in folate deficiency requires knowledge of the role played by folate in normal metabolism. Folate (Fig. 6–3) consists of three parts: a nitrogen-containing ring system known as the *pteridine*, a second ring consisting of p-aminobenzoic acid, and a chain of glutamic acid residues that prevent the vitamin from leaking out of cells. The vitamin itself is metabolically inert; the active form is produced by reduction of the right half of the pteridine to give tetrahydrofolate (THF). This reduction is accomplished by an enzyme called *dihydrofolate reductase*.

The function of THF is to transfer one-carbon fragments from various donors — mostly the amino acid serine — to various acceptors — primarily intermediates of nucleotide biosynthesis. These one-carbon fragments are transferred to and from a very small region of the complex THF molecule. This region, which in a sense is the business end of THF, is a simple chain of four atoms with the so-called N^5 nitrogen at one end and the N^{10} nitrogen at the other (Fig. 6–4).

The main reaction that loads folate with one-carbon fragments is the transfer of the one-

Fig. 6–4. A portion of the tetrahydrofolate (THF) molecule, showing the "business end" (**boldface**) and the partly reduced pteridine.

carbon side chain from serine to THF. This yields glycine together with a form of THF in which N^5 and N^{10} are linked by a —CH_2— bridge: $N^{5,10}$-methylene THF. This bridge may be oxidized to produce the forms of THF that function in purine production; it may be reduced to produce N^5-methyl THF, the major circulating form; or it may be transferred as such to the uracil of deoxyuridine monophosphate (dUMP) to form thymidylic acid (dTMP). These interconversions are summarized in Figure 6–5.

The conversion of dUMP to dTMP is unique among folate one-carbon transfers in that the pteridine is oxidized during the course of the reaction and must be re-reduced before it can participate further in one-carbon metabolism (Fig. 6–6). The product of the thymidylate synthetase reaction is dihydrofolate (DHF); it is reduced back to THF by dihydrofolate reductase. Certain highly effective chemothera-

Fig. 6–5. Interconversions of folate-bound one-carbon fragments. (**Top**) Fully oxidized forms; carbons from the oxidized form are incorporated into the purine ring during purine nucleotide biosynthesis. (**Bottom**) Fully reduced form, the major circulating folate. For the sake of clarity, THF is represented by its "business end" only, and the one-carbon fragments are shown in boldface.

Fig. 6–6. Folate and the synthesis of thymidylic acid (dTMP). Thymidylic acid is synthesized by the transfer of a one-carbon fragment from $N^{5,10}$-methylene tetrahydrofolate (THF) to deoxyuridine monophosphate (dUMP). During this transfer, the folate is oxidized from the tetrahydro- to the dihydro form. This dihydrofolate, a metabolically inert compound, is reduced back to the metabolically active tetrahydrofolate by the enzyme *dihydrofolate reductase*.

peutic agents act by inhibiting dihydrofolate reductase, thereby killing dividing cells by gradually diverting all their metabolically active folates into an inert pool of DHF (see below).

Assimilation

Folate is present in most foods; it is especially abundant in vegetables, where its presence in leafy parts gave it its name. Almost all this folate contains a polyglutamate chain, a structural feature described by the term *conjugated*. During absorption (Fig. 6–7), which can take place throughout the length of the small intestine, the polyglutamate chain is split off by an enzyme known as *deconjugase*, which is present on the brush border of the intestinal epithelial cell. The deconjugated folate moves into this cell, where it is converted to N^5-methyl THF and is then released into the bloodstream. Almost all the circulating folate is in the form of unconjugated (i.e., containing only a single glutamate residue) N^5-methyl THF.

The circulating N^5-methyl THF is taken up into cells by means of a specific THF carrier. Here it rapidly transfers its methyl group to homocysteine to form THF and methionine in a cobalamin-requiring reaction that is catalyzed by an enzyme known in short form as *methyltransferase*. The demethylated THF is then reconjugated by the addition of a chain of glutamate residues (5 to 7 is the normal number) to produce the tissue form of THF, ready to play its role in one-carbon metabolism.

There are two points of interest in regard to the reconjugation reaction: (1) the glutamates are attached to each other by peptide bonds, but these bonds involve the "wrong" carboxyl group and are therefore resistant to hydrolysis by ordinary proteases; and (2) the methyltransferase reaction is an essential preliminary to reconjugation, because N^5-methyl THF is a poor substrate for the conjugating enzyme and must be converted to THF before conjugation can take place.

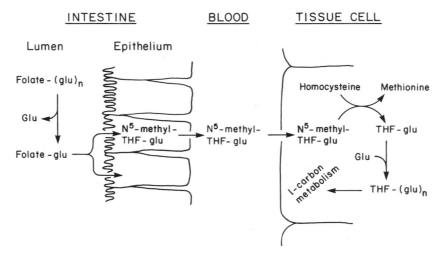

Fig. 6–7. Absorption of folate. Folate is deconjugated in the intestinal lumen, then converted by the intestinal cell to N^5-methyl THF and released into the bloodstream. In this form, it is actively transported into cells. The methyl group is then removed by transfer to homocysteine, and the resulting THF is reconjugated, entering into one-carbon metabolism.

Folate Deficiency

Causes

Folate deficiency usually occurs because folate intake fails to meet needs. Occasionally it is the result of a defect in intestinal absorption.

Folate-Poor Diet

The most common cause of folate deficiency is a folate-poor diet. This is seen in alcoholics, whose customary diet of ethanol and congeners is lacking in folate and many other vitamins, and in the poor, especially the elderly poor, who for financial and other reasons are unable to obtain enough food to stave off malnutrition.

Increased Folate Requirements

Under certain circumstances, folate requirements may increase to the point where an ordinary diet cannot meet the augmented needs of the patient. This occurs in patients in whom for one reason or another cell replication is greatly increased. Folate deficiency resulting from increased requirements is most frequently seen in pregnancy, in which the growing products of conception impose a severe stress on

folate supplies. In pregnant women, the macrocytosis typical of folate-deficient megaloblastic anemia may be offset by microcytosis caused by iron deficiency, so that folate deficiency may be easily overlooked in this circumstance. Routine supplementation of pregnant women with folate as well as iron is a good idea. Other conditions in which increased folate requirements may lead to vitamin deficiency are severe hemolytic anemias and exfoliative dermatitis, with greatly augmented erythropoiesis and epidermal cell production, respectively. Like pregnant women, patients with these conditions may require folate supplementation.

Malabsorption

Certain intestinal diseases are characterized by a reduction in nutrient absorption by the affected bowel. Occasionally, folate absorption is sufficiently impaired in these conditions to lead to folate deficiency. The disease most commonly associated with clinically significant folate malabsorption is tropical sprue.

Manifestations

Megaloblastic Anemia

The most typical manifestation of folate deficiency is megaloblastic anemia, a hematopoietic disorder whose features have already been discussed. The salient molecular abnormality in folate deficency is a marked slowing of DNA synthesis, a defect expressed not only in the characteristic morphological abnormalities of the megaloblastic cells, but also in a marked prolongation of the S (DNA synthetic) phase in replicating cells and in a disruption in chromatin structure detectable as chromosomal tangles and breaks. Despite extensive study, a biochemical explanation for the slowing of DNA synthesis in folate deficiency is not yet

---

Cause of Folate Deficiency

Folate-poor diet
  Alcoholism
  Poverty
Increased folate requirements
  Pregnancy
  Severe hemolytic anemia
Malabsorption

available, although it appears to be somehow related to the defect in dTMP formation seen in folate-deficient cells.

Other Manifestations

Folate deficiency affects other rapidly dividing tissues. A stomatitis characterized by a sore mouth and a smooth, beefy red tongue occurs frequently. It probably results from impaired proliferation of the oral mucosa, which is worn away during eating and must be constantly renewed. The gastric and intestinal mucosa acquire megaloblastic characteristics that can lead to confusion on cytological examination, although functional impairment due to these changes is slight.

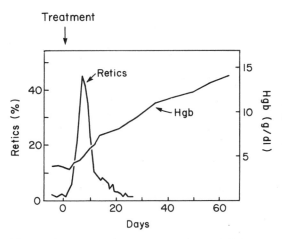

Fig. 6–8. Response of anemia of folate deficiency to treatment. (Redrawn from Wyngaarden, J.B. & Smith, L.H. (1982) Cecil Textbook of Medicine. 16th ed. W.B. Saunders, Philadelphia, with permission.)

Management

The diagnosis of folate deficiency is made by demonstrating reduced levels of folate in the serum. Serum folate responds rapidly to alterations in dietary folate status; hence a reduced serum folate level means that a state of folate deficiency has existed over the previous few days. Red blood cells, on the other hand, contain roughly the quantity of folate they held when they were released from the marrow, so measurement of red cell folate provides an indication of folate status over the preceding weeks. It is sometimes useful to measure the red cell folate in a treated patient if it is desirable to establish the existence of a prior state of folate deficiency.

Folate deficiency is treated simply by giving the vitamin. The response to treatment is striking. The megaloblastic morphology of cells in the bone marrow is gone within 24 to 48 hours. The reticulocyte count begins to rise by 3 to 5 days and rapidly reaches a peak that in severe cases may exceed 50 percent reticulocytes. Concomitantly, there is healing of the stomatitis. The reticulocyte count then begins

to fall and returns to normal with a complete resolution of the anemia. The whole process takes 3 to 6 weeks, depending on the severity of the initial disease. A typical treatment response is shown in Figure 6–8.

COBALAMIN AND MEGALOBLASTIC ANEMIA

Cobalamin has two metabolic functions: (1) it participates in folate metabolism, and (2) it is required for the degradation of certain fatty acids. Megaloblastic anemia and neurological abnormalities are the typical manifestations of cobalamin deficiency. Both appear to be caused by disturbances involving the cobalamin–folate connection.

This vitamin is currently undergoing a change in nomenclature. It was originally called vitamin B_{12}, but cobalamin is now the preferred terminology, the term *vitamin B_{12}* being reserved for the cyanide-containing form of the vitamin (see below). The old terminology, however, is still used from time to time.

Fig. 6–9. Cobalamin. The full structure is cyanocobalamin, one of the four types of cobalamin found in tissues. The three parts of the molecule are indicated in this structure. The partial structures are hydroxocobalamin, methylcobalamin, and adenosylcobalamin, the other cobalamins found in tissues. The nucleoside base in these cobalamins is not the usual purine or pyrimidine, but instead is the rare base, 5,6-dimethylbenzimidazole. Cobalamin is the only biological compound in which this base occurs.

Normal Function of Cobalamin

Metabolic Role

Like folate, cobalamin consists of three basic parts; the corrin ring, a hemelike structure that contains cobalt at its center; the nucleotide, attached to the ring by a side chain and bonded to the cobalt through one of the nitrogens of its base; and the β-group, attached to the cobalt on the opposite side of the ring from the nucleoside (Fig. 6–9). Tissue cobalamins contain four different kinds of β-groups: methyl, adenosyl, OH⁻, and CN⁻ (Fig. 6–9). The methyl- and adenosylcobalamins serve as coenzymes, each working in a different reaction (see below). Hydroxo- and cyanocobalamin have no coenzymatic activity of their own, but are readily converted to the coenzymatically active forms by tissue enzymes.

Cyanocobalamin is the form of the vitamin that is usually sold commercially.

Methylcobalamin is necessary for only one reaction in mammalian systems: the conversion of N^5-methyltetrahydrofolate to tetrahydrofolate (Fig. 6–10). This reaction serves two purposes: (1) to produce methionine by the transfer of a methyl group to homocysteine; and (2) to convert newly acquired cellular folate to a form that can be conjugated to a polyglutamate chain.

Adenosylcobalamin also serves as the cofactor for a single mammalian reaction (Fig. 6–10). This is the rearrangement of methylmalonyl coenzyme A (CoA) to succinyl CoA, catalyzed by the adenosylcobalamin-dependent enzyme methylmalonyl CoA mutase. Methylmalonyl CoA is generated by the addition of CO_2 to propionyl CoA, a compound produced in large quantities by the combustion of valine

Fig. 6–10. Cobalamin-dependent reactions.

and isoleucine, amino acids that serve as important fuels for muscle. The product of the methylmalonyl CoA mutase reaction is a Krebs cycle intermediate that can be burned in the mitochondria to yield energy.

Assimilation

The assimilation of cobalamin is a complex process involving several carrier proteins as well as a series of specialized cellular transport systems (Fig. 6–11 and Table 6–1). As will be seen, defects in one or another of the elements of this process are responsible for most cases of cobalamin deficiency.

The process of assimilation of cobalamin begins in the duodenum. Here the vitamin becomes attached to intrinsic factor (IF), a glycoprotein that is secreted by the parietal cells of the stomach. The cobalamin–IF complex does not form in the stomach because at the low pH of the working stomach, cobalamin is preferentially bound to R binder, a cobalamin-binding protein of unknown function present in all secretions, including saliva and gastric juice. The change in pH that occurs when the gastric contents pass into the duodenum causes the cobalamin to shift from the R binder to intrinsic factor. The R binder is digested, but the cobalamin–IF complex remains intact, because intrinsic factor is highly resistant to proteolysis.

The cobalamin–IF complex passes through the small intestine until it reaches the ileum. Here it attaches to specific receptors and is taken up into the ileal mucosal cells, where the IF is degraded and the cobalamin released. After several hours, the cobalamin passes from the ileal mucosal cell into the portal circulation, now complexed to transcobalamin II (TC II), a protein synthesized by the intestinal epithelium and probably most other tissues.

It is as this complex that cobalamin is taken up into cells. Cells contain surface receptors that bind the TC II–cobalamin complex. Once bound, the complex and its receptor are rapidly carried into the cell by pinocytosis. The

Table 6-1. Cobalamin-binding Proteins

Protein	Source	Required for
Intrinsic factor	Gastric parietal cells	Absorption of cobalamin by intestine
Transcobalamin II	Liver, intestinal mucosa, other	Uptake of cobalamin into cells
R binders	All secretions	Unknown

Fig. 6–11. Assimilation of cobalamin. The stomach secretes two cobalamin-binding proteins: intrinsic factor, which is essential for the absorption of cobalamin, and R binder, whose function is unknown. On entering the stomach, cobalamin forms a complex with R binder. This complex enters the duodenum, where cobalamin is transferred from R binder to intrinsic factor. The intrinsic factor–cobalamin complex passes through the intestine until it reaches the ileum, where the complex attaches to receptors on the ileal mucosal cells. These cells take up the intrinsic factor–cobalamin complex, then release the cobalamin and transport it into the bloodstream, some complexed to a new carrier, transcobalamin II, and the rest as the free vitamin. Once in the bloodstream, the free cobalamin rapidly binds to circulating TC II. The TC II–cobalamin complex then attaches to receptors on the surfaces of cells throughout the body. These cells take up the complex and release the cobalamin for use in their metabolism.

internalized cobalamin is released from TC II, which is degraded. The cobalamin is then converted to its coenzymatically active forms.

Although newly absorbed cobalamin circulates in the form of a TC II complex, most of the cobalamin in the bloodstream is complexed to transcobalamin I (TC I) a circulating member of the R-binder family. Unlike the cobalamin-TC II complex, which circulates for less than an hour before being taken up by the tissues, the cobalamin-TC I complex has a very long survival, with a half-time measured in days. Because of the relative rates of turnover of the TC I and TC II complexes, most of the cobalamin in blood drawn at random is found to be associated with TC I. It is not known how the cobalamin–TC I complex is formed, but it is thought to be eliminated by excretion in the bile.

Cobalamin Deficiency

Causes

Cobalamin deficiency is almost invariably caused by a derangement in absorption. This derangement may result from a failure of intrinsic-factor (IF) secretion by the stomach, from disease or absence of terminal ileum, or from the presence in the small intestine of organisms that trap cobalamin on its way from the stomach to the terminal ileum.

Gastric Failure

The most common cause of cobalamin deficiency is a failure of IF secretion caused by atrophy of the gastric mucosa. This atrophy,

---

Causes of Cobalamin Deficiency

Gastric
   Gastric atrophy (pernicious anemia)
   Total gastrectomy
Ileal
   Disease of terminal ileum (regional enteritis, tropical sprue)
   Ileal resection
Competing organisms
   Bacterial overgrowth (blind loops, intestinal strictures)
   Fish tapeworm

---

currently thought to result from autoimmune destruction, leads to the condition known as *pernicious anemia*. The term "pernicious anemia" is sometimes used as a synonym for anemia caused by cobalamin deficiency from any cause, but it should be reserved for this one specific condition.

Other conditions that lead to the destruction or elimination of the gastric mucosa will also cause cobalamin deficiency of gastric origin. The most common of these conditions is total gastrectomy.

Disease or Absence of the Terminal Ileum

Cobalamin deficiency can result from the destruction or elimination of the terminal ileum, the portion of the small intestine that possesses the capacity to absorb IF cobalamin. Diseases that can affect the terminal ileum so as to cause cobalamin deficiency include regional enteritis (Crohn's disease) and tropical sprue. Absence of the terminal ileum is invariably the result of surgical resection.

Competing Organisms in the Small Intestine

Normally, the small intestine is relatively free of bacteria. However, abnormalities that impede the free flow of material through the organ may permit the accumulation of bacteria in the small intestine in numbers sufficient to cause cobalamin deficiency by taking up the vitamin from the gut before it can reach the terminal ileum. Conditions such as intestinal diverticula or surgically created blind loops contain masses of bacteria that are constantly overflowing into the intestinal lumen, where they can take up the vitamin. Similarly, cobalamin-trapping bacteria will accumulate behind intestinal strictures. Clinically significant cobalamin deficiency is a common complication of these conditions.

The fish tapeworm, *Diphyllobothrium la-*

tum, accumulates cobalamin avidly. Infestation with this worm can result in cobalamin deficiency.

Manifestations

Megaloblastic Anemia

The megaloblastic anemia of cobalamin deficiency is identical to that seen in folate deficiency and in fact arises because of a deficiency in tissue folate that develops in cobalamin-deficient patients (Fig. 6–12). The basis of this anemia is an impairment in the activity of the cobalamin-requiring methyltransferase that occurs in cobalamin deficiency. After entering the cell, N^5-methyl THF, the circulating form of folate, is demethylated to THF by methyltransferase. The THF is then conjugated to a polyglutamate side chain, converting it to a form that can be retained by the cell. In cobalamin deficiency, conjugation is compromised because of an impairment in the conversion of the poorly conjugable N^5-methyl THF to the readily conjugable demethylated form. With the failure of conjugation, there is leakage of folate out of the cell, leading to a deficiency of tissue folate. In this connection it should be pointed out that the megaloblastic anemia of cobalamin deficiency can be fully corrected by the administration of folic acid, though the dose required is several times larger than that necessary to correct the anemia of folate deficiency.

Stomatitis and gastrointestinal mucosal alterations similar to those seen in folate deficiency are also observed in cobalamin deficiency, probably for the same reason.

Neurological Manifestations

A critically important feature of cobalamin deficiency not seen in folate deficiency is neurological disease. The disease is a demyelinating condition that most frequently affects peripheral nerves, presenting as a symmetrical mixed motor and sensory neuropathy, but it may involve the brain and spinal cord as well (Fig. 6–13). Involvement of the brain leads to dementia, psychological disturbances, or both, whereas cord involvement in its most severe form leads to demyelination of the posterior and lateral columns, with spastic paralysis and absent proprioception. The spinal cord disease

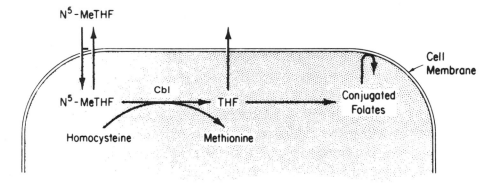

Fig. 6–12. Cobalamin deficiency leading to tissue folate depletion. Folate is taken up by cells as N^5-methyl-THF, an unconjugated form of the vitamin. Once in the cells, the folate must be conjugated (i.e., supplied with a polyglutamate chain) to keep it from leaking out again. Before the folate can be conjugated, however, it must first be demethylated. Cobalamin is required in order for this demethylation reaction to occur. When cobalamin is in short supply, demethylation is impaired. As a result, conjugation is defective, and the cells are unable to retain their folate. (Redrawn from Wyngaarden, J.B. & Smith, L.H. (1982) Cecil Textbook of Medicine. 16th ed. W.B. Saunders, Philadelphia, with permission.)

Fig. 6–13. Spinal cord demyelination in cobalamin deficiency. The myelin stains dark in this section; demyelinated areas appear as white patches. (From Robbins, S.L. (1974) Pathologic Basis of Disease. W.B. Saunders, Philadelphia, with permission.)

is known as *combined system disease*, because demyelination affects both the proprioception and motor-conducting systems of the cord.

Demyelination is currently thought to be caused by a defect in methylation that arises because of diminished methyltransferase activity (Fig. 6–14). The principal biological methylating agent is S-adenosylmethionine, formed from methionine and adenosine triphosphate (ATP). The reduction in methyltransferase activity that occurs in cobalamin deficiency leads to a decrease in methionine production, with an accompanying fall in S-adenosylmethionine formation. The result is an impairment in S-adenosylmethionine dependent methylations —in particular, the methylation of phosphatidylethanolamine to phosphatidylcholine, and the methylation of a critical histidine in myelin basic protein. Demyelination is presumably a consequence of this impairment in methylation.

A crucial feature of this demyelinating condition is that it may be seen in the absence of megaloblastic anemia and under these circumstances is easy to misdiagnose. This is a tragic error, because, unlike the anemia, the neurological disease may not be completely reversed by vitamin replacement therapy. Indeed, neurological disease has been reported to occur after the erroneous treatment of cobalamin-deficient megaloblastic anemia with folate, which will correct the anemia, but will obviously have no effect on the neurological abnormalities of cobalamin deficiency.

Pernicious Anemia

Pernicious anemia has clinical features not seen in other forms of cobalamin deficiency.

Epidemiological. Pernicious anemia is typically a disease of late middle age, although onset in late childhood or adolescence occurs very occasionally. It is seen most frequently in northern Europeans and American blacks.

NORMAL

N^5 – Methyl THF + homocysteine $\Rightarrow$ Methionine $\Rightarrow$ S-adenosylmethionine

Cbl

Protein

Phosphatidylcholine
Methylated DNA
Methylated proteins
Creatine
etc.

COBALAMIN DEFICIENCY

N^5 + Methyl THF + homocysteine $\longrightarrow$ Methionine $\longrightarrow$ S-adenosylmethionine

Cbl

Protein

Phosphatidylcholine
Methylated DNA
Methylated proteins
Creatine
etc.

Fig. 6–14. Deficient methylation in cobalamin deficiency. In cobalamin deficiency, the production of methionine from homocysteine and N^5-methyltetrahydrofolic acid is decreased. As a result, there is an impairment in the biosynthesis of S-adenosylmethionine, the principal biological methylating agent. This leads in turn to a drop in the rates of reactions in which S-adenosylmethionine participates. These reactions include the methylation of DNA, important in the regulation of gene expression, and the production of a large number of essential biochemical materials, including among others phosphatidylcholine, creatine, and methylated proteins. Among the methylated proteins is myelin basic protein, a major myelin constituent that contains a methylated histidine. Could the neuropathy in cobalamin deficiency be caused by a defect in the biosynthesis of myelin basic protein?

Special Features of Pernicious Anemia

Epidemiological
   Most frequent in northern Europeans, American blacks
   Tends to run in families
Gastric
   Achlorhydria
   Increased incidence of gastric cancer
Immunological
   Antibodies against parietal cells and intrinsic factor
   Associated with other autoimmune diseases (e.g., Hashimoto's thyroiditis)

There is a tendency for the disease to run in families.

Gastric. Because of the atrophy of parietal cells, total achlorhydria is a universal feature of pernicious anemia. The frequency of gastric cancer is increased in pernicious anemia, although malignancy generally develops only after many years of disease.

Immunological. Almost all patients with pernicious anemia have a serum antibody against parietal cells, and most show antibodies against intrinsic factor. The antiparietal cell antibodies are currently thought to play a role in the pathogenesis of the condition. Other autoimmune diseases, particularly Hashimoto's thyroiditis, are increased in frequency in pernicious anemia.

Other Manifestations

Manifestations specific for the cause of the vitamin deficiency may be seen. Ileal disease is associated with characteristic gastroenterological signs and symptoms. Bacterial overgrowth may be associated with fat malabsorption, and an anatomical lesion of the small intestine (e.g., intestinal diverticula) may be seen on radiographs. *Diphyllobothrium latum* infestation may be indicated by eggs or macroscopically visible proglottids in the stools.

Management

The existence of a state of cobalamin deficiency can be established by measurements of serum cobalamin levels. To determine the cause of the cobalamin deficiency, however, requires further testing.

A useful test for this purpose is the Schilling test, which measures cobalamin absorption by determining the fraction of an orally administered dose of radioactive cobalamin excreted in the urine over 24 to 48 hours (Fig. 6–15). To carry out this test, radioactive cobalamin is given by mouth. TC I and TC II are then saturated by means of a large parenteral dose of nonradioactive cobalamin. Because of the saturation of the transcobalamins, some labeled cobalamin absorbed from the intestine will be carried in the blood in the unbound form and rapidly cleared by the kidney. Decreased excretion of label in the urine therefore indicates decreased intestinal absorption of the vitamin (assuming normal renal function). This can arise from any of the causes noted above. To distinguish among these causes, the Schilling test is repeated with the modification that intrinsic factor is given by mouth along with the labeled vitamin. Cobalamin malabsorption of gastric origin is corrected by this procedure, whereas cobalamin malabsorption caused by ileal disease is not; cobalamin malabsorption resulting from competition by intestinal organisms may or may not be corrected by oral intrinsic factor.

Other investigations that may be carried out will depend on the whole clinical story. They should be directed toward ascertaining the cause of the condition in the most efficient way.

Cobalamin deficiency is treated by parenteral administration of the vitamin. Depending on whether the cause of the deficiency is re-

Fig. 6–15. Schilling test. A dose of radioactive cobalamin is first given by mouth. The circulating cobalamin binders are then saturated by giving a large dose of unlabeled cobalamin by injection. Because the binders are saturated with unlabeled cobalamin, any free radioactive cobalamin absorbed from the intestine will find nothing to bind to and will have to circulate as the free vitamin, which is rapidly excreted into the urine. The amount of radioactivity appearing in the urine thus indicates how well the vitamin is absorbed from the intestine.

versible, parenteral vitamin therapy may be necessary for the duration of the patient's life. Treatable conditions such as bacterial overgrowth, anatomical abnormalities of the intestine, or fish tapeworm infestation should be corrected where possible by appropriate medical or surgical therapy.

The response of the anemia to treatment is similar to that seen in folate-deficient anemia: reversal of the marrow abnormalities in 1 to 2 days and a reticulocytosis peaking within about 1 week after the start of therapy (Fig. 6–8). Neurological manifestations, however, may correct themselves only partially, or not at all.

Other Causes of Megaloblastic Anemia

Drugs that interfere with DNA synthesis can cause megaloblastic anemia (see also Ch. 31). These drugs fall into two categories: those that interfere with DNA synthesis per se (examples are hydroxyurea, which inhibits ribonucleotide reductase, and cytosine arabinoside, an analogue of cytosine) and those that antagonize folate (examples are the antiprotozoal drugs pentamidine and pyrimethamine, the diuretic triamterine, and the antibiotic trimethoprim). Megaloblastic anemia induced by these drugs is usually mild, occurring as a rather harmless concomitant of their therapeutic action, and generally needs no treatment. If treatment is required, the most effective measure is to eliminate the drug or lower its dose and give supplemental folic acid. Correction of the anemia occurs promptly.

With one drug, however, megaloblastic anemia can represent a very serious problem. This drug is methotrexate, a commonly used chemotherapeutic agent (Fig. 6–16). Methotrexate is an exceedingly powerful inhibitor of dihydrofolate reductase, the enzyme necessary for the regeneration of tetrahydrofolate from the dihydrofolate produced in the thymidylate synthetase reaction. In the presence of toxic concentrations of the drug, this reaction is almost totally blocked, with the result that most of the tissue folate becomes trapped in a metabolically inert pool of dihydrofolate. Folate-

---

Non-nutritional Causes of Megaloblastic Anemia

Drugs
    Inhibitors of DNA synthesis
    Folate antagonists
        Methotrexate
        Other
Idiopathic
    Refractory megaloblastic anemia
    DiGuglielmo's syndrome
    Congenital dyserythropoietic anemia

---

requiring processes such as the biosynthesis of purines and dTMP are thereby brought to a halt, with serious clinical consequences affecting rapidly replicating tissues. A florid megaloblastic anemia quickly develops. A severe and agonizingly painful stomatitis also ensues. The most serious consequence, however, is necrosis of the mucosa of the gastrointestinal tract, with severe nausea and vomiting and fulminant diarrhea that may be grossly bloody.

Fig. 6–16. Methotrexate and its antidote. Methotrexate is a powerful inhibitor of dihydrofolate reductase, blocking the regeneration of THF and bringing to a halt all folate-requiring reactions. Methotrexate blockade can be circumvented by giving N^5-formyl-THF (citrovorum factor), a metabolically functional form of THF that can be given as a drug.

A fatal outcome can be expected in severe methotrexate poisoning.

Fortunately, there exists a specific antidote for methotrexate poisoning: citrovorum factor, or N^5-formyltetrahydrofolate. This compound, unlike other tetrahydrofolate derivatives, is stable in air and consequently can be used to provide an exogenous supply of fully reduced folate. After administration, it is converted in an ATP-requiring reaction to N^{10}-formyl THF, which is freely interconvertible with the other forms of THF that are normally present in tissues. In this manner, the pool of metabolically active folates is replenished, and the clinical manifestations of methotrexate poisoning are rapidly corrected.

Idiopathic

Refractory Megaloblastic Anemia

Refractory megaloblastic anemia is a form of bone marrow failure of unknown cause that occurs generally in patients of late middle age or older. It is characterized clinically by reduced numbers of any or all of the formed elements of the blood, a variable incidence of morphological peculiarities especially among cells of the granulocyte series (e.g., hypogranularity, abnormal nuclear segmentation), and a marrow that is hypocellular and shows megaloblastic changes in the red cell series only (i.e., no giant bands or metamyelocytes). The condition is a form of myelodysplasia (see Ch. 28), with a similarly bad prognosis and a similar tendency to evolve into a particularly intractable form of acute myelogenous leukemia. Treatment is generally supportive, although an occasional patient may respond to pharmacological doses of pyridoxine.

DiGuglielmo's Syndrome

DiGuglielmo's syndrome is a form of leukemia in which malignant red cell precursors are particularly evident. It is mentioned here because megaloblastic red cell precursors are almost invariably seen in the marrow in this condition.

Congenital Dyserythropoietic Anemias

These rare and poorly understood inherited disorders present as an isolated anemia with no other hematological abnormalities. Anemia is present from birth, but may not be picked up for years. The diseases (there are three varieties) are characterized by ineffective erythropoiesis together with abnormalities in the nuclei of red cell precursors, the most obvious of which is multiple nuclei. Megaloblastic changes are seen in the most common of the three disorders. Life expectancy is normal, and treatment is generally not required.

SUGGESTED READINGS

Allen, R.H. (1976) The plasma transport of vitamin B12. Br. J. Haematol. *26*:153–159.

Babior, B.M., ed. (1975) Cobalamin: Biochemistry and Pathophysiology. John Wiley & Sons, New York.

Chanarin, I. (1979) The megaloblastic anemias. 2nd ed. Blackwell Scientific Publishers, Oxford, UK.

Gräsbeck, R. (1984) Biochemistry and clinical chemistry of vitamin B12 transport and the related diseases. Clin. Biochem. *17*:99–107.

Herbert, V. (1985) Megaloblastic anemias. Lab. Invest. *52*:3–19.

Kapadia, C.R. & Donaldson, R.M. Jr. (1985) Disorders of cobalamin (vitamin B12) absorption and transport. Annu. Rev. Med. *36*:93–110.

Lindenbaum, J. & Roman, M.J. (1980) Nutritional anemia in alcoholism. Am. J.. Clin. Nutr. *33*: 2727–2735.

Rosenblatt, D.S. & Cooper, B.A. (1987) Inherited disorders of vitamin B12 metabolism. Blood Rev. *1*:177–182.

Shane, B. & Stokstad, E.L. (1985) Vitamin B12-folate interrelationships. Annu. Rev. Nutr. *5*: 115–141.

Shojania, A.M. (1980) Problems in diagnosis and investigation of megaloblastic anemia. Can. Med. Assoc. J. *122*:999–1004.

Shojania, A.M. (1984) Folic acid and vitamin B12 deficiency in pregnancy and in the neonatal period. Clin. Perinatol. *11*:433–459.

Wickramasinghe, S.N. (1988) Nutritional anaemias. Clin. Lab. Haematol. *10*:117–134.

Hypoproliferative Anemia

In a few conditions anemia develops because of an isolated suppression of erythropoiesis. White cell and platelet production are normal, but red cell production is sluggish and feeble. The clinical picture is almost invariably that of a normochromic, normocytic anemia. The reticulocyte count may be low, normal, or high, but it is always less than expected for the observed hematocrit, and the bone marrow shows a reduction in red cell precursors (Fig. 7–1).

RENAL FAILURE

The most frequent cause of an isolated hypoproliferative anemia is chronic renal failure. Patients with severe chronic renal failure may have hematocrit levels as low as 20 ml/dl solely on the basis of their underlying disease (Fig. 7–2). Other anemia-producing factors are also at work in these patients (e.g., red cell survival is often somewhat decreased, the tendency to bleed from the gastrointestinal tract may lead to iron deficiency, and complications caused by dialysis may also contribute to the anemia), but diminished red cell production caused by renal insufficiency is the baseline on which all these other factors are superimposed.

The anemia of chronic renal failure is generally attributed to the decrease in erythropoietin production that results from the reduced mass of the failing kidney (see Ch. 2). This is clearly part of the story, because erythropoietin levels in patients with chronic renal failure are definitely lower than in patients with equally severe anemias from other causes. Erythropoietin, however, does not disappear from the blood; in fact, in some patients erythropoietin levels are substantially higher than normal, although not as high as would be expected from the degree of anemia. This indicates that the patient with chronic renal failure exhibits not only a deficiency of erythropoietin, but also a deficiency in the response of the bone marrow to such erythropoietin as is present. Apparently a second factor plays a role in the anemia of renal failure, acting directly on the marrow to suppress red cell production. The identity of this second factor is unknown.

Clinically, the anemia is normochromic and normocytic, with a reduction in reticulocytes, just as expected for a hypoproliferative anemia. Under the microscope, the red cells may be normal in shape or they may show knobs distributed in a regular pattern over the red cell surface—the so-called "burr cells" (Fig. 7–3). Functionally, the red cells may show a reduction in oxygen affinity caused by an elevation in red cell 2,3-diphosphoglyceric acid (2,3-DPG), a consequence of the elevation in serum phosphate typical of chronic renal failure. The marrow shows a decreased number of red cell precursors. The spleen is normal in size. Other manifestations are primarily those of chronic renal failure, including elevations of the BUN and creatinine, characteristic electrolyte abnormalities, and abnormal findings on renal radi-

Hypoproliferative Anemias

Renal failure
Endocrine disorders
  Hypothyroidism
  Hypopituitarism
  Pure red cell aplasia

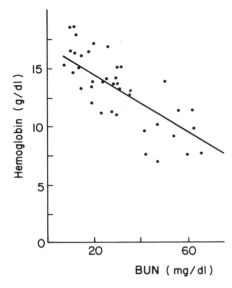

ography, as well as such clinical abnormalities as nausea and vomiting, polyuria, hypertension, eye-ground abnormalities, and cardiac signs and symptoms.

The conventional management of this anemia is largely supportive, with transfusions as necessary to maintain the hematocrit at the lowest level consistent with reasonable function—generally about 25 ml/dl or so. Recently recombinant human erythropoietin has proved to be highly effective in correcting the anemia of chronic renal failure and may in the near future supplant transfusions as standard

Fig. 7–2. Relationship between creatinine and hematocrit levels in chronic renal failure. (Modified from Kaye, M. (1958) The anemia associated with renal disease. J. Lab. Clin. Med. *52*:83–100, with permission.)

therapy. Aggravating factors (e.g., folate deficiency) are corrected. Dialysis is of little benefit—indeed, it can impose problems of its own—but transplantation will generally correct the anemia.

Fig. 7–1. Bone marrow in hypoproliferative anemia. This is a particularly striking example, showing no red cell precursors. (From Marmont, A.M. & Damasio, E. (1981) Aplastic, hypoplastic, and metaplastic myelopathies. Ch. 5. pp. 243–254. In Zucker-Franklin, D. et al. (eds.) Atlas of Blood Cells: Function and Pathology. Edi. Ermes s.r.l., Milan, with permission.)

Factors Contributing to the Anemia in Chronic Renal Failure

Diminished red cell production
  Decreased erythropoietin
  Circulating inhibitor(s) of erythropoiesis
Shortened red cell life span
Chronic gastrointestinal bleeding
Dialysis
  Iron deficiency
  Folate deficiency
  Other

Fig. 7–3. Burr cells in renal failure. (From Erslev, A.J. & Gabuzda, T.G. (1975) Pathophysiology of Blood. W. B. Saunders, Philadelphia, with permission.)

Dialysis

Dialysis has added a number of types of anemia to the standard assortment seen in undialyzed renal failure patients: iron deficiency, folate deficiency, and other dialysis-associated anemias.

Iron Deficiency

Iron deficiency arises with hemodialysis because a certain amount of blood is lost through priming every time the patient is connected to a hemodialysis machine. Iron deficiency may result from this recurrent loss of blood into the machine.

Folate Deficiency

Folate is fully dialyzable, so that folate deficiency can easily arise in patients receiving either hemodialysis or peritoneal dialysis as a result of losses of this vitamin into the dialysis fluid. Patients receiving chronic dialysis should be routinely given folate supplements.

Other Dialysis-Associated Anemias

Aluminum poisoning may be the cause of a microcytic anemia in dialysis patients with normal iron stores. Very occasionally, peculiar anemias have developed in patients because of dialysis against fluids that have been defective in one way or another (e.g., too hot, deficient in a trace element required for hematopoiesis, contaminated with a hemolytic chemical). Identifying the culprit in this sort of situation can require imaginative detective work.

ENDOCRINE DISEASE

Endocrine disorders involving the thryroid and the pituitary can cause isolated hypoproliferative anemias.

Hypothyroidism

An isolated anemia is often seen in hypothyroidism. The anemia may be either normocytic or slightly macrocytic. Other clinical manifestations are those of the underlying disorder, and the anemia remits when the thyroid status is corrected.

The anemia of hypothyroidism is interesting in physiological terms, because in a sense it is not an anemia at all. It represents an appropriate response on the part of the bone marrow to the decreased tissue oxygen consumption in the hypothyroid patient. It is slow to develop and slow to remit; 3 or 4 months may be required from the onset of replacement therapy before the hematocrit returns to normal.

Aside from anemia caused by thyroid disease per se, the possibility of anemia attributable to cobalamin deficiency must be kept in mind in this situation. The incidence of cobalamin deficiency is increased in patients with thyroid disease because of the association between pernicious anemia and autoimmune diseases, of which both hypothyroidism (Hashimoto's) and hyperthyroidism (Graves') are examples.

Hypopituitarism

Anemia is seen in patients with panhypopituitarism. This anemia has several causes. The decrease in thyroid function that occurs in hypopituitary states accounts for some of the anemia. In men, a decrease in androgen production also accounts for some of the anemia, because androgens stimulate erythropoiesis, exerting their effect by promoting erythropoietin formation as well as by a direct effect on the marrow. (It is this action of androgens that explains why men have higher hematocrit levels than do women.) Finally, pituitary deficiency itself has an effect on erythropoiesis over and above that caused by thryoid and gonad hypofunction. This effect is thought to be caused by a deficiency of growth hormone, which has a trophic effect on the bone marrow similar to its effect on other tissues.

The anemia of panhypopituitarism is normochromic and normocytic, with a reduction in reticulocytes and a somewhat hypocellular marrow. It is a minor component of the constellation of manifestations that make up clinical pituitary insufficiency. Treatment of the endocrine disorder is the only therapy required.

PURE RED CELL APLASIA

Pure red cell aplasia is a typical hypoproliferative anemia, with a normochromic, normocytic smear, reticulocytopenia, and a selective reduction in marrow normoblasts. It is usually caused by the immunological destruction of marrow red cell precursors. This anemia is discussed fully in the chapter on immunologically mediated blood cell disorders (see Ch. 29).

Two forms of pure red cell aplasia are seen very young children: Diamond-Blackfan syndrome and transient erythroblastopenia.

Diamond-Blackfan Syndrome

Diamond-Blackfan syndrome, a serious disorder, begins in infancy. Red cell precursors show a decreased sensitivity to erythropoietin, and the red cells themselves are fetal in character, with a high mean cell volume and elevated fetal hemoglobin (see Ch. 10). The anemia, which responds variably to steroids, may last for life.

Transient Erythroblastopenia of Childhood

Transient erythroblastopenia of childhood is a typical pure red cell aplasia of immune origin. The red cells are qualitatively normal. The disorder lasts a few weeks to a few months, then resolves spontaneously.

SUGGESTED READINGS

Ammus, S.S. & Yunis, A.A. (1987) Acquired pure red cell aplasia. Am. J. Hematol. *24*:311–326.

Bailey, R.O., Dunn, H.G., Rubin, A.M. & Ritaccio, A.L. (1988) Myasthenia gravis with thymoma and pure red blood cell aplasia. Am. J. Clin. Pathol. *89*:687–693.

Desforges, J.F. (1975) The role of hemodialysis in the hematological disorders of uremia. Kidney Int. Suppl. *2*:5123–5128.

Eschbach, J.W. & Adamson, J.W. (1988) Modern aspects of the pathophysiology of renal anemia. Contrib. Nephrol. *66*:63–70.

Hocking, W.G. (1987) Hematologic abnormalities in patients with renal diseases. Hematol. Oncol. Clin. North. Am. *1*:229–260.

Schuster, S.J., Caro, J. & Erslev, A.J. (1987) Erythropoietin: current concepts and future prospects. Hematol. Pathol. *1*:193–201.

Hemolytic Anemias: Extravascular Destruction of Red Cells

The accelerated destruction of red cells is referred to as *hemolysis*. A degree of hemolysis is seen in many diseases (e.g., renal failure, cirrhosis of the liver, megaloblastic anemias), contributing to a greater or lesser extent to the clinical manifestations that occur in these disorders. In certain conditions, however, hemolysis is the predominant pathogenetic mechanism. These conditions are known as *hemolytic anemias*.

The hemolytic anemias can be divided into two groups, depending on the predominant site of red cell destruction. In *extravascular* hemolysis, red cells are destroyed primarily by tissue macrophages, especially those in the spleen. In these anemias, red cell destruction can be seen as an exaggeration of the normal mechanisms of red cell disposal. In *intravascular* hemolysis, red cells are destroyed primarily by lysis in the bloodstream. The latter types are discussed in Chapter 9.

EXTRAVASCULAR HEMOLYSIS: GENERAL CONSIDERATIONS

Normal Disposal of Red Cells

Red cells normally live 4 months, then die of old age. The disposal of senile red cells is thought to be handled mainly by the spleen.

To understand how this is accomplished requires some feeling for the anatomy of this complex organ (Fig. 8–1). The spleen contains two regions, the red pulp and the white pulp, surrounded by a fibrous capsule and fed by a vasculature having an unusually complicated organization. By tracing the splenic blood supply from the arterial side to the venous side, the relationship between anatomy and function can be understood.

Arteries enter the spleen from the capsule and from fibrous extensions of the capsule into the splenic pulp. These arteries are surrounded for much of their length by a sheath of lymphoid cells known as the white pulp. The arteries give off branches along their length, some passing through the while pulp and other more remote branches entering the red pulp directly. These branches terminate in two ways:

1. Some expand to form thin-walled sinuses that eventually join to form veins that carry blood out of the spleen. Blood cells can pass through the relatively open structure of the sinus walls, although it is a tight squeeze (Fig. 8–2).

2. Others empty directly into the cords. The cords, so called because of their appearance under the microscope, actually represent a continuous mass of loosely organized tissue composed largely of reticular cells and mononu-

97

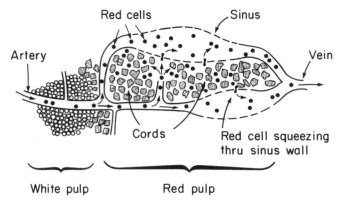

Fig. 8–1. Anatomy of the spleen, bird's eye-view. To understand how the spleen is organized, trace the artery shown by the arrow. It tunnels through a sheath of lymphoid cells, then penetrates into a loosely organized mass of phagocytes and reticular cells known as the splenic cords. All along its course it sends out branches. Some of these branches widen into sinuses that meander through the cords and eventually join to form the splenic veins. Others end as open pipes that empty directly into the splenic cords. The sheath of lymphoid cells is called the white pulp, and the region of cords and sinuses is called the red pulp. Blood flowing through the spleen follows one of two routes. In one route, known as the closed circulation, the blood flows directly from an arterial branch into a sinus. In the other route, known as the open circulation, the blood is first delivered into the splenic cords, where it percolates through the mass of cordal cells. Only then does it enter the sinus, penetrating the sinus wall from the outside. It is while in the cords that the blood is worked on by the spleen.

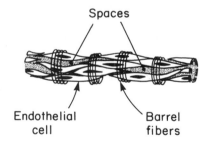

Fig. 8–2. The sinus wall. The sinus is a flattened tube with a wall consisting of a single layer of endothelial cells laid down with their long axes parallel to the direction of blood flow. Along their lateral edges the endothelial cells are only loosely attached to each other, so they are able to separate to form an opening through which blood cells can pass. Wrapped around the sinuses are the barrel fibers, thin strands of collagen that serve to shape and strengthen the sinus wall. The barrel fibers occur only at intervals along the sinus wall; between them, the endothelial cells are in direct contact with the splenic cords. Blood cells squeeze into the sinuses through spaces bounded on the top and bottom by the edges of the separated endothelial cells and on the sides by the barrel fibers.

clear phagocytes, through which the sinuses ramify.

The mass of cordal tissue and associated vasculature constitute the red pulp of the spleen.

Of the blood that enters the spleen, a fraction is delivered directly into the sinuses, where flow is brisk. The remainder is delivered into the cords. Plasma delivered into the cords is able to enter the sinuses freely, but the entry of cells into the sinuses is impeded because of the resistance to passage offered by the sinus wall. The local hematocrit level in the splenic cords therefore rises sharply, and the continuing metabolic activity combined with sluggish flow cause the local oxygen tension, pH, and glucose concentration levels to drop. Normal red cells can resist these metabolic assaults and will eventually make their way into the sinuses and out into the general circulation. Senile or defective cells have impaired resistance to these stresses and sooner or later are destroyed in the splenic cords with the aid of the resident mononuclear phagocyte system.

It is not known how the mononuclear phagocytes recognize susceptible red cells. Once recognition occurs, however, the phagocytes appear to dispose of each defective red cell piecemeal, like a school of hungry piranhas. Fragments of the red cell are ingested and degraded in a characteristic way. Most of the components, including the globin portion of the ingested hemoglobin, are degraded to their constituent building blocks (e.g., amino acids), which can then be used for other purposes. Heme, however, is lost almost completely, only the iron being saved for reuse.

The disposal of heme is of clinical significance, because the accumulation of the products of heme degradation is responsible for some important signs of hemolysis. The following are the steps in heme degradation (Fig. 8–3):

1. *Cleavage of porphyrin ring.* The porphyrin ring is opened by the oxidation of the α-methene bridge (the one-carbon bridge between the two vinyl-bearing pyrrole rings). This oxidation is catalyzed by the microsomal enzyme, heme oxygenase. The products of this reaction are iron, the linear tetrapyrrole biliverdin, and a molecule of carbon monoxide that

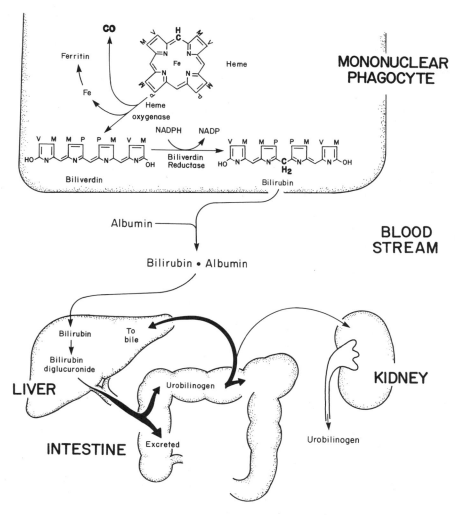

Fig. 8–3. Degradation of heme.

represents the oxidized α-methene bridge. Heme degradation is virtually the only endogenous source of carbon monoxide in humans.

2. *Disposal of cleavage products.* The liberated iron is incorporated into ferritin, while the biliverdin is reduced to bilirubin and then released into the bloodstream. Here it binds tightly to albumin and is carried in this form to the liver for final elimination.

3. *Bilirubin in the liver.* On reaching the liver, bilirubin dissociates from its albumin carrier and enters the hepatocyte. In this cell it is converted to a highly water-soluble derivative, bilirubin diglucuronide, through a reaction known as *conjugation*. Finally, the conjugated bilirubin is excreted through the bile into the intestine.

4. *Urobilinogen.* On reaching the intestine, a portion of the bilirubin is acted on by bacteria, which further reduce it to urobilinogen. The urobilinogen is absorbed into the bloodstream but is then rapidly re-excreted, most by the liver but some by the kidneys.

Phagocytes are messy eaters. As a result, extravascular hemolysis, whether normal or pathological, is always accompanied by the spillage of some hemoglobin into the plasma. This free hemoglobin is not handled by the mononuclear phagocytes, but is dealt with instead by the hepatocytes, which take it up with the aid of a circulating protein known as *haptoglobin* (Fig. 8–4). This protein is avid for hemoglobin, forming a very tight 1:1 complex with the hemoglobin tetramer. The release of hemoglobin into the plasma is followed almost instantly by the formation of the hemoglobin–haptoglobin complex. This complex is rapidly transported into the hepatocytes (the half-life for the disappearance of the circulating complex is about 10 minutes). Once there, the hemoglobin is degraded just as it would be in the mononuclear phagocytes; that is, the protein is digested, the iron is deposited as ferritin, and the porphyrin ring is converted to bilirubin and excreted.

Asplenia (Absence of the Spleen)

In the absence of the spleen, screening for defective erythrocytes is impaired and red cells with characteristic morphological abnormalities appear in the circulation. Many of the cells are misshapen, whereas others may contain nuclear remnants, such as Howell-Jolly bodies and Cabot rings (Fig. 8–5), or precipitates of denatured hemoglobin (not seen on routine smears, but visible as Heinz bodies when the blood is stained with crystal violet). These abnormal red cells are not seen in normal blood, presumably because they are rapidly recognized and destroyed by the spleen after release into the bloodstream. Howell-Jolly bodies and Cabot rings are so typical of asplenia that their presence in a blood smear strongly suggests that the spleen is either absent or nonfunctional.

Asplenia also causes a rise in both the white count and the platelet count (especially the latter) and induces an unusual susceptibility

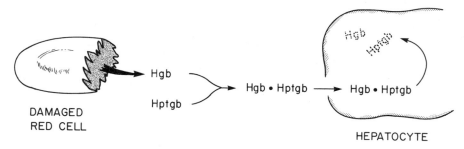

Fig. 8–4. Haptoglobin removal of free hemoglobin from the bloodstream.

A   B

Fig. 8–5. Howell-Jolly bodies and a Cabot ring. (**A**) Howell-Jolly bodies are small, round, darkly-stained nuclear fragments. (**B**) The Cabot ring is a thin, darkly-stained ring that follows the margin of the red cell. (From Castodli, G.L. (1981) Erythrocytes. Ch. 3. In Zucker-Franklin D. et al. (eds.) Atlas of Blood Cells: Function and Pathology. Edi. Ermes s.r.l., Milan, with permission.)

to certain types of infections. The red cell life span is not altered by the absence of the spleen, probably because the liver and other mononuclear phagocyte-containing organs are able to take over the spleen's job of destroying senile red cells.

Manifestations of Extravascular Hemolysis

Accelerated extravascular hemolysis, of whatever origin, always leads to (1) hypertrophy of the spleen, to handle the increased red cell load; (2) a compensatory increase in red cell production on the part of the marrow; (3) increased hemoglobin breakdown, associated with a rise in the consumption of haptoglobin and an increased bilirubin load for the liver to excrete (Table 8–1). Many of the signs and symptoms of hemolysis reflect these secondary consequences of red cell destruction. Others,

caused by the anemia itself, are ordinarily not prominent unless the condition is severe in degree or abrupt in development.

Splenic Hypertrophy

Enlargement of the spleen is one of the most constant clinical findings in extravascular hemolysis.

Increased Red Cell Production

Signs of increased red cell production include the release of young erythrocytes into the peripheral blood and an increase in marrow cellularity as red cell precursors expand in response to need. A reticulocytosis is therefore an almost invariable consequence of hemolysis. The release of younger forms is unusual, but if hemolysis is both severe and acute, nor-

Table 8-1. Principal Manifestations of Extravascular Hemolysis

Mechanism	Clinical	Laboratory
Splenic hypertrophy Increased red cell production	Splenomegaly	Reticulocytosis Marrow red cell hyperplasia
Increased hemoglobin breakdown Red cell destruction	Jaundice Gallstones Pallor and faintness Cardiac symptoms Aggravation of underlying vascular disease	Indirect bilirubinemia Decreased serum haptoglobin Anemia

moblasts may appear. With increased red cell production comes an increased need for iron by the marrow, leading to a rise in the plasma iron turnover (PIT).

Normal marrow can increase its red cell production as much as eightfold. Anemia occurs when the marrow's ability to manufacture red cells is outstripped by the hemolytic process. In some cases the marrow can keep up; under such circumstances anemia does not develop, although other manifestations of hemolysis (e.g., reticulocytosis) are still evident.

Increased Hemoglobin Breakdown

The rise in bilirubin production leads to an increase in serum bilirubin concentration. This condition can be detected at the bedside as well as in the laboratory, because excess bilirubin is deposited in the skin and sclerae, where it gives rise to jaundice. In uncomplicated hemolytic anemia, the bilirubin that accumulates in the bloodstream is in the unconjugated form, because a normal liver can conjugate and excrete bilirubin as fast as it can be taken up. Unconjugated bilirubinemia is reported by the laboratory as an increase in *indirect bilirubin*, a term referring to a method for

measuring that detects mostly the unconjugated form. If there is liver damage along with hemolytic anemia, both unconjugated and conjugated bilirubin appear in the blood, the latter leaking into the bloodstream from the damaged liver cell before it can be excreted in the bile. Conjugated bilirubinemia is reported as an increase in *direct bilirubin*.

Products of bilirubin metabolism can also be detected in the urine. The increase in bilirubin delivered to the intestine leads to an increase in urobilinogen production and consequently to the delivery of more urobilinogen into the urine, where it is detected both as such and as its product of oxidation, urobilin. Conjugated bilirubin will also be excreted in the urine if it is present in the blood in significant concentrations; the highly water-insoluble unconjugated bilirubin never appears in the urine.

Another sign of increased hemoglobin breakdown is an alteration in iron kenetics (Fig. 8–6). Red cell iron leaves the bloodstream with unusual speed and accumulates in the spleen in greater than normal amounts as the short-lived red cells are trapped and destroyed in the splenic pulp. There is also an increase in haptoglobin consumption, as haptoglobin molecules capture the hemoglobin spilled into the plasma during hemolysis and carry it to the liver. The result is a fall in serum haptoglobin levels.

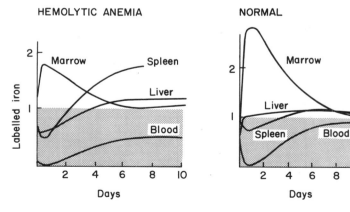

Fig. 8–6. Ferrokinetics of hemolytic anemia. (**Left**) Hemolysis. (**Right**) Normal. (Right: From Finch, C.A. et al. (1970) Ferrokinetics in man. Medicine *49*:17, with permission.)

Anemia

Pallor, faintness, signs of cardiac dysfunction, and appearance of manifestations localized to areas in which the blood supply has previously been compromised by vascular disease may be indicators of anemia.

Special Problems

Adding to all the forgoing are two special problems that can cause trouble in patients with extravascular hemolysis, especially if their condition is chronic and severe: gallstones and aplastic crises.

Gallstones

The increased load of excreted bilirubin may lead to the precipitation of bilirubin stones in the gallbladder. These stones tend to be multiple and small and are sometimes radiopaque because of their calcium content. Gallstones in an adolescent or young adult should suggest a hemolytic anemia of long duration.

Aplastic Crises

Aplastic crises are characterized by the disappearance of reticulocytes from the blood and a plummeting hematocrit count. Aplastic crises occur in association with other illnesses (particularly, parvovirus infections) and are caused by acute marrow suppression secondary to the intercurrent illness. Illness-related marrow suppression also occurs in persons with normal red cell survival, but it usually goes unnoticed because marrow function returns before the uncompensated loss of senile red cells from the circulation has had a chance to produce a significant degree of anemia. When the red cell life span is short, however, a cutoff of red cell production can cause an abrupt drop in the hematocrit level as a result of uncompensated

hemolysis. Despite their transiency, aplastic crises may result in life-threatening degrees of anemia.

Measuring Red Cell Survival

It is possible to establish the diagnosis of a hemolytic state by measuring the red cell life span. This measurement is generally made by labeling red cells with radioactive chromium and following the disappearance of the tagged cells from the blood over a period of time. Labeling is accomplished by withdrawing whole blood from the patient and incubating it with $Na^{51}CrO_4$. The label is taken up by the red cells, reduced to $^{51}Cr^{3+}$, and fixed to protein. Cells are then reinfused, and blood samples are obtained at intervals for measurements of ^{51}Cr levels.

A normal survival curve is shown in Figure 8–7. Because red cells of all ages are labeled by the ^{51}Cr tagging procedure, and because red cells die at about age 120 days, it would be expected that the survival curve of ^{51}Cr-tagged red cells would be a straight line, reaching zero at 120 days. What is seen, however, is a nonlinear disappearance curve with the 50 percent survival point at about 25 days, not the 60 days expected from what is known about red cell kinetics. This deviation from ex-

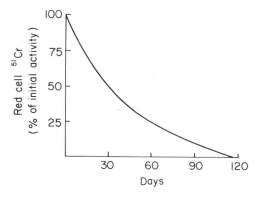

Fig. 8–7. Survival of ^{51}Cr-tagged red cells. (Redrawn from Wintrobe, M.M. et al. (1974) Clinical Hematology. 7th ed. Lea & Febiger, Philadelphia, with permission.)

pected results occurs because ^{51}Cr is lost from the blood through leaching from the cells as well as through destruction of the cells, making absolute red cell survival difficult to measure by this method. Red cell survival relative to normal, however, can be measured reliably with this technique and has proved useful for demonstrating accelerated red cell destruction in anemic patients.

The site of red cell destruction (i.e., spleen versus other mononuclear phagocyte-containing organs, particularly the liver) can also be determined using ^{51}Cr-tagged red cells. For this determination, the amount of radioactivity taken up by the organ in question is measured by scanning. This method has been used to try to predict the usefulness of splenectomy in patients with extravascular hemolysis, but without much success.

EXTRAVASCULAR HEMOLYTIC ANEMIAS

Hemolytic anemias in which red cell destruction is accomplished primarily by the mononuclear phagocyte system are listed below.

Extravascular Hemolytic Anemias

Autoimmune hemolytic anemia
Diseases of the red cell membrane
    Hereditary spherocytosis
    Others
Spur cell anemia
    Liver disease
    Abetalipoproteinemia (very rare)
Congenital nonspherocytic hemolytic anemia
    Pyruvate kinase deficiency
    Others
Unstable hemoglobin disease

Autoimmune Hemolytic Anemia

The most common cause of extravascular hemolysis is autoimmune hemolytic anemia. This disease results from the presence of an antibody that binds to autologous red cells, marking them for destruction by phagocytes. See Chapter 29 for a full discussion of this anemia.

Hereditary Spherocytosis and Other Diseases of the Red Cell Membrane

Certain inherited red cell disorders result in a characteristic abnormality of red cell shape. These disorders are thought to be caused by an abnormality of one or another of the constituent proteins of the red cell membrane. In all but one of these disorders, extravascular hemolysis is an invariable feature.

The Red Cell Membrane

Like all cells, the red cell is enclosed within a plasma membrane composed of lipids and proteins. The lipids, which consist principally of cholesterol and phospholipids, are arranged in a bilayer in which the membrane proteins are embedded. The plasma membrane can thus be characterized as a sort of two dimensional solution of proteins in lipid. Some of the proteins are free to move, floating about in the bilayer like icebergs in the sea; others are anchored more or less firmly in place.

Lying immediately beneath the plasma membrane is the cytoskeleton, a network of structural proteins that confers on the red cell its unique discoid shape. The most characteristic protein of the cytoskeleton is spectrin, a large (MW of about 10^6) tetramer unique to red cells. The spectrin tetramers are long and flexible and form a fibrous mesh that lines the inner surface of the membrane. The flexibility of the spectrin strands give the mesh a rubberlike elasticity. This elasticity is what makes the red cell able to deform reversibly when passing through narrow spaces in capillaries and the spleen.

Othe cytoskeletal components include actin, band 4.1, band 4.9, and ankyrin, a protein associated with both the cytoskeleton and the plasma membrane, anchoring the former to the latter through an interaction with a plasma membrane protein known as band 3. (Band 3 is an example of a plasma membrane protein that is unable to move freely in the plane of the bilayer.) The way these proteins are assembled to form the cytoskeleton is shown in Figure 8–8.

Between them, the plasma membrane and the cytoskeleton contain dozens of proteins. Apart from those proteins that are components of the cytoskeleton, however, few have been assigned a function. Of those few, the most important in clinical terms is the Na^+/K^+ adenosine triphosphatase (ATPase), the ion pump that maintains the Na^+ and K^+ gradi-

ents across the red cell membrane. In the normal erythrocyte, the intracellular Na^+ concentration is about 15 mEq/L, and the K^+ concentration 85 mEq/L. By contrast, in the plasma, the Na^+ and K^+ concentrations are 140 and 5 mEq/L, respectively. This disparity between the intracellular and extracellular ion concentrations passively drives Na^+ into the red cell and K^+ out. Although these passive ionic movements are very slow because of the low permeability of the plasma membrane, there is nevertheless a steady trickle of ions that has to be counteracted if the difference between the intracellular and extracellular ion concentrations is to be maintained. The agent responsible for counteracting this slow tendency to ionic equilibration is the membrane Na^+/K^+ ATPase. This enzyme, a multisubunit protein that completely traverses the plasma membrane, catalyzes an ion exchange reaction in which Na^+ is pumped out of the red cell in exchange for K^+ or H^+, which is pumped in. In this uphill process, energy is

Fig. 8–8. The red cell cytoskeleton. Shown are four major cytoskeletal proteins: spectrin, actin, and the coupling proteins ankyrin and band 4.1. Ankyrin (the anchor) attaches the cytoskeleton to the plasma membrane by coupling spectrin to band 3, a plasma membrane protein. Band 4.1 couples spectrin to actin. (From Lux, S.E. (1979) Dissecting the red cell membrane skeleton. Nature *281*:426–429, with permission.)

Fig. 8–9. Gel electrophoresis of red cell membrane proteins. (From Steck, T.L. (1974) The organization of proteins in the human red blood cell membrane. J. Cell. Biol. *62*:1–19, with permission.)

obtained from the hydrolysis of ATP, one molecule for each exchange reaction. This is thought to be the major ATP-consuming reaction of the red cell.

Much of the information on red cell membrane proteins has been obtained through gel electrophoresis of purified red cell membrane preparations. Protein patterns obtained by this technique are shown in Figure 8–9. The protein bands, which are highly reproducible from sample to sample, are numbered according to

molecular weight, the bands of highest molecular weight (those migrating the smallest distance into the gel) being given the lowest numbers. This numbering pattern provides the basis for the numerical terminology referred to above. Names and functions have been assigned to a few of the numbered proteins (Table 8–2), but most have neither.

Hereditary Spherocytosis

Hereditary spherocytosis (HS) is the most common of the inherited disorders of red cell shape. In this disorder, cells have a smaller surface-to-volume ratio than normal; they are thicker than the normal red cell and on the peripheral smear they lack the normal area of central pallor, resulting in the spherical appearance that has given the disease its name (Fig. 8–10). The abnormality in cell shape in HS strongly suggests that the condition is caused by a defect in the cytoskeleton. Recent studies have borne this out, showing that in most HS patients, the disease results from a defect in band 4.1 that leads to an abnormally low level of red cell spectrin. Moreover, clinical severity correlates with the red cell spectrin content: the lower the spectrin, the worse the disease. This correlation between the red cell spectrin levels and the severity of the disease explains the peculiar genetics of HS, which in milder forms is transmitted as an autosomal recessive trait but in severe forms becomes autosomal dominant. It is likely that in mild HS, the genetic defect causes only a modest decline in spectrin production, so that a double dose of the defective gene is necessary to reduce red cell spectrin to

Table 8-2. Names and Functions of Some Red Cell Membrane Proteins

Band	Name	Function
1, 2	Spectrin monomers	Network-forming component of the cytoskeleton
2.1	Ankyrin	Couples spectrin to band 3
3	Anion channel	Facilitates passage of Cl^- in and out of the cell
4.1		Couples spectrin to actin
5	Actin	A component of the cytoskeleton
6	Glyceraldehyde 3-phosphate dehydrogenase	Glycolytic enzyme
PAS-1, PAS-2[a]	Glycophorin	Function unknown; carries the MN antigen system

[a] These proteins are designated PAS-1 and PAS-2 because they are stained by periodic acid-Schiff, indicating that they are glycoproteins.

Fig. 8–10. Red cells in hereditary spherocytosis. (**A**) Blood smear, showing the typical spherocytes. (**B**) Spherocytes as seen by scanning electron microscopy. (A: From Lessin, L.F. & Bessis, M. (1972) Morphology of the erythron. In Williams, W.J. et al. Hematology. McGraw-Hill, New York, 1982. Used with permission of the McGraw-Hill Book Co. B: From Castoldi, G.L. (1981) Erythrocytes. Ch. 3 in Zucker-Franklin, D. et al. (eds.) Atlas of Blood Cells: Function and Pathology. Edi. Ermes s.r.l., Milan, with permission.)

a clinically significant level (autosomal recessive transmission); but in severe HS, spectrin production is so seriously impaired by the genetic defect that only a single defective gene is needed to produce clinically significant spectrin deficiency (i.e., autosomal dominant transmission).

The other important problem with the HS cell is its abnormal permeability to Na^+. This ion leaks into the HS cell at about 10 times the normal rate. The leak is compensated for by a proportionate increase in the activity of the membrane Na^+/K^+ ATPase, but this requires an increase in energy production to supply the ATP necessary for ion pumping. Glucose metabolism is therefore substantially accelerated in HS cells.

The combination of abnormal shape and the permeability defect account for the increase in the destruction of HS cells by the spleen. Because of their spherical shape, these cells lack the flexibility of normal cells, causing them to become trapped in the cords of the spleen because of the difficulty they have squeezing into the sinuses. The increased ion pumping caused by their Na^+ leak forces them to burn more

glucose; this accelerated rate of glucose metabolism works against them, and they quickly run out of fuel in the glucose-poor environment of the splenic cords. Energy production ceases, and the cells are destroyed.

The manifestations of HS are attributable to the destruction of the defective cells in the spleen. These manifestations are often detected in childhood, but sometimes are not picked up until later in life. Presenting findings include an anemia of variable severity, plus the big three of extravascular hemolysis: splenomegaly, reticulocytosis, and indirect bilirubinemia. In addition, gallstones and aplastic crises are particularly common in HS.

HS should be suspected in a patient with a hemolytic anemia and an appropriate family history whose blood smear contains spherocytes (Fig. 8–10). The presence of spherocytes and reticulocytosis on smears from family members provides even stronger evidence of HS. The diagnosis of HS is usually made by the *osmotic fragility* test, which depends on the fact that the thicker shape of HS cells makes it difficult for them to increase their volume to the same extent as normal cells. In this test, red cells are incubated in hypotonic saline at various concentrations. The cells imbibe water and increase their volume until their internal osmolarity is reduced to that of the saline, or until they burst. Because of their shape, normal cells are able to tolerate much lower osmolarities than HS cells (Fig. 8–11); the latter are therefore said to exhibit increased osmotic fragility. Incubation for a day at 37°C greatly increases the susceptibility of HS cells to osmotic stress and can be used to bring out the defect if the osmotic fragility of fresh red cells from a suspected HS patient is ambiguous.

As to therapy, the anemia virtually always responds to splenectomy, making it the treatment of choice. In considering splenectomy, however, three points should be borne in mind: (1) splenectomy should not be done unless warranted by the degree of anemia; (2) splenectomy should be avoided if possible in children younger than the age of 5 or 6, because of the risk of fulminant septicemia in splenectomized children; (3) in patients with gallstones, the spleen should be removed along with the gallbladder, to prevent stone formation in the bile ducts caused by the continued excretion of excessive amounts of bilirubin by the liver. Folate supplements should be given to meet the increased folic acid requirements

associated with long-term hemolysis. Aplastic crisis is managed by supportive therapy, primarily transfusions as necessary.

Related Disorders

Other disorders of red cells shape thought to be caused by defective proteins in the cytoskeleton or plasma membrane are hereditary elliptocytosis and hereditary stomatocytosis. The red cell morphology in these two conditions is shown in Figure 8-12. The important points to remember are that (1) they are quite rare; (2) in hereditary elliptocytosis, the more common of these conditions, the red cell life span is usually normal or only modestly decreased; and (3) an acquired form of stomatocytosis is seen in alcoholics.

Spur Cell Anemia

Spur cells are red cells whose shape is altered because of an increase in the area of the red cell membrane without an accompanying increase in red cell volume. This increase usually results from the uptake of cholesterol by the cell membrane. The cholesterol in red cell membranes exchanges freely with the cholesterol in plasma lipoproteins; when the concentration of these proteins change, so does the amount of cholesterol in the red cell membrane. Under normal circumstances, the variations in lipoprotein concentration are small enough that the accompanying fluctuations in red cell membrane cholesterol do not cause a detectable change in red cell shape. At sufficiently high lipoprotein concentrations, however, enough cholesterol is transferred to the red cell membrane that changes in shape become evident. Modest increases lead to flattened red cells that appear on smears as target cells. Sufficiently large increments of cholesterol cause the membrane to be thrown up into spikes, forming spur cells (Fig. 8–13).

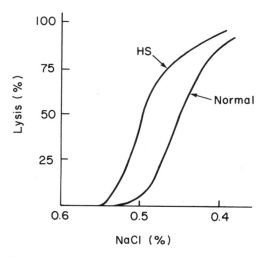

Fig. 8–11. Osmotic fragility in HS.

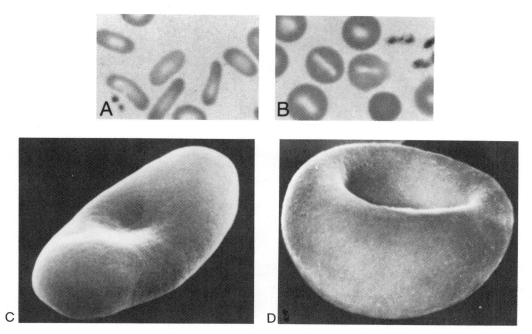

Fig. 8–12. Red cell morphology in two other disorders of the red cell membrane. Hereditary elliptocytosis: (**A**) blood smear; (**C**) scanning electron micrograph. Hereditary stomatocytosis: (**B**) blood smear; (**D**) scanning electron micrograph. The diseases are named for the morphology of the red cells. The origin of "elliptocyte" is obvious. "Stomatocyte" is a fanciful term derived from the mouth (*stoma*)-like appearance of these cells on the smear. (A, B: From Lessin, L.F & Bessis, M. (1972) Morphology of the erythron. In Williams, W.J. et al. Hematology. McGraw-Hill, New York, 1982, with permission. C, D: From Bessis, M. (1973) Living Blood Cells and Their Ultrastructure. Springer-Verlag, New York, with permission.)

Liver Disease with Hypercholesterolemia

By far the most common cause of spur cell anemia is severe liver disease, especially alcoholic cirrhosis. In this condition, serum lipoproteins typically increase, leading to the transfer of cholesterol to the red cell membrane and the appearance of target cells and spur cells in the blood smear. The spur cells are subject to destruction in the spleen. Here phagocytes first nip off some of the projecting spurs, accounting for the irregular shape of most of the spur cells. (The nibbling away of defective parts of red cells by splenic phagocytes is termed *pitting* or *conditioning*. It is also seen in autoimmune hemolytic anemias and in diseases associated with intracellular precipitation of denatured hemoglobin.) This process is soon followed by the elimination of the cells, an event that takes place in the spleen as well. It is obvious that the spleen is important in the pathogenesis of the anemia, though not the spurs, in spur cell disease. The fact that this organ is enlarged in liver disease makes its role in spur cell anemia all the more important.

Splenectomy has in fact been shown to ameliorate hemolysis in this condition and to regularize the appearance of the spur cells on the smear (Fig. 8–13). Nevertheless, this operation is hazardous in liver disease and should

Normal → Membrane lipid uptake → Target cells

Further lipid uptake

Spur cells → Spleen → Conditioned spur cells

Fig. 8–13. Formation of spur cells. Spur cells develop when the area of the red cell membrane increases without an increase in the red cell volume. With a modest increase in membrane area, the erythrocyte appears on the smear as a target cell. As the area increases further, the erythrocyte becomes a spur cell, with long spikes projecting uniformly in all directions. Finally, some of the spikes are amputated in the spleen, causing the spur cell to acquire an irregular, asymmetric appearance. Spur cells are sometimes called acanthocytes (*acantho-*, "thorn"). They are distinguished from the knob-covered burr cells of renal failure by the length and shape of the spikes. (Bottom: From Cooper, R.A. (1980) Hemolytic syndrome and red cell membrane abnormalities in liver disease. Semin Hematol. *17*:103, with permission. Top: From Lessin, L.F. & Bessis, M. (1972) The morphology of the erythron. In Williams, W.J. Hematology. McGraw-Hill, New York, 1972, with permission.)

therefore be undertaken only after the most careful evaluation. Fortunately, it is rarely necessary in this condition.

Hereditary Abetalipoproteinemia

Spur cells are also seen in abetalipoproteinemia, a very rare inherited abnormality of lipid metabolism. Sphinogomyelin accumulation seems to be the culprit in this condition; red cell cholesterol levels are normal. Hemolysis is negligible in abetalipoproteinemia.

Disorders of Red Cell Adenosine Triphosphate Production

Pyruvate Kinase Deficiency

Pyruvate kinase deficiency is one of the group of inherited conditions known as the congenital nonspherocytic hemolytic anemias (CNSHAs). These conditions are characterized by the presence from birth of hemolytic anemia; a smear showing variable numbers of irregularly shaped cells but few spherocytes (the absence of spherocytes distinguishes them from hereditary spherocytosis, which they otherwise closely resemble); and typical manifestations of extravascular red cell destruction (reticulocytosis, marrow hyperplasia, splenomegaly, and indirect bilirubinemia). The CNSHAs described to date are all caused by inherited deficiencies of enzymes involved in either glycolysis or the protection of the red cell against oxidative damage. The CNSHAs are very rare; pyruvate kinase deficiency, although an unusual disease, is observed with greater frequency than the others.

The problem in pyruvate kinase deficiency is a defect in energy production. This defect is less of a problem in reticulocytes than in older cells, because reticulocytes still contain mitochondria and can therefore make much more ATP than older cells can produce from the trickle of pyruvate that seeps past the block. The defect in energy production leads to a marked shortening of red cell survival. A minor but interesting abnormality in pyruvate kinase deficiency is an increase in red cell 2,3-DPG, leading to a reduction in oxygen affinity of uncertain clinical significance.

The diagnosis of pyruvate kinase deficiency is made by measuring the level of pyruvate kinase in the red cell. The mainstay of therapy is folic acid supplements and transfusion as necessary. Splenectomy generally leads to some improvement and reduces the transfusion requirement, but it does not completely correct the anemia. This is surprising in view of the fact that most of the red cell destruction in this condition occurs extravascularly; it probably reflects the fact that in pyruvate kinase deficiency, the liver and other organs containing large numbers of mononuclear phagocytes can take up the slack when the spleen is removed. Another unexpected feature of pyruvate kinase deficiency is that after splenectomy, the reticulocyte count rises, even though the improvement in the anemia that follows the operation would be expected to result in decreased red cell production by the marrow. It would appear that pyruvate kinase-deficient reticulocytes, although metabolically healthier than mature red

cells, are nevertheless subject to destruction by the spleen, accounting for their improved survival once this organ is removed. No one knows why this is so.

Other Disorders of Adenosine Triphosphate Production

In *severe hypophosphatemia*, red cell glycolysis may be impeded by very low intracellular phosphate levels, leading to a hemolytic anemia with acquired spherocytosis and very low erythrocyte ATP levels. Levels of 2,3-DPG also fall sharply, resulting in impaired oxygen release by these cells. The anemia is cured by correcting the serum phosphate imbalance.

Inherited *pyrimidine-5'-nucleotidase deficiency* causes a hemolytic anemia associated with prominent basophilic stippling of the affected red cells. The hemolysis is thought to result from abnormal ATP generation, whereas basophilic stippling reflects impaired RNA degradation. Both have been attributed to the inhibition of red cell enzymes by undegraded pyrimidine nucleotides.

Unstable Hemoglobin Diseases

Unstable mutant hemoglobins that denature and precipitate in the circulating red cell are another cause of extravascular hemolysis. These are almost always the result of amino acid alterations that weaken the interaction between the heme and the globin chain.

More than 75 unstable hemoglobins have been identified to date. In most instances these hemoglobins have been found in only one family, but hemoglobin Köln ($\beta^{98val \rightarrow met}$), by far the most common of the unstable hemoglobins, has been found in more than 10 kindreds. Unstable hemoglobin disease is inherited as an autosomal dominant trait—not surprising, because the unstable variant will amount to roughly one-half the hemoglobin in the red cell of a heterozygote, and the denaturation of this fraction of the cell's hemoglobin would be bound to cause symptoms.

The sequence of events involved in the pathogenesis of unstable hemoglobin disease is straightforward (Fig. 8–14). The key event is the denaturation of the unstable hemoglobin by some sort of oxidative process. The denatured hemoglobin forms an intracellular precipitate that causes the red cell to be held up and destroyed in the spleen (in severe cases, the liver and other macrophage-containing organs participate in red cell destruction as well). In most patients with unstable hemoglobin disease, the red cells are destroyed in a perfectly conventional manner, their heme going to bilirubin and storage iron. In a few patients, however, only part of the heme goes to bilirubin; the rest is converted by a poorly understood series of reactions to highly colored dipyrroles (Fig. 8–14), which are for the most part excreted in the urine.

The clinical manifestations of unstable hemoglobin disease are those of an extravascular hemolytic anemia. The hematocrit may be normal or reduced, depending on the severity of the disease, but a reticulocytosis is generally present. Jaundice or splenomegaly may be seen, and gallstones may appear at an early age. In a small minority of patients the urine is intermittently dark, sometimes nearly black, a very unusual feature in extravascular hemoly-

sis. The urinary pigment in these patients is not bilirubin, which in any case would not be expected to appear in the urine of a patient with uncomplicated hemolysis because it would be in the unconjugated form; rather, the pigment consists of the dipyrroles referred to above (Fig. 8–14). The anemia is typically episodic, with acute attacks precipitated primarily by infections and by certain drugs that impose an oxidant stress on red cells.

The severity of the disease varies widely from patient to patient, depending on the nature of the unstable hemoglobin. In the most severe cases, a profound anemia is present from early childhood. The mildest forms have no clinical manifestations whatsoever. Most patients have a disease of intermediate severity, displaying a modest reticulocytosis with or without anemia. In these patients the disease is usually detected in adolescence or early adulthood, although it was present since birth.

There are two characteristic tests for unstable hemoglobin disease:

1. *Heinz bodies.* When red cells containing precipitates of denatured hemoglobin are stained with crystal violet, the denatured protein, undetectable on a routine smear, takes up the dye and becomes visible as a small, round, purple-staining mass. This precipitate is the Heinz body (Fig. 8–15). It appears in the

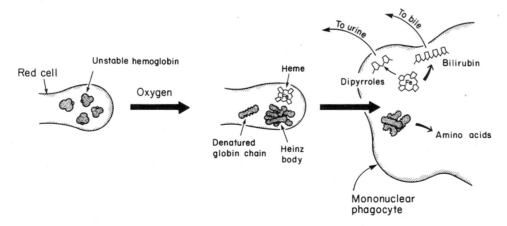

Fig. 8–14. Pathogenesis of unstable hemoglobin disease.

Fig. 8–15. Heinz bodies in crystal violet-stained red cells. (From Kapff, C.T. & Jandl, J.H. (1981) Blood: Atlas and Sourcebook of Hematology. Little, Brown, Boston, with permission.)

three varieties of red cells disease in which hemoglobin denaturation is a prominent feature: unstable hemoglobin disease, oxidant hemolysis, and thalassemia. Because red cells containing precipitates of denatured hemoglobin (i.e., Heinz body positive cells) are ordinarily removed from the circulation by the spleen, Heinz bodies are particularly prominent in splenectomized patients with unstable hemoglobin diseases.

2. *Hemoglobin precipitation.* Because of the ease with which unstable hemoglobins undergo denaturation, they will precipitate in response to stresses that have no effect on normal hemoglobin. The formation of a precipitate when a hemolysate is gently heated (50°C for a few minutes) or mixed with dilute isopropyl alcohol is so characteristic of an unstable hemoglobin that either one of these tests can be used to make the diagnosis of unstable hemoglobin disease.

It may be possible to detect the presence of an abnormal hemoglobin by electrophoresis, but this test cannot always be done, and in any case hemoglobin electrophoresis can offer no conclusive evidence as to whether the abnormal hemoglobin is unstable. Once an unstable hemoglobin is detected, it can be characterized further to determine the precise nature of the molecular defect, but this is a complicated undertaking generally carried out for research purposes only.

The treatment of unstable hemoglobin disease is similar to that of other hemolytic diseases: folate supplements and transfusions as required. Oxidant drugs should be avoided. Splenectomy has been useful in some cases.

SUGGESTED READINGS

Berlin, N.I. & Berk, P.D. (1981) Quantitative aspects of bilirubin metabolism for hematologists. Blood *57*:983.

Beutler, E. (1978) Hemolytic anemia in disorders of red cell metabolism. Topics in Hematology, Plenum, New York.

Beutler, E. (1979) Red cell enzyme defects as diseases and non-diseases. Blood *54*:1.

Cooper, R.A. (1980) Hemolytic syndromes and red cell membrane abnormalities in liver disease. Semin. Hematol. *17*:103.

Dacie, Sir John (1985) The Haemolytic Anaemias. Churchill Livingstone, Edinburgh.

Lande, W.M. & Mentzer,, W.C. (1985) Haemolytic anaemia associated with increased cation permeability. Clin. Haematol. *14*:89–103.

Milner, P.F. & Wrightstone, R.N. (1981) the unstable hemoglobins: a review. Prog. Clin. Biol. Res. *51*:197–222.

Miwa, S. (1981) Pyruvate kinase deficiency and other enzymopathies of the Embden-Myerhoff pathway. Clin. Haematol. *10*:57.

Paglia, D.E. & Valentine, W.N. (1981) Haemolytic anaemia associated with disorders of the purine and pyrimidine salvage pathways. Clin. Haematol. *10*:81–98.

Palek, J. (1987) Hereditary elliptocytosis, spherocytosis and related disorders: consequences of a deficiency or a mutation of membrane skeletal proteins. Blood Rev. *1*:147–168.

Palek, J. & Lux, S.E. (1983) Red cell membreane

skeletal defects in hereditary and acquired hemolytic anemias. Semin. Hematol. *20*189–224.

Schacter, B.A. (1988) Heme catabolism by heme oxygenase: physiology, regulation, and mechanism of action. Semin. Hematol. *25*:349–369.

Sills, R.H. (1987) Splenic function: physiology and splenic hypofunction. CRC Crit. Rev. Oncol. Hematol. *7*:1–36.

Smith, M.A. & Ryan, M.E. (1988) Parvovirus infections. From benign to life-threatening. Postgrad. Med. *84*:127–128, 131–134.

Valentine, W.N., Tanaka, K.R. & Paglia, D.E. (1985) Hemolytic anemias and erythrocyte enzymopathies. Ann. Intern. Med. *103*: 245.

Woods, C.M. & Lazarides, E. (1988) The erythroid membrane skeleton: expresssion and assembly during erythropoiesis. Annu. Rev. Med. *39*:107–122.

Hemolytic Anemias: Intravascular Destruction of Red Cells

The second mechanism for the pathological destruction of erythrocytes is intravascular hemolysis, a process in which the cells rupture during circulation, spilling their hemoglobin into the plasma. Some hemoglobin is normally released into the plasma during the course of extravascular red cell destruction (both normal and pathological), simply because mononuclear phagocytes are messy eaters. In diseases associated with major intravascular hemolysis, however, almost all the hemoglobin in the lysed red cell is released into the plasma. The presence of this hemoglobin aids in the detection of these conditions, although their diagnosis usually depends on more specific investigations.

INTRAVASCULAR HEMOLYSIS: GENERAL CONSIDERATIONS

Disposal of Plasma Hemoglobin

Mechanism for clearing hemoglobin from the plasma can be divided into two classes: (1) a haptoglobin-dependent mechanism (recall that haptoglobin is the hemoglobin-scavenging protein of the plasma), and (2) a group of haptoglobin-independent mechanisms. Normally, the haptoglobin mechanism is the only one in operation, because free hemoglobin is cleared so rapidly that nothing is left behind to be disposed of by the other mechanisms. The haptoglobin mechanism, however, can only handle a limited amount of hemoglobin at a time, because there is only a small quantity of haptoglobin in the blood to begin with (equivalent to about 1 mg hemoglobin/ml whole blood), and this haptoglobin is used up in the hemoglobin-clearing reaction. In clinically significant intravascular hemolysis, the limited capacity of the haptoglobin mechanism is almost always exceeded, either because of the sudden release of large amounts of hemoglobin by a major hemolytic event or because ongoing intravascular hemolysis consumes haptoglobin faster than it can be replaced. Under these circumstances, haptoglobin vanishes from the bloodstream and free hemoglobin appears. The second class of mechanisms now takes over the disposal of the hemoglobin.

One of these mechanisms involves the kidney (Fig. 9–1). In the plasma, free hemoglobin will dissociate to a limited extent into $\alpha\beta$-dimers. These dimers are small enough to pass freely into the glomerular filtrate. In the nephron, the hemoglobin dimers are rapidly resorbed by the proximal tubular cells, where they are degraded in the usual way; the protein is destroyed, the iron is deposited as hemosid-

115

Mechanisms for Clearing Hemoglobin from the Plasma

Haptoglobin dependent
Haptoglobin independent
   Clearance by the kidney
   Destruction in the plasma

---

erin, and the heme is converted to bilirubin, which is released into the bloodstream and eventually excreted in the bile. The proximal tubular cell, however, has only a limited capacity to take up hemoglobin dimers; if this capacity is exceeded, hemoglobin appears in the urine.

The other mechanism involves the oxidation of the iron of the circulating hemoglobin (Fig. 9–2). This is a fairly rapid reaction that may take place before the hemoglobin is lost through the kidney. The product is methemoglobin, which quickly dissociates into ferriheme (heme in which the iron is trivalent), and

Fig. 9–1. How hemoglobin is handled by the kidney. (From Bunn, H.F. & Jandl, J.H. (1969) The renal handling of hemoglobin. II. Catabolism. J. Exp. Med. *129*: 925–934, with permission.)

the apoproteins. Some of the ferriheme is taken up by the heme-binding protein hemopexin, which carries it to the liver for the usual processing to iron and bilirubin. The rest is taken up by albumin to form methemalbumin; this ferriheme eventually ends up in the liver as well, where it suffers the same fate. What happens to the apoproteins is not known.

Manifestations of Hemoglobinemia

There are many ways to demonstrate that hemoglobin has been released into the plasma (Table 9–1), all of which depend on measuring hemoglobin itself or the traces it leaves behind as it is degraded.

1. *Fall in haptoglobin*. The most sensitive indicator of hemoglobin release into the plasma is a fall in haptoglobin. In extravascular hemolysis, haptoglobin levels will vary from near normal to zero, depending on the severity of the condition. With intravascular red cell destruction, however, haptoglobin almost always disappears completely. A point to remember is that haptoglobin levels rise during illness, so that a "normal" level in a sick patient in whom hemolysis is suspected might actually be the result of the offsetting effects of the hemolytic process (causing a fall) and the illness (causing a rise).

2. *Free hemoglobin in the plasma or urine*. Straightforward evidence of intravascular hemolysis is provided by the finding of free hemoglobin itself, in either the plasma or the urine. Hemoglobinemia leads to red plasma, a bedside indicator of intravascular hemolysis, although the clinical impression must be confirmed by a laboratory measurement. Because of the rate at which hemoglobin is cleared from the plasma, the red color disappears within a few hours after the cessation of hemolysis. Sometimes, but not always, the red is replaced by the brown of methemalbumin, which persists for a day or two after the episode of hemolysis. Hemoglobinuria results in

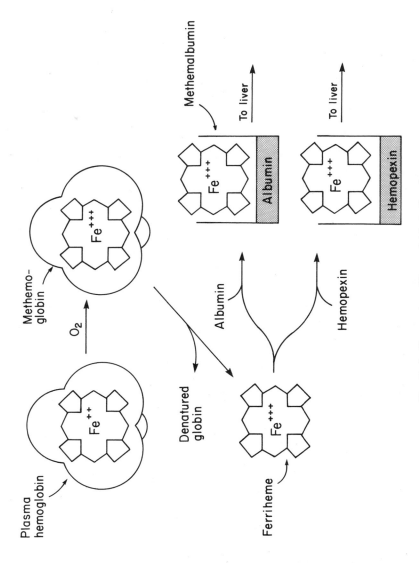

Fig. 9–2. Destruction of hemoglobin in the plasma.

Table 9-1. Detecting the Release of Hemoglobin in the Plasma

Sign	Remarks
Haptoglobin absent	Most sensitive test: occurs in all intravascular hemolysis, as well as in brisk extravascular hemolysis (e.g., sickle cell disease, immune hemolytic anemia)
Hemoglobinemia and hemoglobinuria	Red plasma, red urine: indicates active release of hemoglobin into plasma and disappears a few hours after cessation of hemolysis
Methomoglobinemia	Brown plasma: disappears 2 to 3 days after cessation of hemolysis
Hemosiderinuria	Lasts a few weeks after hemolysis ends: a good sign of prior or chronic release of hemoglobin into the plasma

dark urine that gives a positive test for blood. Laboratory confirmation is essential here too, because myoglobin and red blood cells also produce dark urine that tests positive for blood.

3. *Hemosiderinuria.* Free hemoglobin also gives rise to hemosiderinuria. The proximal tubule cells that have taken up hemoglobin dimers converts the iron to hemosiderin. These cells are shed over the course of a few weeks and are excreted in the urine, carrying their load of hemosiderin with them. The presence of these hemosiderin-containing cells in the urine is therefore a strong indication of intravascular hemolysis.

In applying these findings to the diagnosis of intravascular hemolysis, their transitory nature must be kept in mind. After a bout of intravascular hemolysis, hemoglobin can be detected in the blood and urine for only a few hours, haptoglobin is depressed for a couple of days, and hemosiderin is detected in the urine for at most a few weeks. It is easy to see how a single episode of acute intravascular hemolysis could be missed by these tests. Chronic intravascular hemolysis, however, is another story. Hemoglobinemia and hemoglobinuria may be hard to detect in chronic intravascular hemolysis because they are intermittent and low grade, but the haptoglobin is usually low, and hemosiderinuria is virtually always present because of the steady processing of free hemoglobin dimers by the kidney. Persistent hemosiderinuria is probably the best single clue to the diagnosis of chronic intravascular hemolysis.

Clinical Features of Intravascular Hemolysis

The general clinical features of intravascular hemolysis are identical to those of extravascular hemolysis, except for two points: splenomegaly does not occur and plasma hemoglobin is seen. The features are summarized in Table 9–2.

INTRAVASCULAR HEMOLYTIC ANEMIAS

Traumatic Hemolysis ("Waring Blender" Syndrome)

Traumatic hemolytic anemia is a form of intravascular hemolysis caused by the mechanical destruction of red cells in the circulation. It occurs under three types of circumstances.

1. *When red cells pass at high velocity through regions of turbulent flow.* The cells break under these conditions by smashing against rigid obstructions in their path or by stretching past their limit of deformability, tearing themselves apart. Such flows are produced (1) in malignant tumors, in which the blood vessels tend to be highly tortuous and irregular; (2) in malignant hypertension, because of rapid flow produced by the extreme degree of vasoconstriction characteristic of this condition, and (3) in tight aortic stenosis and prosthetic valve leaks, where blood flows with great velocity through a narrow opening past

Table 9-2. Principal Manifestations of Intravascular Hemolysis

Mechanism	Clinical Findings	Laboratory Findings
Increased red cell production		Reticulocytosis
		Marrow red cell hyperplasia
Plasma hemoglobin	Dark urine	Absent serum haptoglobin
	Red plasma	Hemoglobinemia and hemoglobinuria
		Hemosiderin in urine
Increased hemoglobin	Jaundice	Indirect bilirubinemia
breakdown	Gallstones	
Red cell destruction	Pallor and faintness	Anemia
	Cardiac symptoms	
	Aggravation of underlying vascular disease	

rigid walls. The anemia in giant hemangioma of childhood (Kasabach-Merritt syndrome) is caused by red cell damage that occurs as blood passes through the deformed vessels of the tumor.

2. *When red cells pass through regions of intravascular coagulation.* Although blood normally does not clot in the vascular tree, there are conditions in which coagulation takes place within blood vessels. In two of these conditions, disseminated intravascular coagulation and thrombotic thrombocytopenia purpura, clotting occurs within capillaries, which may fill with a mesh of fibrin strands through which the blood must flow (fibrin is the protein, generated at sites of coagulation, whose polymerization produces the solid clot). Red cells rupture as they are clotheslined by the fibrin strands (Fig. 9–3). Traumatic hemolytic anemia is therefore characteristic of these two clotting disorders.

3. *When red cells pass through vessels in the soles of the feet.* Some people have red cells that are unusually susceptible to mechanical damage. Every time such persons take a step, a few of the red cells in the soles of their feet are broken. With sufficient vigorous activity, this sort of red cell damage may increase to the point at which it becomes clinically evident as a traumatic hemolytic anemia. This condition tends to be seen in athletes and in soldiers after a long march, hence the name *march hemoglobinuria*. It has also been reported in bongo drummers and martial artists, in whom the damage is inflicted as the blood passes through the palms of the hands.

Fig. 9–3. Red cell clotheslined by a fibrin strand. (From Bull, B.S. & Kuhn, I.N. (1970) The production of schistocytes by fibrin strands (a scanning electron microscope study). Blood *35*:104–111, with permission.)

Conditions Producing Traumatic Hemolysis

Rapid turbulent blood flow
   Malignant tumors
   Malignant hypertension
   Tight aortic stenosis
   Prosthetic valve leaks
Intravascular coagulation
"March hemoglobinuria"

The clinical manifestations of traumatic hemolytic anemia are those of intravascular hemolysis together with the signs and symptoms of the underlying disorder. Anemia, reticulocytosis, and indirect bilirubinemia are seen, the hallmarks of hemolysis, but the spleen tends not to be palpable in this and other intravascular hemolytic anemias. If the hemolysis is mild, the haptoglobin is low, but evidence of free plasma hemoglobin is lacking. More severe hemolysis results in hemoglobinemia. This is most likely to be detected only through hemosiderinuria, but there may be enough hemoglobin in the plasma to be found by laboratory tests. Frank hemoglobinemia and hemoglobinuria, detectable at the bedside in the form of red plasma and dark urine, are unusual in traumatic hemolysis and are seen only in the most severe cases.

In a patient with chronic traumatic hemolytic anemia, enough iron may be lost through hemosiderinuria to lead to a superimposed iron deficiency anemia. In such patients, the morphological abnormalities resulting from the iron deficiency may mask the characteristic changes seen in the underlying hemolytic condition, so that they are missed unless looked for after the iron-deficient state is corrected. In patients with iron deficiency unexplained by menses, pregnancy, or gastrointestinal bleeding, the urine should not be overlooked as a source of iron loss.

The diagnostic feature of traumatic hemolytic anemia is found in the blood smear (Fig. 9–4). Here, red cell fragments are seen in the form of helmet cells, triangles, and other oddly deformed pieces of erythrocyte. These shapes are produced when the membrane of a red cell fragment reseals before all the hemoglobin is lost. Such fragments are not seen in every case of traumatic hemolysis—they are generally absent, for instance, in march hemoglobinuria, a condition in which only a small number of red cells are damaged—but in severe traumatic hemolytic anemia, these fragments may represent more than 10 percent of the cells on the smear.

Treatment is aimed primarily at the underly-

Fig. 9–4. Blood smear in traumatic hemolysis. Red cell fragments are abundant. (From Kapff, C.T. & Jandl, J.H. (1981) The anemias. Ch. 3. In Blood: Atlas and Sourcebook of Hematology. Little, Brown, Boston, with permission.)

ing disease. The anemia itself may be treated with transfusions if sufficiently severe. If the condition is chronic, folate should be given to prevent a deficiency that might otherwise result because of the increased erythropoiesis. Iron supplements may also be needed to offset iron losses in the urine.

Glucose-6-Phosphate Dehydrogenase Deficiency and Oxidant Hemolysis

Oxidant Defense in the Red Cell

The function of the red cell is to transport oxygen from the lungs to the tissues. Ordinarily, oxygen is picked up and released by the red cell without undergoing any chemical changes; it is transported as inert cargo. Occasionally, however, an oxygen molecule will be converted to a more reactive oxidizing species such as superoxide (O_2^-) or hydrogen peroxide (H_2O_2). O_2^- is produced when oxyhemoglobin is converted to methemoglobin:

$$Hb(Fe^{2+})-O_2 \rightarrow Hb(Fe^{3+}) + O_2^-$$

H_2O_2 is also produced from the aberrant dissociation of oxyhemoglobin; it arises as well from additional sources, the latter not well characterized. These two compounds represent

Oxidant Defenses in the Red Cell

Glutathione-dependent system
  Glutathione peroxidase/reductase
  Hexosemonophosphate shunt
Superoxide dismutase
Catalase

a potent oxidizing threat and must be destroyed, or they will destroy the red cell.

The red cell has several ways of dealing with these oxidizing species. It contains superoxide dismutase, an enzyme that represents the major defense against O_2^-, converting it to H_2O_2 and oxygen. It also contains catalase, which eliminates H_2O_2 by converting it to oxygen and water. The most important defense against H_2O_2, however, is a glutathione-requiring system. Defects in this system cause clinically important intravascular hemolytic conditions.

The glutathione antioxidant system consists of glutathione itself; two enzymes, namely glutathione peroxidase and glutathione reductase; and a source of reducing power. The destruction of H_2O_2 is accomplished by glutathione peroxidase, which catalyzes its reduction to water by glutathione:

$$2GSH + H_2O_2 \rightarrow GSSG + 2H_2O$$

The oxidized glutathione formed in this reaction is converted back to the reduced state by NADPH in a reaction catalyzed by glutathione reductase:

$$GSSG + NADPH \rightarrow 2GSH + NADP$$

Thus in the glutathione antioxidant system, glutathione cycles between its reduced and oxidized forms, converting one molecule of H_2O_2 to water with each turn of the cycle. Because NADPH is consumed by this system, this reducing agent has to be regenerated to maintain the system's capacity to destroy H_2O_2.

In the red cell, the sole source of NADPH is the hexosemonophosphate shunt. The NADPH-producing producing reactions in this metabolic path are the glucose 6-phosphate dehydrogenase (G6PD) reaction:

$$\text{Glucose 6-phosphate} + \text{NADP}$$
$$\rightarrow \text{6-phosphogluconate} + \text{NADPH}$$

and the 6-phosphogluconate dehydrogenase reaction:

$$\text{6-Phosphogluconate} + \text{NADP}$$
$$\rightarrow \text{ribulose 5-phosphate} + CO_2 + \text{NADPH}$$

It is clear that the normal operation of the hemosemonophosphate shunt, particularly its first reaction, is essential if the antioxidant defenses of the red cell are to retain their effectiveness.

Glucose 6-Phosphate Dehydrogenase Deficiency

G6PD deficiency is the most common inherited enzyme deficiency affecting red cells. The gene that encodes G6PD is on the X chromosome, so the deficiency is inherited as an X-linked trait. From the foregoing discussion, it is apparent that G6PD is critical for the antioxidant defenses of the red cell. It is therefore not surprising that G6PD deficiency leads to an anemia associated with an increase in the susceptibility of the cell to injury by oxidants.

Oxidants cause two kinds of damage to red cells: damage to hemoglobin and damage to the membrane (Fig. 9–5). The attack of oxidants on hemoglobin may result first in the production of methemoglobin, which accumulates because it is generated faster than it can be reconverted to hemoglobin. From the methemoglobin, the oxidized heme dissociates, leaving behind the free globin, which is destroyed by further oxidation. Alternatively, the initial damage may be sustained by the globin protein, which is destroyed without losing its heme. In either case, the denatured hemoglobin eventually precipitates as an intracellular mass of agglutinated protein. These masses are

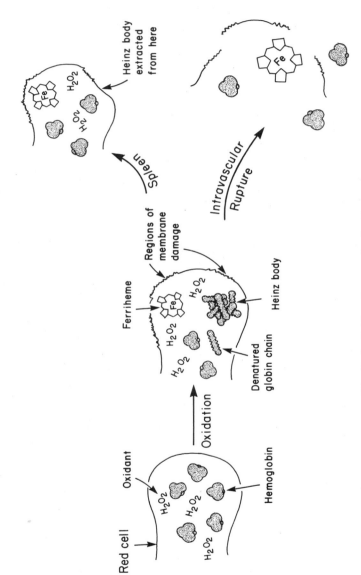

Fig. 9–5. Oxidant damage of red cells.

extracted when damaged red cells pass through the spleen, another version of splenic "conditioning" or "pitting" of defective erythrocytes (compare the amputation of projections from spur cells by splenic macrophages). The extraction of the hemoglobin precipitate results in a reduction in the size of the red cell and an alteration in its shape, which becomes more spherical than before. At the same time, the oxidants attack the red cell membrane, destroying its integrity. It is probably membrane damage, rather than hemoglobin denaturation, that is responsible for the intravascular hemolysis characteristic of G6PD deficiency.

Hemolysis in G6PD deficiency is precipitated when the red cells are exposed to an oxidant stress. The two most common stress-inciting agents are infections and oxidant drugs. Just how infections impose an oxidant stress on red cells is unclear, but it is certain that they do, because hemolysis is a common occurrence in infected patients with G6PD deficiency. With oxidant drugs, the mechanism is better understood: These drugs enter the red cell and then function as artificial electron carriers, passing electrons from endogenous reductants (e.g., NADH) to oxygen to produce H_2O_2. A large variety of drugs are able to precipitate oxidant hemolysis in G6PD-deficient red cells; those most commonly associated with this problem are the antimalarials and the sulfonamides. Finally, a particularly serious hemolytic event that has led to a number of fa-

---

Clinical Manifestations of G6PD Deficiency

X-linked inheritance
Most common in blacks
Precipitated by
    Infections
    Drugs
Signs and symptoms
    Hemolysis
        Primarily intravascular
        Usually episodic, occasionally chronic
    Enlarged spleen
    Gallstones

---

talities will occur when certain patients with an unusually severe form of G6PD deficiency eat broad beans (fava beans), which contain pyrimidine derivatives having potent oxidant properties.

The clinical manifestations of G6PD deficiency are primarily those of intravascular hemolysis. There is an acute fall in the hematocrit, accompanied by a reticulocytosis and an increase in indirect bilirubin. Haptoglobin falls sharply, and signs of hemoglobin release into plasma are often seen (i.e., hemoglobinemia, hemoglobinuria, hemosiderinuria). Some extravascular red cell destruction also takes place because of the presence of hemoglobin precipitates in cells that have not been damaged enough to rupture in the bloodstream. This occurs in the spleen, which enlarges through a sort of work hypertrophy as it conditions the red cells by extracting the precipitated hemoglobin. Evidence of conditioning may be seen in the smear as misshapen red cells and microspherocytes (the latter to be distinguished from spherocytes of normal size, which are seen in hereditary spherocytosis). Often, however, the smear shows no abnormal findings. As with all congenital hemolytic anemias, there is a tendency to gallstone formation.

This bare listing of signs and symptoms gives a qualitative idea of the clinical picture

---

Oxidant Drugs

Antimalarials
    Chloroquine
    Primaquine
Dapsone
Sulfonamides
Nitrofurantoin
Antipyretics (only at very high doses)
    Aspirin
    Phenacetin

in G6PD deficiency. What cannot be gathered from this list is a feel for the quantitative aspects of the disease. As it happens, G6PD deficiency is one of the most variable of the inherited red cell disorders. The anemia in this condition can range from a form so mild as to be apparent only during the most rigorous oxidant stress to a form so severe that it has caused death from massive acute hemolysis. What accounts for this variability is the difference from patient to patient in the proportion of red cells destroyed during a hemolytic event. This in turn is directly related to the properties of the defective enzyme.

More than 100 different forms of the human enzyme have been described to date. Two of these forms are found in normal persons: the B form, present in normal whites and in most normal blacks, and the A (or A$^+$) form, present in about 30 percent of normal black men and 55 percent of normal black women, most of whom are AB heterozygotes. These normal forms are easy to distinguish by electrophoresis (Fig. 9–6). Virtually all the other forms of the enzyme have been isolated from patients with clinical G6PD deficiency.

These different forms of G6PD have been found to vary widely in their properties. Of particular importance is the variation in stability among these enzymes, because it is this as much as anything that determines the clinical severity of the disease. The relationship between stability and clinical severity is best explained by considering the two extreme forms of G6PD deficiency: the very common mild form seen in blacks, and the rare severe form found in people from the Mediterranean basin (Table 9–3).

1. *G6PD Type A$^-$ form.* By far the most common form of G6PD deficiency is caused

Fig. 9–6. Electrophoresis of G6PD, showing three patterns (**Left**) Black subject with the A type. (**Center**) White subject with the B type. (**Right**) Black subject with both types. The enzyme is detected by an activity stain. (From Giblett, E.R. (1969) Genetic Markers in Human Blood. Blackwell Scientific Publishers, Oxford, with permission.)

by G6PD type A$^-$, a low-activity variant of the type A enzyme (G6PD A$^{202val \rightarrow met}$). The condition is seen exclusively in blacks. The gene for the A$^-$ enzyme is carried by about 20 percent of black women, so roughly 10 percent of black males have the disease.

The important property of the A$^-$ enzyme is its reduced stability compared with the normal enzyme. Red cells containing the A$^-$ enzyme have adequate levels of G6PD when they are released from the marrow, but activity declines as the enzyme decays, so that by the time the cells are 1 month old they no longer contain any G6PD. When these cells are stressed, as by the ingestion of an oxidant drug, cells old enough to have lost their G6PD will be lysed, but the younger cells will survive; only a fraction of the red cell population is therefore lost, and the resulting anemia is mild. It is important to remember that a second oxidant challenge will have little effect if it occurs shortly after the initial exposure, because

Table 9-3. Two Extremes of G6PD Deficiency

	G6PD$_{A-}$	G6PD$_{Mediterranean}$
Instability of enzyme	Mild	Severe
Deficiency seen in	Old red cells	All red cells
Clinical severity	2+	4+
G6PD levels immediately after attack	May be normal	Always low

the cells that survived the first oxidant exposure and the new cells released from the marrow in response to the initial hemolytic event will contain enough G6PD to fend off the second challenge. Furthermore, the diagnosis of G6PD deficiency may be difficult to make immediately after a hemolytic event, because the deficient cells will have been swept from the bloodstream; it may not be possible to diagnose the disease until several weeks have elapsed, during which the deficient population will reaccumulate as the surviving cells age and lose their G6PD.

2. *G6PD*$_{Mediterranean}$ *form.* A much more severe hemolytic disease is caused by G6PD$_{Mediterranean}$. This rare variety occurs in whites from the Mediterranean basin: Italians, Greeks, persons from the Near East and North Africa, and those from the Mediterranean islands (e.g., Sicily, Sardinia). The enzyme is extremely unstable, so G6PD activity is greatly diminished in all red cells, even those newly released from the marrow. As a result, virtually all red cells are susceptible to oxidant hemolysis, and an oxidative challenge of sufficient magnitude will cause hemolysis of the most severe degree, with gross hemoglobinemia and hemoglobinuria and a sudden fall in the hematocrit to life-threatening levels. In this form of the disease there is no resistance to a susbequent oxidative challenge, and the diagnosis can always be made because G6PD-deficient red cells are always present in the bloodstream.

A feature of G6PD and other X-linked diseases (Fig. 9–7) is that female heterozygotes (i.e., females who inherited a defective X chromosome from one parent and a normal one from the other) always contain two populations of cells: one that is completely normal, and another that expresses the inherited defect in its full-blown form. Affected males, however, contain only a single population of cells, all defective. The duality of population in female heterozygotes is known as mosaicism. As a result of this mosaicism, female heterozygotes show much less hemolysis than do affected males, simply because female heterozy-

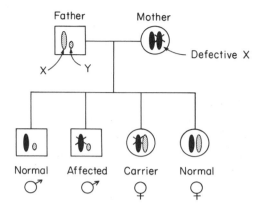

Fig. 9–7. X-linked transmission. X-linked diseases are transmitted primarily by female carriers. In such carriers, one X chromosome has a defective gene, the other X chromosome is normal. The child of a carrier mother has a 50:50 chance of inheriting the defective X chromosome. If a male child inherits the defective chromosome, he will have the disease in its full-blown form, because the only X chromosome in his cells is the defective one received from his mother. In contrast, a female who inherits the defective chromosome will be clinically normal, or at worst will have a milder form of the disease, because she will have inherited a second X chromosome from her father that can compensate for the defect in her maternal X chromosome; she will herself, however, be a carrier of the disease.

gotes always have some normal red cells in their circulation. In the rare female homozygote (one who has inherited G6PD deficiency from both her parents), homolysis is just as severe as in the male.

Mosaicism results from the fact that early in female embryogenesis, one of the two X chromosomes loses its capacity to code for protein synthesis. The loss of function is referred to as X-chromosome inactivation (Fig. 9–8). Inactivation is a random process in that each of the two X chromosomes in a given cell is equally likely to become inactivated. In the case in which one of the X chromosomes contains a defective gene, the effect of random inactivation will be to create a fetus containing some cells in which the functioning X chromosome is normal and others in which the functioning X chromosome is defective. The cells

Fig. 9–8. X-chromosome inactivation. When the founder cell that gives rise to the blood-forming tissues starts to differentiate in a female embryo, both X chromosomes are active. After the newly established blood-forming tissue has reached the 16- or 32-cell stage, however, one of the two X chromosomes in each cell undergoes inactivation, losing its capacity to code for proteins, but retaining its ability to duplicate itself when the cell divides. In a given cell, the choice as to which of the two X chromosomes will undergo inactivation is completely random. Once that cell has made its choice, however, all its descendents will inherit the same pattern of X-chromosome inactivation.

will breed true thereafter with respect to the functioning X chromosome, accounting for the mosaicism in adult female carriers of X-linked diseases.

The diagnosis of G6PD deficiency is made by measuring the level of G6PD in the red cell. It will be very low in patients having severe disease and a badly defective enzyme (e.g., G6PD$_{Mediterranean}$), but it may be moderately decreased in patients with enzymes whose properties are closer to normal (e.g., G6PD A$^-$), especially if the measurement is made shortly after an episode of hemolysis. The disease can also be diagnosed by staining a blood smear for G6PD (Fig. 9–9); a population of cells that lacks the enzyme is seen in G6PD-deficient patients. The enzyme can be characterized by electrophoresis of hemolysates followed by an activity stain (Fig. 9–6) as well as by more detailed enzymological studies (e.g., K$_m$, stability) that are usually carried out only in research laboratories.

Although the definitive diagnosis requires measurements of G6PD levels, the presence of Heinz bodies can furnish a valuable clue to the existence of the disease in a patient with an undiagnosed acute hemolytic anemia. Heinz bodies are intracellular precipitates of dena-

tured hemoglobin that become visible when the cell is stained with crystal violet. Heinz bodies are typically seen in oxidant hemolysis, unstable hemoglobin disease, and thalassemia. In oxidant hemolysis, they are present only transiently, appearing at the onset of an attack and disappearing with the elimination of the last damaged red cells. If they are seen in the blood of a patient with an acute hemolytic anemia, G6PD deficiency should be strongly suspected, and drugs that precipitate hemolysis in this condition should be scrupulously avoided until the diagnosis is confirmed or refuted by direct measurement of the enzyme.

G6PD deficiency is managed primarily through the avoidance of agents known to provoke hemolysis. Antimalarials are particularly hazardous in this regard. Other drugs represent less potent oxidant challenges and can be used in patients with mild G6PD deficiency if given with great care, but it is best to avoid all oxidant drugs in G6PD deficiency if at all possible. The eating of fava beans by a person with severe G6PD deficiency can be catastrophic. An acute attack is treated supportively with fluids to maintain urine flow and transfusions as required. A few patients with severe G6PD deficiency may have CNSHA: in

Fig. 9–9. Blood smears stained for G6PD. (**A**) Normal. (**B**) Affected male. (**C**) Female heterozygote, showing mosaicism. (From Gall, J.C., Jr., Brewer, G.J. & Dern, R.T. (1965) Studies of glucose-6-phosphate dehydrogenase activity of individual erythrocytes: The methemoglobinelution test for identification of females heterozygous for G6PD deficiency. Am. J. Human Genet. *17*:359–370, with permission.)

these, splenectomy may be of some help, although it is usually of little value in this condition.

Other Enzyme Deficiencies

Deficiencies of enzymes involved in glutathione metabolism may lead to oxidant hemolysis. Deficiency of 6-phosphogluconate dehydrogenase, the second enzyme of the hexosemonophosphate shunt, does not cause anemia.

Immune Hemolytic Anemias

Intravascular hemolysis is characteristic of certain types of immune hemolytic anemias. Intravascular hemolysis is typically seen in transfusion reactions caused by ABO incompatibility. A very rare but potentially fatal cause of intravascular hemolysis is the so-called Donath-Landsteiner antibody, which

causes red cells to lyse when they are transiently cooled below body temperature and is responsible for the condition known as paroxysmal cold hemoglobinuria. These conditions are discussed in full in Chapters 29 and 30.

Infections

Intravascular hemolysis is a prominent feature of a few infectious diseases, some rare and some not so rare. *Clostridium perfrigens*

Other Enzyme Deficiencies That Cause Oxidant Hemolysis

Glutathione reductase
γ-Glutamylcysteine synthetase
Glutathione synthetase

secretes a toxin that can cause intravascular hemolysis by breaking down phospholipids in the red cell membrane. *Bartonella bacilliformis* is the cause of the rare Andean disease known as Oroya fever, one of whose manifestations is an intravascular hemolytic process of a few weeks' duration. The most common infections causing intravascular hemolysis, however, are those caused by *Plasmodia*; malaria is one of the most prevalent infections in the world and is responsible for hundreds of thousands of deaths yearly.

Paroxysmal Nocturnal Hemoglobinuria

Paroxysmal nocturnal hemoglobinuria is a stem-cell disease of unknown etiology in which the abnormal marrow cell line produces, among other things, a population of red cells that are unusually susceptible to lysis by complement. Chronic recurrent intravascular hemolysis is one of the hallmarks of this disease. Paroxysmal nocturnal hemoglobinuria is discussed in detail in Chapter 28.

SUGGESTED READINGS

Beutler, E. (1971) Abnormalities of the hexose-monophosphate shunt. Semin. Hematol. *8*:311.

Bunn, H.F. & Forget, B.D. (1984) Human Hemoglobins. 2nd Ed. W.B. Saunders, Philadelphia.

Dacie, Sir John (1985) The Haemolytic Anaemias. Churchill Livingstone, Edinburgh, UK.

Gordon-Smith, E.C. (1980) Drug-induced oxidative haemolysis. Clin. Haematol. *9*:557.

Luzzatto, L. & Battistuzzi, G. (1985) Glucose-6-phosphate dehydrogenase. Adv. Hum. Genet. *14*:217–329, 386–388.

McClung, J.A., Stein, J.H., Ambrose, J.A., Herman, M.V. & Reed, G.E. (1983) Prosthetic heart valves: a review. Prog. Cardiovasc. Dis. *26*:237–270.

Morgan, E.H. & Baker, E. (1986) Iron uptake and metabolism by hepatocytes. Fed. Proc. *45*:2810–2816.

Morse, E.E. (1988) Toxic effects of drugs on erythrocytes. Ann. Clin. Lab. Sci *18*:13-18.

Murgo, A.J. (1987) Thrombotic microangiopathy in the cancer patient including those induced by chemotherapeutic agents. Semin. Hematol. *24*:161–177.

Weatherall, D.J. & Abdalla, S. (1982) The anaemia of Plasmodium falciparum malaria. Br. Med. Bull. *38*:147–151.

Reider, R.F. (1974) Human hemoglobin stability and instability: Molecular mechanisms and some clinical correlations. Semin. Hematol. *11*:423.

Schulman, J.D., Mudd, S.H., Schneider, J.L. et. al. (1980) Genetic disorders of glutathione and sulfur amino acid metabolism. Ann. Intern. Med. *93*:330.

Valentine, W.N., Tanaka, K.R. & Paglia, D.E. (1985) Hemolytic anemias and erythrocyte enzymopathies. Ann. Intern. Med. *103*:245–257.

Vennerstrom, J.L. & Eaton, J.W. (1988) Oxidants, oxidant drugs, and malaria. J. Med. Chem. *31*:1269–1277.

10

Hemoglobin Biosynthesis: Thalassemia and Hemoglobin E

At first glance, it would appear that hemoglobin biosynthesis should be a straightforward, uncomplicated matter. Hemoglobin A is by far the predominant protein in the red cell, and its production should proceed smoothly along the path defined by the so-called "central dogma" of molecular biology:

$$gene \rightarrow messenger \rightarrow protein$$

In fact, though, many hemoglobins besides hemoglobin A occur normally in red cells. These are particularly prominent in the very young, and their proportions change extensively during fetal development and the first 6 months or so of postnatal life. The biosynthesis of these hemoglobins involves (1) the activation and inactivation of more than a dozen genes distributed between two pairs of chromosomes, (2) the production of highly complex messenger RNA precursors that undergo extensive post-transcriptional processing to yield the templates on which the hemoglobin chains are assembled, and (3) the synthesis of different types of hemoglobin chains at rates that are somehow balanced so that they are all used up in the assembly of the final hemoglobin tetramers.

Thalassemia results when there is an impairment in the biosynthesis of one of the two constituent chains of hemoglobin A, the major

adult hemoglobin. Because of what has been learned about hemoglobin biosynthesis, it is probably fair to say that thalassemia is as well understood at a molecular level as any human disease.

NORMAL HEMOGLOBIN PRODUCTION

Normal Hemoglobin Species: The Ontogeny of Hemoglobin

During the course of our lifetime, we manufacture six different normal hemoglobins (Table 10–1). These hemoglobins are assembled from two families of chains: the α-family, containing the α-chain itself and the ζ-chain, and the β-family, containing the β-, γ-, δ-, and ε-chains. The prototype hemoglobin, hemoglobin A, is a tetrameric protein composed to two α-chains and two β-chains (see Ch. 3). Each of the other five normal hemoglobins is also a tetramer containing a pair of α-family chains and a pair of β-family chains.

The amount of a given chain that occurs in the red cells is not constant throughout life, but varies with age in a manner that is characteristic for each type of chain (Fig. 10–1). As a consequence, different hemoglobins are

129

Table 10-1. Normal Human Hemoglobins

Hemoglobin	Chain Composition
Embryonic	
Gower I	$\zeta_2\epsilon_2$
Gower II	$\alpha_2\epsilon_2$
Portland	$\zeta_2\gamma_2$
Fetal	
Hemoglobin F	$\alpha_2\gamma_2$
Adult	
Hemoglobin A	$\alpha_2\beta_2$
Hemoglobin A_2	$\alpha_2\delta_2$

There are two families of globin chains: the α-family and the β-family. The α-family contains the α- and ζ-globin chains; these are coded for by genes on chromosome 16. The β-family contains the β-, γ-, δ-, and ϵ-chains; the genes for these are on chromosome 11. Each normal hemoglobin species contains a pair of chains from each family.

found in the human at different ages. Three of the six hemoglobins are normally found only in the embryo, whereas the other three are present at birth and remain present throughout the lifetime of the individual. This will all become clear as the individual hemoglobins are discussed.

Embryonic Hemoglobins

The first red cells that appear during fetal development arise from the blood vessels of the embryo. These vessels begin as clusters of

mesodermal cells known as blood islands that appear on the yolk sac during the first week of development. These blood islands send out cords that join and hollow out to form the primitive vascular network. The cells at the periphery of these cords differentiate into the blood vessel walls, whereas those in the center form the large, nucleated, hemoglobin-filled cells that constitute the embryonic erythrocytes. Yolk sac erythrocytes appear in the embryo about the third week of gestation and remain for about 10 weeks. They then disappear, never to return.

The major hemoglobins of these primitive erythrocytes are the Gower hemoglobins, of which there are two, both containing ϵ, the embryonic β-family chain. One, Gower I, also contains ζ, the embryonic member of the α-family; its complete composition is $\zeta_2\epsilon_2$. The other, Gower II, contains the adult α-chain ($\alpha_2\epsilon_2$). The Gower hemoglobins, the first that can be detected in the developing embryo, decline as yolk sac erythropoiesis is overtaken by hepatosplenic erythropoiesis and are gone by 10 weeks.

The third embryonic hemoglobin, hemoglobin Portland, is present only in traces. It resembles Gower I in containing the embryonic

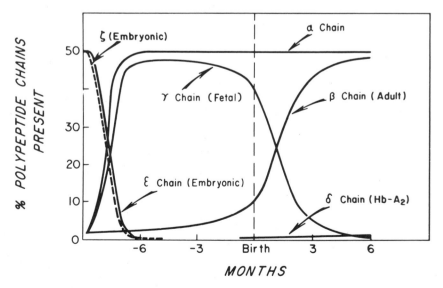

Fig. 10-1. Hemoglobin composition of red cells during fetal development and the first year after birth. (From Bunn, H.F., Forget, B.G. & Ranney, H.M. (1977) Hemoglobin biosynthesis. Ch. 4. In Human Hemoglobins. W.B. Saunders, Philadelphia, with permission.)

α-family chain ζ, but instead of the very primitive β-family chain ε, it contains its ontogenic successor, the γ-chain. Accordingly, the composition of hemoglobin Portland is $\zeta_2\gamma_2$. This hemoglobin can be detected in tiny amounts throughout fetal life.

Hemoglobin F

At about 6 weeks, a new population of hematopoietic cells begins to express itself. These cells will be responsible for hematopoiesis during the rest of the individual's life. They appear first in the liver and spleen, which rapidly become the major source of blood cells in the developing fetus. After about the fourth month, blood formation begins in the bone marrow, and the liver and spleen decline in importance as hematopoietic organs until by the time of birth they no longer make blood. However, they retain the memory of their former hematopoietic role and in certain pathological states will once again make blood cells, an activity known as *extramedullary hematopoiesis.*

From the time the permanent hematopoietic line takes over until several weeks past birth, the major hemoglobin in the red cell is hemoglobin F, or fetal hemoglobin. The β-class chain of this hemoglobin is the γ-chain; its composition is $\alpha_2\gamma_2$. Hemoglobin F actually consists of several closely related species: (1) there are two types of γ-chains in hemoglobin F, one containing a glycine at position 136 ($^G\gamma$) and the other alanine ($^A\gamma$). All hemoglobin-F-containing red cells have some of each; and (2) about one-half the hemoglobin F is acetylated at the N-terminus of the γ-chain. All these species behave similarly, however, so that in functional terms there is only one kind of hemoglobin F.

As the predominant hemoglobin in fetal red cells, hemoglobin F bears the major responsibility for delivering oxygen to the fetal tissues. To obtain this oxygen, it must steal from the maternal bloodstream. This act of theft is made easier by the difference in the way the oxygen affinities of fetal (Hb F) and maternal

---

Properties of Hemoglobin F

Structure

$\alpha_2\gamma_2$

Two types of γ-chains: $^G\gamma$ (γ^{136gly}) and $^A\gamma$ (γ^{136ala})

Partly acetylated

Function

Oxygen affinity similar to hemoglobin A

2,3-DPG has little effect on oxygen binding

(Hb A) hemoglobin are regulated by 2,3-disphosphoglyceric acid (2,3-DPG). Although the inherent oxygen affinities of these two hemoglobins are about equal, Hb A is much more sensitive than Hb F to the oxygen unloading effect of 2,3-DPG. The effect of this difference is to lower the oxygen affinity of the Hb-A-containing maternal red cells with respect to the Hb-F-containing fetal red cells, because 2,3-DPG is a major regulator of oxygen affinity in intact erythrocytes. As a result, it is easy for the fetal red cells to strip oxygen from the maternal red cells as these two red cell populations flow past each other in the placenta.

Hemoglobin F begins to decline about the 30th week of gestation and is nearly gone by 6 months of age (Fig. 10–1). Unlike the case of the embryonic hemoglobins, however, a small amount of hemoglobin F persists in the circulation throughout life. This trace of hemoglobin F is not uniformly distributed among the red cells, but is found mainly in a minor population known as F cells, each of which contains some 10 percent or so of hemoglobin F. These F cells can be detected by a special procedure in which blood smears are treated with acid before staining (Fig. 10–2). The acid pretreatment leaches hemoglobin A from the red cells; but hemoglobin F, which is relatively acid resistant, remains behind and is visualized by the subsequent staining procedure.

Fig. 10–2. F cells in a blood smear. The F cells take up stain because of their hemoglobin F, which stays behind during the staining procedure while hemoglobin A is washed away. The F cells stain darkly. The F-cell stain is sometimes called the Betke-Kleihauer stain. (From Castoldi, G.L. (1981) Erythrocytes. Ch. 3. In Zucker-Franklin, D. et al. (eds.) Atlas of Blood Cells: Function and Pathology. Edi. Ermes s.r.l., Milan, with permission.)

Hemoglobin A and A$_2$

The hemoglobins of the adult red cell are hemoglobin A $(\alpha_2\beta_2)$ and hemglobin A$_2$ $(\alpha_2\delta_2)$. Hemoglobin A replaces hemoglobin F during late gestation and infancy, reaching adult levels by 6 months of age or so (Fig. 10–1). In the adult, hemoglobin A constitutes more than 95 percent of the hemoglobin in the red cell. Hemoglobin A$_2$ begins to appear at birth and increases over the first year or two of life. It never amounts to much more than 1 percent of the total hemoglobin in normal red cells. Because it is present in such low concentrations, it is of no practical use as an oxygen-carrying protein. It does, however, provide physicians with a useful diagnostic tool for evaluating patients with thalassemia.

Genetics of Hemoglobin Production

The genes that code for the hemoglobin chains have been identified on chromosomes 11 and 16 (Fig. 10–3). Chromosome 16 carries the α-family genes, two coding for the α-chain and one for the ζ-chain. Between the ζ-gene and the two α-genes is a long stretch of DNA of unknown function. Reading from 5' to 3', the direction of DNA transcription, the genes are lined up as follows: ζ, space, α, α. The β-family genes are on chromosome 11. These are arranged in three groups with two long stretches of DNA between them. The order is as follows: ϵ, space, $^G\gamma$, $^A\gamma$, space, δ, β. It is curious that the order of the genes on the chromosomes is the same as the order in which the chains appear during fetal development.

The genes themselves have a complex structure (Fig. 10–4). The template for the globin chain is present in the gene as a sequence of nucleotides arranged in a particular order. The template sequence, however, is not present as a continuous stretch of nucleotides; instead, it is present in segments interrupted by stretches of DNA whose nucleotide sequences are never translated into protein. The segments of template are known as *exons*, because they are *ex-*

Fig. 10–3. Arrangement of globin genes on chromosomes 11 and 16.

Fig. 10–4. Diagram of a globin gene. Exons are shown in black. The *arrow* shows the location of the "cap" site, the point at which messenger RNA transcription begins. Rates of messenger transcription are controlled by untranslated stretches on both sides of the exon/intron portion of the gene. The lengths of these controlling stretches are not known, although on the 5′ untranslated side they extend to the left of the "cap" site.

pressed in the final globin product; the untranslated stretches are known as *introns*, because they are *inter*vening sequences that separate the template segments from each other. Finally, there are untranslated regions on both 5′ (left) and 3′ (right) sides of the exon/intron portion of the gene that are involved in the regulation of gene expression.

From this gene, the messenger RNA is produced (Fig. 10–5). Transcription begins at the "cap" site in the 5′ untranslated region, continues straight through the exon/intron region, and terminates somewhere in the 3′ untranslated region. The initial RNA product is thus a faithful copy of a stretch of an entire gene sequence, containing introns, exons, and all.

Fig. 10–5. Production of the globin messenger. The initial transcription product is a complete copy of the globin DNA gene from the "cap" site to the termination site. It includes exons (*thick black*), introns (*thin*), and flanking sequences, the portions of the transcript lying outside the exon/intron region (*stippled*). The initial transcript is converted to mature globin messenger RNA by splicing out the introns, adding a 7-methyl G cap to the end of the 5′ flanking sequence, and adding a poly-A chain to the end of the 3′ flanking sequence.

This product is not translated directly, but is first converted to the true messenger RNA by post-transcriptional modifications. These modifications include (1) the excision of the introns to fuse the exons into a continuous stretch of message for translation, a process known as splicing; (2) the attachment of a 7-methyl G cap to the 5′ end of the messenger (this is why the transcription initiation site is called the "cap" site); and (3) the addition of a poly-A chain to the 3′ end of the messenger. This mature messenger RNA is then used as the final template for globin chain synthesis.

Evaluating Hemoglobin Biosynthesis

With current techniques, it is possible to evaluate hemoglobin biosynthesis from the finished product back to the level of the gene.

Hemoglobin Electrophoresis

Abnormalities in hemoglobin biosynthesis often alter hemoglobin proportions or cause the appearance of a hemoglobin not normally found in the red cell. Accordingly, the simplest way to evaluate hemoglobin biosynthesis is to measure the proportions of the various hemoglobins in the circulating red cells. This is most often done by hemoglobin electrophoresis.

Hemoglobin electrophoresis is usually carried out at pH 8.6 on cellulose acetate strips or starch gels. Under these conditions, hemoglobin A, A_2, and F are separated and abnormal hemoglobins whose electrophoretic mobilities differ from those of the normal species appear as bands distinct from the normal hemoglobins. The separated hemoglobins are quantified by staining and measuring the intensity of color. A normal hemoglobin electrophoresis pattern is shown in Figure 10–6.

Origin A₂   F A

Fig. 10–6. Normal hemoglobin electrophoresis. The major band is hemoglobin A. Running slightly behind this is the faint band of hemoglobin F. Much slower than either of these is hemoglobin A_2.

FRACTION NUMBER

Fig. 10–7. Globin chain synthesis in normal reticulocytes. Whole blood is first incubated with radioactive leucine. Labeled globin chains are then separated by column chromatography, and the amount of radioactivity in each of the chains is determined by counting the fractions from the column, using authentic α- and B-globin chains to mark the locations of the labeled chains. The α- and B-chain peaks are seen to contain about the same number of counts, indicating that in these reticulocytes the two chains were synthesized at equal rates. (It is not necessary to correct for differences in the leucine content of the two chains, because they contain the same number of leucines). (From Bunn, H.F., Forget, B.G. & Ranney, H.M. (1981) The thalassemias. Ch. 5. In Human Hemoglobins. W.B. Saunders, Philadelphia, with permission.)

Globin Chain Synthesis

Reticulocytes newly released from the marrow retain their ability to synthesize protein for 24 to 48 hours. The protein manufactured by these cells is almost entirely hemoglobin. Reticulocytes thus provide an easily obtained system in which to examine globin chain synthetic rates.

These rates are measured as follows. Radioactive leucine is incubated for a short time (1 to 2 hours) with whole blood, which serves as the source of the reticulocytes. During the incubation, the labeled amino acid becomes incorporated into the globin chains. These chains are then isolated, separated chromatographically into the individual species, and counted. The number of counts incorporated into a given chain is directly proportional to the rate at which that chain was synthesized in the reticulocytes.

The results from a typical study of normal blood are shown in Figure 10–7. It can be seen that the ratio of counts incorporated into the α- and β-chains is close to 1.0. A deviation from this value suggests the diagnosis of thalassemia.

Molecular Genetics

Gene Mapping

The human genome consists of 3 billion pairs of nucleotides lined up in a precisely ordered sequence. Somewhere in this chain of nucleotides are the stretches corresponding to the globin genes. To map these genes in the sense of defining their precise locations within the entire genome has not yet been accomplished. It has been possible, however, to break up the genome into fragments of sharply defined length and then determine which of these fragments contain the globin genes. This procedure, known as *restriction mapping*, has yielded important information concerning the pathogenesis of the thalassemias.

Restriction mapping is performed as follows (Fig. 10–8). The DNA is first split into fragments of defined length by a restriction endonuclease, an enzyme that recognizes a particular short sequence of nucleotide pairs and cuts double-stranded DNA wherever this sequence occurs (Fig. 10–9). The resulting restriction fragments are separated according to size by gel electrophoresis, and the sized fragments are blotted onto a nylon sheet. The fragments

5' – ATCC'GGGTAAACGCC'GGCATA
 TAGG'CCCATTTGCGG'CCGTAT – 5'

|

Hpa I

↓

ATCC   GGGTAAACGCC   GGCATA
TAGG   CCCATTTGCGG   CCGTAT

Fig. 10–8. Mechanics of a restriction enzyme. The restriction enzyme Hpa I, which is specific for the C—G bond in CCGG, will split a stretch of double-standard DNA into fragments of precisely defined size.

(one or more) containing the globin gene are located on the blot by soaking it in a solution containing a radioactively labeled probe consisting of a short length of DNA that includes part of the globin gene sequence. This probe will hybridize to any DNA that contains a complementary sequence; in particular, it will hybridize to those fragments on the blot that contain regions of globin gene corresponding to those in the probe. Finally, the globin gene-containing fragments are visualized by autoradiography of the blot and their size is determined by comparison with standards.

DIGESTION   ELECTROPHORESIS

BLOTTING   BINDING OF PROBE

RADIOAUTOGRAM

Fig. 10–9. Restriction mapping. DNA is chopped up into fragments of defined size by a restriction enzyme. These fragments are separated according to molecular weight by gel electrophoresis. The separated fragments are blotted onto a nitrocellulose sheet, which is then soaked in a solution of radioactive globin DNA probe. This probe will bind to the blot whenever it meets a fragment of DNA containing a sufficiently large part of the globin gene. The locations of these fragments are then determined by autoradiography.

Any cell in the body can be used as a source of DNA for mapping the globin genes, because every gene is present in the DNA of every cell; in contrast, tests that assay globin proteins (hemoglobin electrophoresis and measurements of globin chain synthesis) can only be carried out on erythroid cells, because only those cells make those proteins. Typical restriction maps of the α- and β-globin genes in the normal genome are shown in Figure 10–10. A map obtained with the restriction endonuclease EcoRI shows a single α-globin gene-containing fragment 23 kilobases (kb) in size. Using other restriction enzymes, this fragment has been shown to contain both α-globin genes. These two genes therefore lie within 23 kb of each other. The map of the β-globin gene was also obtained with EcoRI. This enzyme splits the β-globin gene such that part of it is found in one fragment (5.2 kb) and part in another (3.6 kb). The 2.2-kb band is a δ-gene containing fragment picked up by a stretch of δ-gene sequence present in this particular β-globin probe.

Gene Sequencing

It is possible not only to map a patient's globin genes, but to determine their nucleotide sequence as well. The sequencing of globin genes has made it possible to pinpoint the mutations responsible for the defects in hemoglobin production in many patients with thalassemia.

Polymerase Chain Reaction

The polymerase chain reaction, familiarly known as "PCR," is a recently developed technique for amplifying selected DNA sequences more than a billion-fold by repeated cycles of DNA replication. The technique employs primers consisting of two oligonucleotides: one (the Watson primer) exactly complementary to a short DNA sequence on the Crick strand of the double helix, and the other (the Crick primer) exactly complementary to a short stretch of DNA a short distance (≈ 1000

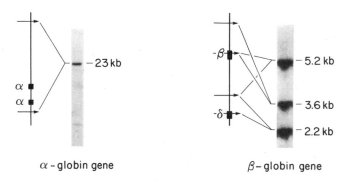

α – globin gene   β – globin gene

Fig. 10–10. Restriction maps of the α- and β-globin genes. (**Left**) α-Globin genes mapped using EcoRI. Both genes are found in a single 23-kb fragment. (**Right**) The β-globin gene mapped using EcoRI. This enzyme cuts the β-globin gene in two, so part is found in one fragment (5.2 kb) and part in another (3.6 kb). The 2.2-kb fragment contains part of the δ-globin gene. The *arrows* show the locations of the EcoRI cuts. (Left: Modified from Kan, Y.W. et al. (1979) Molecular basis of hemoglobin-H diseases in the Mediterranean population. Blood *54*:1434–1438, with permission. Right: Modified from Orkin, S.H. et al. (1980) Cloning and direct examination of a structurally abnormal human β⁰-thalassemia globin gene. Proc. Natl. Acad. Sci. *77*:3558–3562, with permission.)

base pairs or less) downstream from the first primer, but on the opposite (Watson) strand of the double helix. The reaction mixture for the polymerase chain reaction starts with the DNA to be amplified, together with large excesses of these two primers. The reaction then proceeds as follows:

1. *The first cycle of DNA replication.* In the first cycle of DNA replication, two new strands are synthesized from each DNA molecule to be amplified. The strands synthesized in this first cycle of replication (hereafter referred to as "second" strands) are of variable lengths, but one strand begins with the Watson primer and the other with the Crick primer. The DNA duplexes are then separated by heat and allowed to reanneal. Because of the large excess of primers initially added to the reaction mixture, this annealing process results in the uptake of Watson primers by the newly synthesized Crick strands, and Crick primers by the Watson strands.

2. *The second cycle of DNA replication; initial synthesis of the defined DNA segments.* With the second cycle of DNA replication, the original strands and the second strands are all copied. The original strands once again yield copies that are variable in size. Copies of the second strands, however, consist of DNA segments of precisely defined length. Each starts with the primer (say, the Watson primer) that annealed to the second strand, which is now the template; and each terminates opposite the second strand's 3′ end, which actually consists of the Crick primer that was incorporated into the second strand during the first cycle of DNA synthesis. Heating and cooling then causes new primers to hybridize to these short but precisely defined second strand copies. It is these defined segments that are amplified in the key event of the polymerase chain reaction.

3. *The subsequent cycles of DNA replication: amplification of the defined DNA segments.* During the third cycle of DNA replication, the second strand copies are themselves copied, yielding defined segments of double-

stranded DNA, each running from the Watson primer to the Crick primer. Heating and cooling then melts these short double helixes to produce single strands of the defined DNA, each annealed to its complementary primer (these primers are still present in vast excess). Each new cycle of DNA replication now doubles the number of these defined segments of DNA, all of identical length and sequence.* After 30 to 35 cycles of DNA synthesis, melting and annealing, the DNA segment between the two primers has been amplified to the point where it can be seen on gel electrophoresis even without a radioactive probe, and can be sequenced and otherwise manipulated with ease.

Many genetic questions can be answered by the polymerase chain rection in just a fraction of the time taken by classical cloning methods. To identify a new β-thalassemia mutation by classical cloning technolgy, for example, it would be necessary to isolate DNA from the thalassemic patient and fragment that DNA with an appropriate restriction endonuclease; to insert the DNA fragments into an appropriate bacteriophage (the bacteriophages that contain these DNA fragments are known collectively as a genomic library); to grow the recombinant bacteriophage library on a lawn of bacteria, and then screen tens of thousands of individual bacteriophage plaques by hybridization with a suitable probe to find one that contains β-globin gene sequences; and finally, to purify and amplify the β-globin gene-containing recombinant bacteriophage and sequence its DNA insert. In contrast, it is possible through PCR to amplify the genomic region of interest without ever isolating it. Amplification by PCR followed by the sequencing of the amplified products then gives the desired information in just a few days, instead of the months that might be required using traditional meth-

---

* In this context, a given DNA sequence is considered identical to its complementary sequence, since both contain exactly the same information.

ods. Other situations in which this technique could be of use are easy to imagine.

THE β-THALASSEMIAS

The β-thalassemias are a group of inherited disorders in which the synthesis of the β-globin chain is impaired for one reason or another. Anemia is the rule in all but one of these conditions. In the homozygous state, the anemia is so severe that affected patients commonly die in their teens or early twenties.

Pathogenesis

The fundamental problems in β-thalassemias is the uncoupling of α- and β-chain synthesis. Normally, these chains are made in almost equal quantities. In β-thalassemias, however, β-chain production is depressed— moderately in the heterozygous form (β-thalassemia minor or trait), and very severely in the homozygous state (β-thalassemia major). The depression in β-chain synthesis has two adverse consequences. First, there is a reduction in total red cell hemoglobin. This is partly offset by increases in hemoglobins containing other β-class chains (hemoglobins F and A_2), but these do not compensate fully for the decreased quantity of hemoglobin A in thalassemia cells. Second, and more importantly, there is an accumulation of free α-chains in the red cells.

It is the free α-chains that do most of the damage. The free α-chains are very unstable and denature rapidly to form precipitates within the red cells. In β-thalassemia minor, in which a relatively small proportion of the red cell hemoglobin is lost as denatured α-chain, these precipitates are pitted out by mononuclear phagocytes, leaving behind oddly shaped red cells of diminished size. In β-thalassemia major, however, denatured α-chains represent the bulk of the hemoglobin in the red cell. Most of these precipitate-filled red cells are destroyed in the marrow before they are

Pathogenesis of β-Thalassemia[a]

Ineffective erythropoiesis
Hemolysis
Increased red cell production
    In the bone marrow
    In the liver and spleen (extramedullary hematopoiesis)

---

[a] Diminished production of β-globin chains leads to a surplus of α-globin chains, which denature and precipitate, causing the manifestations listed.

ever released into the bloodstream; this ineffective erythropoiesis is the major factor responsible for the anemia of β-thalassemias. A substantial portion of the cells released from the marrow are destroyed prematurely in the spleen, but this hemolytic process is relatively low grade and contributes in only a small way to the anemia of β-thalassemia. Finally, there is a phenomenal increase in erythropoiesis, represented not only by a vast expansion of marrow red cell production, but also by the persistence of erythropoiesis in the spleen and liver (extramedullary hematopiesis).

In molecular terms, there are several varieties of β-thalassemia. All are characterized by sharp reductions in β-chain synthetic rates in the homozygote. They differ in the extent to which β-chain synthesis is blocked, in the amounts of other hemoglobins present in the affected red cells, and, most fundamentally, in the nature of the genetic defect responsible for the disease. These varieties are listed in Table 10–2. Two deserve special comment.

Hemoglobin Lepore Disease

This disease is a form of β-thalassemia in which an abnormal β-family chain is produced. This chain is a hybrid in which the

Table 10-2. Varieties of β-Thalassemia

Variety	Defect in Globin Chain Production
β⁺-Thalassemia	Diminished β-chain
β⁰-Thalassemia	No β-chain
δβ-Thalassemia	No β- or δ-chain
Hemoglobin Lepore	No β-chain; δ-chain replaced by δβ hybrid
Hereditary persistence of fetal hemoglobin (HPFH)	No β- or δ-chain; defect fully compensated by increased γ-chain production

amino end of a normal δ-chain has been fused to the carboxy-terminal end of a β- chain. Hemoglobin Lepore is hemoglobin A in which the two β-chains have been replaced by the hybrids.

The fused chains appear to have arisen through a defect in chromosome recombination during meiosis. It may be recalled that before the division that reduces the number of chromosomes in a sperm or ovum to 23, an active exchange of material takes place between the two members of the chromosome pair. What seems to happen is that homologous portions of the two chromosomes pair up, break at equivalent sites, and then exchange partners (Fig. 10–11). These homologous portions usually represent corresponding regions in each of the two chromosomes (e.g., the β-globin gene regions). Occasionally, however, a mismatch will occur, so that exchange takes place not between corresponding regions, but between noncorresponding regions having sufficiently similar molecular structures. The β-globin and δ-globin genes represent such structurally similar noncongruent regions. It is thought that the hemoglobin Lepore gene is the product of an aberrant recombination event between these two regions, the event resulting in a shortened

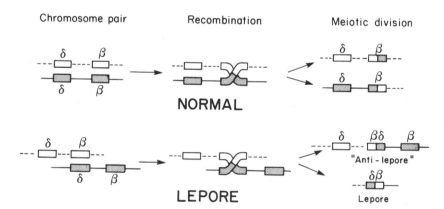

Fig. 10–11. Origin of hemoglobin Lepore. Hemoglobin Lepore is thought to arise through a chromosomal deletion that occurs during meiosis. In meiosis, a cell divides without duplicating its chromosomes. During this division, the pairs of chromosomes in the parent cell are split up, one member of each pair going to each of the two daughter cells. Just before this division takes place, the pairs of chromosomes exchange pieces, an event known as recombination. The pieces exchanged are almost always from chromosomal regions that correspond exactly to each other (e.g., the β-globin gene regions might exchange places). Occasionally, however, the pieces will be from noncorresponding regions having similar structures. The effect will be to delete material from one chromosome of the pair and give it to the other. Hemoglobin Lepore results when the β-chain region of one chromosome exchanges material with the δ-chain region of the other; the deletion resulting from this abnormal exchange gives rise to a new gene that codes for a hybrid globin chain that is δ at the amino end and β at the carboxyl end. Other thalassemia-causing gene deletions are thought to occur in the same way.

chromosome in which the upstream portion of the δ-gene has been fused to the downstream portion of the β-gene, with a deletion of the remaining portions of the two genes together with the intergenic region.

Hereditary Persistence of Fetal Hemoglobin

Although technically a form of β-thalassemia, hereditary persistence of fetal hemoglobin (HPFH) is clinically very different from the classic forms of the disease, because it involves an increase in γ-chain production sufficient to compensate almost fully for the defects in β- and δ-chain synthesis, defects that are total in homozygous HPFH. As a result, there is no accumulation of denatured α-chain precipitates in affected red cells, and anemia is mild in the homozygote and absent in the heterozygote. Red cells from homozygotes contain 100 percent hemoglobin F, whereas heterozygote red cells contain 10 to 30 percent hemoglobin F, which is distributed uniformly throughout the population of cells, not concentrated preferentially in F cells as normally the case.

HPFH represents an important but as yet undeciphered message about red cell development. Whereas γ-chain production in other forms of thalassemias occurs only at a low rate (the adult pattern), rates of production of α- and γ-chains are almost equivalent in HPFH (the fetal pattern). The genetic lesion in HPFH has somehow inactivated the "switch" responsible for the change in the pattern of hemoglobin synthesis around the time of birth. The nature of this switch remains to be elucidated.

Clinical Manifestations

The clinical manifestations of all the various forms of β-thalassemias are similar (except for HPFH). The disease occurs primarily in persons of Mediterranean European descent (e.g., Italian, Greek, Sardinian), in Arabs, and in blacks. In the heterozygote (thalassemia minor or thalassemia trait) it presents as a mild to moderate anemia associated with splenomegaly (Fig. 10–12). The red cells are very small, the MCV averaging 65 femtoliters (fl) compared with a normal of about 95 fl (it is important to recognize that thalassemia and iron deficiency anemia are the two major causes of microcytic anemia). The microcytosis is confirmed on the smear (Fig. 10–13), which shows small red cells that vary widely in size and shape, occasional basophilic stippling, and a reticulocytosis whose severity depends on the degree of anemia. Other manifestations are those of ineffective erythropoiesis: a serum iron on the high side, slight indirect bilirubinemia, and a juicy hypercellular marrow with hyperplasia of the red cell precursors and an increase in iron. Perhaps the most important point about β-thalassemia heterozygotes is that they are for the most part clinically well, but their children are at risk for homozygous β-thalassemia.

Patients with homozygous β-thalassemia (β-thalassemia major) are generally seriously ill (Fig. 10–12). At the root of their problems is an exceedingly severe anemia. The degree of anemia in these patients places such heavy burden on the cardiovascular system that death in childhood from high-output congestive failure used to be the typical outcome in β-thalassemia major; most patients now receive long-term transfusion therapy, so life expectancy has increased by a decade or two, and the mode of death has changed from high-output failure to hemochromatosis. Growth and maturation in these patients is retarded, and they develop a greatly enlarged liver and spleen along with a characteristic facial deformity ("chipmunk facies," Fig. 10–14) caused by bones that have expanded to accommodate the greatly increased amount of hematopoietic tissue that fills their marrow cavities.

The blood and marrow picture is similar to that seen in thalassemia trait, but much more severe (Fig. 10–13). Microcytosis and gross deformities of the red cells are seen on the smear, together with a marked reticulocytosis and prominent basophilic stippling. Nucleated

MAJOR

Severe anemia and
retarded growth,
plus –

MINOR

Mild anemia,
plus –

"Chipmunk facies"

Cardiac failure

Hepatosplenomegaly

Splenomegaly

Fig. 10–12. Clinical manifestations of thalassemia.

red cells are common. The exceedingly hyperplastic marrow, which is packed with red cell precursors and loaded with iron, fills and expands the marrow cavity of every bone; this is strikingly evident on radiographs, which show distended bones crisscrossed with hyperplastic trabeculae (the remarkable "hair-on-end" picture of the skull) (Fig. 10–15). Extramedullary hematopoiesis is prominent in the liver and spleen.

The diagnosis of thalassemia is established by showing the typical quantitative abnormalities in the hemoglobin content of the red cells. This is usually accomplished by hemoglobin electrophoresis. The usual finding in β-thalassemia trait is a modest increase in the minor hemoglobins whose pattern is a logical consequence of the genetic defect (e.g., in $\delta\beta$-thalassemia, hemoglobin F is elevated, but hemoglobin A_2

is normal or decreased, because the genetic lesion in this condition involves the δ-chain as well as the β-chain). Hemoglobin A remains the predominant hemoglobin in β-thalassemia trait, despite the impairment in β-chain production in this condition. In thalassemia major, however, hemoglobin A is greatly decreased (β^+-thalassemia) or absent (other forms of thalassemia). The major hemoglobin in the red cell is hemoglobin F, whereas the amounts of other hemoglobins in the cell depend on the nature of the genetic defect. The red cell hemoglobin patterns in the three classic varieties of β-thalassemia (i.e., all but HPFH) are shown in Table 10–3.

Hemoglobin electrophoresis is usually all that is necessary to establish a diagnosis of β-thalassemia. The only situation in which hemoglobin electrophoresis fails is when it is neces-

Fig. 10–13. Blood smear in thalassemia. **(A)** Normal. **(B)** Thalassemia minor. **(C)** Thalassemia major. Thalassemia shows microcytosis, target cells, deformed red cells, basophilic stippling, and (in thalassemia major) nucleated red cells. (From Kapff, C.T. & Jandl, J.H. (1981) The anemias. Ch. 3. In Blood: Atlas and Sourcebook. Little, Brown, Boston, with permission.)

sary to make the diagnosis in a fetus at risk for β-thalassemia major (a fetus is at risk if both parents have some form of β-thalassemia). This problem is discussed below.

ical forms of α-thalassemia. These range from a form that is totally asymptomatic to one that is invariably fatal during gestation or early infancy.

THE α-THALASSEMIAS

Inherited impairment of α-chain synthesis leads to the group of diseases known as the α-thalassemias. This group contains four clin-

Pathogenesis

α-Thalassemia is caused by a functional abnormality in one or more of the four α-globin genes on the chromosome 16 pair. In most

Table 10-3. Hemoglobins A and A$_2$ in β-Thalassemia[a]

Variety	Major		Minor	
	Hb A	Hb A$_2$	Hb A	Hb A$_2$
β$^+$-Thalassemia	Sharply ↓	↑	Slightly ↓	↑
β^0-Thalassemia	Absent	↑	Slightly ↓	↑
δβ-Thalassemia (and Hemoglobin Lepore)	Absent	Absent	Slightly ↓	Not ↑

[a] All β-thalassemia patients have elevated hemoglobin F. The different kinds of β-thalassemia can be distinguished by looking at the percentages of hemoglobins A and A$_2$.

Fig. 10–14. "Chipmunk facies" of thalassemia major. Gross marrow hyperplasia has expanded the facial bones. (From Weatherall, D.J. & Clegg, J.B. (1972) Disorders resulting from defective B- or δ-chain synthesis: the B- and δβ-thalassemias. Ch. 4. In The Thalassemia Syndromes. Blackwell Scientific Publishers, Oxford, with permission.)

Fig. 10–15. "Hair-on-end" skull of thalassemia major. (From Weatherall, D.J. & Clegg, J.B. (1972) Disorders resulting from defective β- or δ-chain synthesis. The β- and δβ-thalassemias. Ch. 4. In The Thalassemia Syndromes. Blackwell Scientific Publishers, Oxford, with permission.)

Consequences of Decreased α-Chain Production in α-Thalassemia

Reduced concentrations of all normal hemoglobins (A, A_2, and F)
Assembly of excess β-class chains into abnormal hemoglobin tetramers
  Hemoglobin H (β_4)
  Hemoglobin Bart's (γ_4)
Hemoglobin Portland ($\zeta_2\gamma_2$) in cells that completely lack α-chains

---

cases, the disease results because the affected genes are no longer able to code for the globin chain, hence their contribution to total α-chain production is lost altogether. In the Far East, however, there is a common form of α-thalassemia caused by a mutant gene that codes for the production of an abnormal α-chain known as α Constant Spring. For some reason, α Constant Spring cannot be synthesized except at exceedingly low rates, so that patients carrying the Constant Spring gene show a deficit in α-chain production nearly as severe as that in patients with a total failure of α-gene function. (The analogy is clear between Hb Constant Spring versus classic α-thalassemia as compared with β^+- versus β'-thalassemia.)

The decrease in the rate of α-chain synthesis has three consequences. First, there is a reduction in the concentration of all α-chain-containing hemoglobins in the α-thalassemic red cell. This includes all three hemoglobins normally present in the adult erythrocyte. Second, there is an accumulation of free β-family chains, resulting from the imbalance between α- and β-chain production in α-thalassemia. These associate to form hemoglobins consisting of four identical β-class chains; hemoglobin H, from the β-chains (β_4), and hemoglobin Bart's (discovered in St. Bartholomew's Hospital in London), from the γ-chains (γ_4). In the α-thalassemic patient, hemoglobins Bart's and H show the same pattern of changes with age that hemoglobins F and A show in the normal person, and for the same reason: the changes in the rates of production of the γ- and β-chains as fetal and infant development proceeds. The changes in the concentrations of these hemoglobins in the α-thalassemic patient are of considerable clinical importance, as will be seen. Finally, if α-chain synthesis is lacking altogether, the ζ-globin gene, which codes for the production of the embryonic α-class ζ-chain, retains its activity, so hemoglobin Portland ($\zeta_2\gamma_2$) remains a component of the red cell throughout fetal life.

α-Thalassemia occurs in four degrees of severity, depending on the number of malfunctioning genes in the patient. These forms are listed in Table 10−4. Varieties in which one or two genes are defective are mild or asymptomatic. Characteristic diseases, however, are caused by the lack of three or four of the α-globin genes. The problems associated with these diseases are attributable more to the behavior of the hemoglobins formed from the surplus β-class chains than to the deficit in total hemoglobin production (Table 10−5).

The dysfunction of three of the α-globin genes causes hemoglobin H disease. As the name implies, this disease features the accumulation of substantial quantities of hemoglo-

Table 10-5. Properties of the Abnormal Hemoglobins in α-Thalassemia

Hemoglobin	Property
Hemoglobin H (β_4)	Unstable
Hemoglobin Bart's (γ_4)	Very high oxygen affinity

bin H in the erythrocyte—never the majority of the hemoglobin, but always enough to cause serious damage to the red cells. The full-blown disease is not seen until the patient is a few months of age, the time it takes for the concentration of hemoglobin H to rise to adult levels. Problems arise because this hemoglobin is unstable, forming precipitates of denatured protein in affected red cells. These precipitates are pitted out, leading to small, malformed red cells. Ineffective erythropoiesis results because of the destruction of the abnormal cells in the bone marrow; it is never as severe as in β-thalassemia, however, because enough normal hemoglobin is present as a result of the single functioning α-globin gene to moderate the destruction of red cells in the marrow. On the other hand, hemolysis is brisk and contributes substantially to the anemia in patients with hemoglobin H disease.

When all the α-globin genes are out of commission, no α-chains can be made. This situation leads to a fatal clinical syndrome called *hydrops fetalis*. The total absence of α-chain synthesis means that in the fetus, the red cells contain no hemoglobin F. They are filled instead with hemoglobin Bart's (γ_4), a hemoglobin whose oxygen affinity is so high that for practical purposes it is unable to release oxygen to tissues. Death from tissue anoxia is the inevitable outcome in hydrops fetalis.

Clinical Manifestations

α-Thalassemia is primarily a disease of Far Eastern and black populations, although it occurs to a slight extent among Mediterranean Europeans. The severe forms occur almost exclusively among Orientals, because chromosomes carrying two defective α-globin genes are restricted almost entirely to that population

Table 10-4. Varieties of α-Thalassemia

Variety	α-Globin Genes Out of Commission (No)
α_2-Thalassemia trait ("silent carrier")	1
α_1-Thalassemia trait (α-thalassemia minor)	2
Hemoglobin H disease	3
Hydrops fetalis	4

ORIENTAL   BLACK

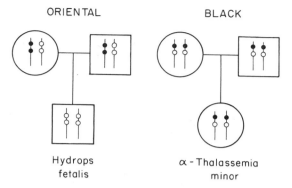

Hydrops   α-Thalassemia
fetalis   minor

Fig. 10–16. Example showing why α-thalassemia is worse in Orientals than in blacks. Each parent has α-thalassemia minor because of two defective α-globin genes. In blacks, the defective genes are on different chromosomes, so their offspring have at worst α-thalassemia minor. In Orientals, the defective genes are on the same chromosome, so an unfortunate pairing can produce a fetus with hydrops fetalis.

(Fig. 10–16). In other populations subject to α-thalassemia, the genetic lesion almost always involves only one of the two α-globin genes, hence the generally mild form of the disease in these populations.

Mild α-Thalassemia

The mild forms of α-thalassemia result from the malfunction of one or two genes. The condition in which a single gene is defective is called α_2-thalassemia trait, or silent carrier α-thalassemia. The term "silent carrier" is highly appropriate, because most of these patients are completely asymptomatic; slight microcytosis is all that is seen, and even this subtle manifestation is often missing. The major clue to the silent carrier state is the presence of more severe forms of α-thalassemia in family members.

When two genes are out of commission, α_1-thalassemia trait, or α-thalassemia minor, is the disease that results. The signs and symptoms are virtually identical to those of β-thalassemia minor: (1) anemia, generally mild, with very small red cells; (2) a blood smear showing small, misshapen red cells, target cells, basophilic stippling, and reticulocytosis; (3) a marrow showing hyperplasia of the red cell series and increased iron; and (4) modest splenomegaly.

In adults, it is difficult to make the diagnosis of α-thalassemia trait (either variety). Hemoglobin electrophoresis, the mainstay of the workup in β-thalassemia trait, is always normal in α_2-thalassemia trait and is often normal in α_1-thalassemia trait, although the presence of some hemoglobin H in the latter may permit the diagnosis to be made (Table 10–6). In newborns, the diagnosis is somewhat easier, as slight elevations in hemoglobin Bart's are seen

Table 10-6. Manifestations of a α-Thalassemia

| Disorder | Findings | |
	Clinical	Hemoglobin Electrophoresis
α_2-Thalassemia trait	None	Normal
α_1-Thalassemia trait	Like β-thalassemia minor	Normal or a trace of hemoglobin H
Hemoglobin H disease	Like mild β-thalassemia major	Hemoglobin H
Hydrops fetalis	Swollen, pale infant, stillborn or dying shortly after birth	Hemoglobin Bart's and Portland (cord blood); no hemoglobin A

in cord blood in both forms of α-thalassemia trait. If necessary, the diagnosis can be established by measuring globin chain production to look for a decrease in the α:β synthetic ratio, or by performing DNA restriction mapping with an α-gene probe, looking for patterns previously found in patients known to have α-thalassemia.

Measurements of globin chain production and analysis of DNA are expensive to perform; these tests are carried out only in a few institutions, usually in connection with research on the molecular biology of thalassemia. When should these tests be done? They are indispensable for prenatal diagnosis in pregnant women with either α- or β-thalassemia trait and cannot be replaced by any other procedure. They are unnecessary in adults with β-thalassemia trait, because this diagnosis can always be established by hemoglobin electrophoresis. What about adults suspected of having α-thalassemia trait in whom hemoglobin electrophoresis is normal? Family studies can sometimes establish a diagnosis with certainty; for instance, the symptomless father of a patient with hemoglobin H disease whose mother has α₁-thalassemia trait would have to be a silent carrier on genetic grounds (Fig. 10–17). When the diagnosis cannot be established by simple means, however, the decision as to whether to carry out these highly specialized tests should be based on whether making the

diagnosis will be of sufficient benefit to the patient to warrant the trouble and expense involved in carrying them out.

Hemoglobin H Disease

The clinical manifestations of hemoglobin H disease are closely similar to those of β-thalassemia major, although the condition tends to be milder than the average case of β-thalassemia major. Anemia is moderate to marked; the smear shows the typical abnormalities of severe thalassemia. The liver and spleen are enlarged, and the marrow undergoes the same expansion in erythropoiesis as seen in β-thalassemia major, leading to the same bony abnormalities.

The diagnosis is made by finding hemoglobin H in the red cells of patients with the clinical picture of thalassemia. This can be done by staining a blood smear with cresyl violet, a procedure that causes the unstable hemoglobin H to precipitate as small clumps of uniform size that fill all the red cells and that are easily seen under the microscope (Fig. 10–18). Hemoglobin H may also be demonstrated by electrophoresis, where it is easily detected as a rapidly moving band that migrates well ahead of hemoglobin A (Fig. 10–18). Electrophoresis also illustrates the point that most of the hemoglobin in hemoglobin H disease erythro-

Fig. 10–17. Diagnosing the silent carrier state. The child with hemoglobin H disease has three defective α-globin genes. Two were inherited from his mother, who has α-thalassemia trait. The third must have come from his symptomless father, who has to be a silent carrier.

Fig. 10–18. The diagnosis of hemoglobin H disease. (**A**) Hemoglobin H stain. The red cells contain small uniform clumps of hemoglobin H. (**B**) Hemoglobin electrophoresis. Hemoglobin H moves ahead of hemoglobin A. Hemoglobin A is the major hemoglobin in these red cells. (A: From Castoldi, G.L. (1981) Erythrocytes. Ch. 3. In Zucker-Franklin, D. et al., (eds.) Atlas of Blood Cells: Function and Pathology. Edi. Ermes s.r.l., Milan, with permission. B: Modified from Pressley, L. et al. (1980) Gene deletions in thalassemia prove that the 5′ζ locus is functional. Proc. Natl. Acad. Sci. 77:3586–3589, with permission.)

tion mapping, are not necessary for the diagnosis of hemoglobin H disease in a patient with clinical thalassemia. They are required, however, for prenatal diagnosis.

Hydrops Fetalis

Hydrops fetalis is the clinical picture caused by fulminant intrauterine congestive heart failure. The affected fetus has a grossly enlarged heart and liver together with edema and massive ascites. In the severest form of α-thalassemia, in which there is total absence of α-chain synthesis, hydrops is the result. Red cells in this condition contain primarily hemoglobin Bart's, which releases its oxygen only with great difficulty, leading to oxygen-starved tissues. In an attempt to compensate for this tissue anoxia, cardiac output increases to the point of congestive heart failure, which also has highly deleterious effects on fetal development. The consequences are so serious that this form of hydrops is always fatal, either in utero or shortly after birth.

The diagnosis, usually postmortem, is made by electrophoresis of cord blood. The only hemoglobins present on electrophoresis are hemoglobin Bart's and a small amount of hemoglobin Portland ($\zeta_2\gamma_2$). Because of the seriousness of the disease, prenatal diagnosis should be strongly considered in any pregnant woman whose fetus is at risk for this form of α-thalassemia.

MOLECULAR GENETICS OF THALASSEMIA

The thalassemias are all caused by mutations in the region of the globin genes. The study of these disorders by molecular genetic techniques has made it clear that the mutations responsible for the thalassemias are highly diverse, involving all regions of the α- and β-globin gene clusters and ranging from simple nucleotide substitutions to huge deletions affecting thousands of bases. A great many of

cytes is hemoglobin A, not hemoglobin H. Indeed, in newborns with hemoglobin H disease, the red cells may contain little hemoglobin H, because of the low β-chain synthetic rate at this time of life; the tip-off to hemoglobin H disease in these patients is a major elevation of hemoglobin Bart's in cord blood.

More sophisticated tests, such as globin chain synthetic measurements and gene restric-

Fig. 10–19. Types and locations of mutations that cause β-thalassemia. IVS: intervening sequence (= intron). (From Orkin, S.H. (1987) Disorders of hemoglobin synthesis. p. 108. In Stomatoyannopoulos, G., Nienhuis, A.W., Leder, P., Majerus, P.W. (eds.) The Molecular Basis of Blood Diseases. W.B. Saunders, Philadelphia, with permission.)

these mutations have been characterized at a molecular level (Fig. 10–19), and their effects on messenger RNA formation and catabolism have been analyzed.

The effect of a mutation depends in part on which region of the gene is involved. Mutations in an intron can slow or stop messenger RNA production by disrupting the splicing process. Mutations in the 3′ or 5′ untranslated regions can decrease messenger RNA production by (1) delaying or preventing the transcription of the messenger RNA from the DNA template; (2) altering post-transcriptional processing of the message (splicing, polyadenylation, export from the nucleus); or (3) decreasing the life of the message in the cytoplasm. Mutations in an exon may (1) impair messenger RNA production; (2) produce a messenger RNA that codes for an abnormal globin (a chain with amino acid substitutions, or one that is shortened or lengthened because of abnormal termination); or (3) produce a messenger RNA that uses a slightly altered code to make a perfectly normal globin. Among the dozens of mutations responsible for the thalassemia phenotype, examples of all these effects have been found.

For reasons that are not clear, there is a crude relationship between thalassemia types and the nature of the responsible mutations. Many of the α-thalassemias, the δβ-thalassemias,

and HPFH are due to gene deletions of major size. On the other hand, most β°- and β⁺-thalassemias seem to be caused by genetic defects that are much more localized: substitutions or small deletions. Large deletions routinely cause abnormalities in restriction maps because of the changes in restriction fragment size that result from the loss of major quantities of DNA from the globin gene region (Fig. 10–20). Localized mutations, however, will cause changes in the restriction map only if they accidentally generate or eliminate a restriction enzyme recognition site. This is rather unlikely, so in most instances, restriction maps from patients with thalassemia caused by a localized mutation have been perfectly normal.

Prenatal Diagnosis

When a pregnant woman and her husband both come from thalassemic families, their fetus is at risk for high-grade thalassemia. In such cases, prenatal testing is often used to determine whether or not the fetus actually has the disease. The prenatal diagnosis is usually made by molecular genetic techniques.

In families with β-*thalassemia*, prenatal diagnosis is usually accomplished by an approach in which the sequences of the defective parental β-globin genes are used to design

Fig. 10–20. Restriction mapping in α-thalassemia caused by deletion of a major gene. The patient has hemoglobin H disease as a result of the deletion of three of the four α-globin genes. The restriction map of the remaining α-globin gene region (**right**) is different from normal (**left**) because the deletion of a 3-kb portion containing one of the two α-globin genes has changed the size of the α-globin restriction fragments obtained from his DNA. (Modified from Kan, Y.W. et al. (1979) Molecular basis of hemoglobin diseases in the Mediterranean population. Blood *54*:1434–1438, with permission.)

priate sequences in the DNA sample; analysis of the amplified products will then furnish the information required.

The serious forms of α-*thalassemia* (hemoglobin H disease and hydrops fetalis) can also be diagnosed prenatally in a fetus at risk. This diagnosis is usually made by DNA restriction mapping, because α-thalassemia often results from major gene deletions that cause obvious abnormalities in α-globin gene restriction maps. The first step is to make a restriction map of DNA from the parents, using α-globin DNA as the probe. If the analysis of these restriction maps confirms that the fetus is at risk (i.e., if one parent is missing two α-globin genes from a single chromosome and the other lacks at least one α-globin gene), the fetal DNA is mapped. A comparison of the fetal map with maps from the parents will make the diagnosis by establishing the number of α-globin genes the fetus inherited from each parent.

Often the restriction map of a defective gene is normal and an oligomer probe to identify the defective gene is unavailable. Under these circumstances, a prenatal diagnosis may still be achieved by taking advantage of *restriction fragment length polymorphisms* (RFLPs, sometimes pronounced "ruflups"). RFLPs appear as differences in the size of a fragment carrying a given piece of genetic material in restriction maps of DNA from different normal subjects. The RFLPs arise because of small interindividual differences in DNA sequence. As an example, if a sequence difference involves an EcoRI site near the β-globin gene (EcoRI is a restriction enzyme from *Escherichia coli* that recognizes the sequence GAATTC), so that DNA from some persons contains that site whereas DNA from others does not, αβ RFLP will be seen when the DNA is mapped with EcoRI and a β-globin gene probe. The fragments obtained from DNA samples isolated from different persons will be of two different sizes, one size generated from DNA that contains the EcoRI site and the other size from DNA that does not. (If two or more nearby EcoRI sites are affected, fragments of several

pairs of short DNA oligomers (one pair for each parent), one of which will bind selectively to the normal gene and the other to the abnormal gene. DNA is then isolated from amniotic fluid cells, which are of fetal origin and are safely and easily obtained by amniocentesis, or by biopsy of a chorionic villus, a technique that can be used to obtain fetal DNA before amniotic fluid appears. The amniocyte DNA is probed with the oligomers to find out which of the parental genes are carried by the fetus. From this the fetal phenotype (normal, carrier, thalassemic) can be predicted. Alternatively, PCR can be used to amplify the approdifferent sizes may be seen.) DNA from a single individual may show both fragments, if one of his chromosomes contains the restriction site and the other does not.

In a family carrying both β-thalassemia and an RFLP linked to the defective globin gene, analysis of restriction maps from enough family members may reveal that the size of the fragment carrying the defective globin gene is different from that of the fragment carrying the normal gene. If so, the RFLP may be used as a marker to establish the presence or absence of the thalassemic gene in a fetus. For example, if in such a family the mother of a fetus at risk has β-thalassemia trait, the restriction map of her DNA should show two β-globin gene-bearing fragments: one (say, a larger fragment) carrying the thalassemic gene and another (a smaller fragment) carrying the normal gene. If the restriction map of the fetal DNA shows the smaller fragment, it can be concluded that the fetus has inherited the normal gene from its mother and is therefore not at risk for β-thalassemia major. If suitable RFLPs occur in both parents' families, it may be possible by this approach to make a complete and accurate prenatal diagnosis of β-thalassemia. Furthermore, it is clear that this type of analysis may be used for prenatal diagnosis of any disease in which the defective gene is linked to a particular RFLP.

MANAGEMENT OF THALASSEMIA

Thalassemia major is usually a fatal disease. The child with untreated thalassemia major is weak and wasted, showing stunted growth, poor development, and the characteristic bony deformities of the disease. The most serious problems involve the cardiovascular system. The chronic high-output state resulting from this anemia causes the heart to fail after only a few years, so that by the time the child is 5 or 6 years old, he has all the signs and symptoms of congestive heart failure and is usually dead from this cause before reaching his teens.

The solution to all these problems should be

> ## Management of Thalassemia
>
> Blood transfusions
> Iron chelation therapy
> Splenectomy
> Bone marrow transplantation
> Prenatal diagnosis

---

blood transfusion. In principle, transfusion to a normal hematocrit should lift the burden from the cardiovascular system and cause the hyperplastic marrow to return to its normal state, fully correcting the functional disorders of thalassemia. Unfortunately, however, blood transfusion has proved to be a two-edged sword, inducing iron overload and hemochromatosis at the same time that it corrects the anemia. Because of this, the management of thalassemia has become a balancing act in which the benefits of transfusion are weighed against the costs, the goal being to optimize the life expectancy of the patient.

The major approach to achieving this goal has been to give patients enough blood to reduce the strain on their hearts to a tolerable state. This is generally accomplished by transfusing to a hematocrit of 20 to 25 ml/dl. Transfusions are obviously unnecessary in patients with thalassemia trait, whose degree of anemia poses no threat to their life expectancy. There are also a few patients with thalassemia major whose anemia, although marked, is not severe enough to warrant transfusion; these patients are described as having thalassemia intermedia.

Transfusion, the mainstay of therapy in thalassemia major, can be supplemented by two measures designed to minimize its risks:

1. *Splenectomy.* Splenectomy is often carried out in thalassemic patients to reduce the transfusion requirement. To the extent that thalassemic red cells are damaged by the spleen, its removal will increase their survival, thereby decreasing the need for transfusions. It

is a useful procedure in treating this condition, yet it generally results in only a modest reduction in the transfusion requirement and puts the patient at increased risk for certain bacterial infections.

2. *Iron chelation therapy.* Because of the iron burden imposed by long-term transfusion therapy, hemochromatosis leading to fatal congestive failure with death in the teens has until recently been the usual outcome for thalassemic patients receiving this form of treatment. This complication has now been largely eliminated through the concurrent use of the iron chelator *desferrioxamine* (see Ch. 4). By binding the excess iron and allowing it to be excreted by the kidneys, desferrioxamine has been able to prevent the hemochromatosis that was formerly such a difficult problem for these patients.

Currently under investigation is a treatment program in which iron chelation is combined with hypertransfusion (i.e., transfusion to a hematocrit of 35 ml/dl, to correct all manifestations of thalassemia). If this program works, it can potentially turn thalassemia major from a fatal disease to nothing more than an expensive nuisance.

A few patients with very severe thalassemia major have been cured by *bone marrow transplantation.* This risky form of treatment should be considered only as a last resort.

The other major aspect of management in thalassemia is prenatal diagnosis (see above). Safe and effective techniques are now available for making the diagnosis of thalassemia major in a fetus at risk for the disease. Thalassemic families should be informed of the availability of these techniques. Whether these families should use these techniques, and what they should do if their fetus proves to have thalassemia major, are matters beyond the scope of this book.

HEMOGLOBIN E

Hemoglobin E disease is a form of β-thalassemia in which the underproduced β-chain (designated β^E) contains the amino acid substitution $\beta^{26:glu \to lys}$. It is caused by a β-globin gene mutation that has a remarkable dual effect. The first and most obvious effect is the alteration in the amino acid sequence of the β-globin chain at position 26. The second effect—much more subtle—is a disturbance in the processing of the β-globin messenger RNA. It is the second effect that explains why hemoglobin E disease is a form of thalassemia.

What the mutation does to RNA processing is to create a false splicing site within an exon of the β^E messenger RNA transcript (Fig. 10–21). This false splicing site leads to defective post-transcriptional modification of the messenger transcripts. Some of the transcripts are processed normally, but others are processed in such a way that exon fusion takes place, not after the coding triplet for amino acid 30, the normal splicing site, but in the middle of the mutated coding triplet for amino acid 26, some dozen nucleotides upstream from the normal splicing site. From this abnormally processed messenger no β-chain is synthesized. The result is an underproduction of β-chain, the hallmark of β-thalassemia.

Hemoglobin E is second only to sickle cell hemoglobin in its worldwide prevalence. It occurs primarily in Asia, where it is exceedingly common in certain population groups. Among Southeast Asians in particular, it is present in more than 10 percent of the population.

Persons with hemoglobin E have no symptoms, no anemia, and little or no shortening of the red cell life span. Blood smears from both heterozygotes (A/E) and homozygotes (E/E) show microcytosis, but target cells are only seen in the homozygote. The diagnosis is made by hemoglobin electrophoresis, in which hemoglobin E is seen to run well behind hemoglobin A. The difference between the electrophoretic mobilities of the two hemoglobins can be explained by the reduction in the overall negative charge of the hemoglobin E molecule that results from the glutamate → lysine substitution.

In contrast to the mildness of A/E and E/E is

Fig. 10–21. A false splicing site in the hemoglobin E gene. The mutation that gives rise to hemoglobin E is located in the first exon of the gene coding for the β-globin chain. This mutation creates a false splicing site in the β^E-chain messenger RNA. As a result, much of the β^E-chain message is processed abnormally, with excision of the first intron occurring, not at the normal location, but at the site of the mutation, which lies several nucleotides upstream from the normal splice site. Globin chains cannot be made from this abnormally spliced message.

the severity of the disease caused by combining hemoglobin E with another form of β-thalassemia. The combination produces thalassemia major; E/β-thalassemia patients are very sick, as opposed to those with minimal disease or thalassemia minor. It seems that the decrease in β-chain synthesis that occurs when the mildy defective β^E-gene is combined with a grossly defective β^+ or $\beta^°$-gene is large enough to cause serious clinical illness.

REFERENCES

Alter, B.P. (1988) Prenatal diagnosis: general introduction, methodology, and review. Hemoglobin *12*:763–772.

Bunn, H.F. & Forget, B.G. (1984) Human Hemoglobins. 2nd Ed. W.B. Saunders, Philadelphia.

Fantoni, A., Farace, M.G. & Gambari, R. (1981) Embryonic hemoglobins of man and other mammals. Blood *57*:623.

Graham, J.B., Green, P.P., McGraw, R.A. & Davis, L.M. (1985) Application of molecular genetics to prenatal diagnosis and carrier detection in the hemophilias: Some limitations. Blood *66*:759.

Gusella, J.F. (1986) Recombinant DNA techniques in the diagnosis of inherited disorders. J. Clin. Invest. *77*:1723.

Higgs, D.R. & Weatherall, D.J. (1983) Alpha-thalassemia. Curr. Top. Hematol. *4*:37–97.

Lachant, N.A. (1987) Hemoglobin E: an emerging hemoglobinopathy in the United States. Am. J. Hematol. *25*:449–462.

Ohene-Frempong, K., Rappaport, E. & Schwartz, E. (1987) Thalassemia syndromes. Recent advances. Hematol. Oncol. Clin. North Am. *1*:503–519.

Orkin, S.H., Disorders of hemoglobin synthesis, in Stamatoyannopoulos, G., Nienhuis, A.W., Leder, P. and Majerus, P.W., eds., Molecular Basis of Blood Diseases, Saunders, 1987, p. 106.

Schwartz, E., Cohen, A. & Surrey, S. (1988) Overview of the beta thalassemias: genetic and clinical aspects. Hemoglobin *12*:551–564.

Weatherall, D.J. (1985) The new genetics and clinical practice. Oxford University Press, Oxford, UK.

Weatherall, D.J. (1986) The regulation of the differential expression of the human globin genes during development. J. Cell Sci. Suppl. *4*:319–336.

Weatherall, D.J. & Clegg, J.B. (1981) The thalassemia syndromes, 3rd Ed. Blackwell Scientific Publications, Oxford, UK.

Wood, W.G., Clegg, J.B. & Weatherall, D.J. (1979) Hereditary persistence of fetal hemoglobin (HPFH) and γβ-thalassemia. Br. J. Haematol. *43*:509.

Sickle Cell Anemia and Related Hemoglobinopathies

The functionally abnormal hemoglobins discussed up to now fall into three categories: those with an altered oxygen affinity, those that remain perpetually in the methemoglobin form, and the unstable hemoglobins. Patients with these hemoglobins, however, constitute only a tiny minority of all patients with functional hemoglobinopathy. By far, most patients with symptomatic functional hemoglobinopathy suffer from sickle cell anemia or one of its variants.

THE SICKLE CELL

Sickle cell diseases are caused by the presence in the red cell of a mutant hemoglobin that forms rigid aggregates when in the deoxy form. Red cells containing such aggregates are stiff and cannot change shape as easily as normal cells when forced to pass through blood vessels smaller than their own diameter (i.e., arterioles and capillaries). As a result, the cells tend to plug these blood vessels. Most of the signs and symptoms of the sickle cell diseases are thought to result from this microvascular blockage.

Hemoglobin S

The mutant hemoglobin of sickle cell anemia is known as hemoglobin S. Like hemoglobin A, it is a tetramer composed of two α-chains and two β-chains. The β-chains, however, are abnormal, containing a valine instead of a glutamate at position 6. These abnormal chains are designated β^S, so the subunit composition of hemoglobin S is written $\alpha_2\beta^S_2$.

There is a general tendency for hemoglobin molecules in the deoxy form to polymerize. This tendency is exaggerated in hemoglobin S, presumably because the substitution of an oil-like valine for a charged glutamate residue makes for a very close fit between the two aggregating hemoglobin molecules (Fig. 11-1). Deoxyhemoglobin S molecules readily assemble into long, stiff bundles composed of 14-strand fibers packed tightly side by side, each strand consisting of thousands of hemoglobin S molecules lined up in single file (Fig. 11-2). The fibers are formed spontaneously within a hemoglobin-S-containing red cell when the cell is placed in an environment in which the hemoglobin loses its oxygen. When they pack into bundles, they deform the cell into an elon-

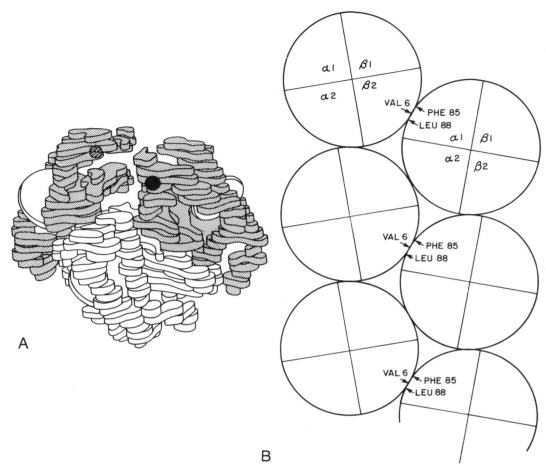

A

B

Fig. 11-1. Location of the mutation in sickle hemoglobin. (**A**) The hemoglobin tetramer. In sickle hemoglobin, a valine is substituted for the glutamate normally found in position 6 of the β-subunit. This valine is seen to lie on the outer surface of the mutant subunit. (**B**) Part of a polymerized sickle hemoglobin strand. Because of its exposed location, the β6-valine of sickle hemoglobin is able to interact strongly with the oil-like β85-phenylalanine and β88-leucine residues on the surface of the adjacent hemoglobin tetramer.

gate irregular rod or crescent (Fig. 11-3). Reoxygenation causes the bundles to melt. This ordinarily restores the cell to its disclike form, but a few cells will remain misshapen even under these circumstances, probably because they have gone through so many cycles of deformation that their membranes have become damaged and can no longer spring back to their original shape. It is the crescent shape of many of the deformed cells that gives the

name "sickle" to the disease and to the cells themselves.

The polymerization of hemoglobin S takes place in three stages (Fig. 11-4). The first stage is called nucleation. It begins with the aggregation of hemoglobin molecules into small clusters. These clusters grow by random collison with molecules in solution until they reach 15 molecules or so in size. At this point they are able to serve as nuclei on which the

X - section

Fig. 11-2. The 14-strand fiber of deoxyhemoglobin S. (Left: From Dykes, G., Crepeau, R. & Edelstein, S.J. (1978) Three-dimensional reconstruction of the fibers of sickle-cell haemoglobin. Nature *272*: 500–510, with permission.)

remaining hemoglobin molecule can assemble. The stage of polymerization now begins. Using the nuclei as starting points, the remaining deoxyhemoglobin S molecules rapidly polymerize into thousands of 14-strand fibers. By the end of the polymerization stage, most of the deoxyhemoglobin S molecules will have been incorporated into fibers, with just a few remaining in solution. At this point, the red cell contains what amounts to a saturated solution of deoxyhemoglobin S in contact with the polymerized hemoglobin fibers. Finally comes the stage of alignment, when the 14-strand fibers assemble into fiber bundles.

Each of these stages has its counterpart in the intact red cell. The nucleation stage is an interval during which nothing seems to happen; the red cell behaves in an almost completely normal fashion. This interval is known as the *lag period*. It is terminated abruptly by a sudden increase in the viscosity of the red cell contents as the deoxyhemoglobin S polymerizes into 14-strand fibers. It is this sharp rise in viscosity that causes the cell to lose the flexibility it needs to make its way through small blood vessels. Finally, the cell acquires its sickle shape as the 14-strand fibers align into bundles.

The time required for the completion of these stages of polymerization is the key to the clinical severity of sickle· cell disease in a given patient. Sickle cells making their circuit through the blood vessels contain significant amounts of deoxyhemoglobin S only during the relatively short interval they spend in the capillaries and veins. For this hemoglobin to polymerize into fibers, the first two stages must be complete before the hemoglobin is reoxygenated in the lungs; for sickling to occur, all three stages must be complete before reoxygenation takes place. The time required for the polymerization and alignment stages is relatively fixed: seconds for polymerization, accounting for the suddenness in the change in viscosity of deoxyhemoglobin-S-containing red cells, and minutes for alignment. The time for nucleation, however, is highly variable, ranging from a few milliseconds to more than an hour, depending on local conditions such as pH (which acts through the Bohr effect), oxy-

Fig. 11-3. A sickle cell. (From Bessis, M. (1973) Living Blood Cells and Their Ultrastructure. Springer-Verlag, New York, with permission.)

NUCLEATION

GROWTH

ALIGNMENT

Fig. 11-4. The three stages in the polymerization of deoxyhemoglobin S. (From Dean, J. & Schechter, A.N. (1978) Sickle-cell anemia: Molecular and cellular bases of therapeutic approaches. N. Engl. J. Med. *299*:752–763, with permission.)

gen tension, and the intracellular concentration of deoxyhemoglobin S. Because of its variability, the time required for nucleation is probably the most critical factor affecting the degree of severity of sickle cell disease. When conditions are such that nucleation is fast, permitting deoxyhemoglobin S to polymerize in the brief time the red cell is deoxygenated, serious clinical problems result; conversely, slow nucleation means less severe clinical disease.

The polymerization of deoxyhemoglobin S is disturbed by the presence of other types of hemoglobin. This is a matter of great clinical significance, because in the red cell, hemoglobin S is always mixed with other types of hemoglobin, and the extent to which these interfere with polymerization profoundly influences the severity of the clinical disease. Other hemoglobins interfere with polymerization by

acting as Trojan horses, in a manner of speaking. Because of their structural resemblance to hemoglobin S, they are incorporated into the hemoglobin S fiber as polymerization takes place. They fit imperfectly into the fiber, however, weakening its structure. Fiber structure is weakened in a particularly effective way by the incorporation of hemoglobin hybrids, asymmetric tetramers containing two different types of β-chains (e.g., $\alpha_2\beta^A\beta^S$). These structural weaknesses disrupt polymerization to a greater or lesser extent. The degree to which polymerization is disrupted will depend of course on how closely the non-S deoxyhemoglobin molecule resembles deoxyhemoglobin S. Certain hemoglobins fit well into the deoxyhemoglobin S polymer, so polymerization is only slightly impaired; others fit very poorly, causing a substantial reduction in the tendency of hemoglobin S to polymerize. Moreover, the concentration of the non-S hemoglobin will also influence polymerization; the higher the non-S concentration, the less the likelihood that polymerization will occur.

Pathophysiology of Sickle Cell Disease

It is the polymerization of deoxyhemoglobin S within the red cell that is responsible for the clinical manifestations of sickle cell disease. Almost all the hemoglobin polymerizes on complete deoxygenation of the red cell, which then deforms into the typical sickle cell. Polymerization, however, is not an all-or-none phenomenon in which hemoglobin S is either fully polymerized or completely in solution. Rather, it seems that whatever quantity of deoxyhemoglobin is present in the red cell at a given time is incorporated into fibers, so that even normal-appearing red cells contain stiff inclusions of polymerized hemoglobin that grow or shrink as the cell gives up or takes on its load of oxygen. Two effects result from these stiff inclusions of polymerized deoxyhemoglobin: extravascular hemolysis and microvascular blockage.

Extravascular Hemolysis

The hemoglobin S-containing cell is conditioned, and eventually destroyed, by the mononuclear phagocyte system. In the very young, this occurs mainly in the spleen, where the cells are trapped in the cords because the inclusions that grow in the oxygen-depleted splenic environment prevent the cells from squeezing through into the sinuses. By late infancy, the spleen has usually lost its function, and other components of the mononuclear phagocyte system, such as the bone marrow macrophages and the Kupffer cells of the liver,

take over the destruction of the red cells. In any case, the result is extravascular hemolysis, the primary cause of the anemia in patients with this condition.

Microvascular Blockage

The most important effect of these inclusions is to impede the flow of blood through the microvasculature of the tissues (Fig. 11-5). This could occur by the following sequence of events, which, though hypothetical, is entirely plausible on the basis of what is known about the behavior of hemoglobin S. As the hemoglobin S-filled red cell passes through the capillary network, it will unload part of its oxygen to the tissues, leaving deoxyhemoglobin S behind. This will polymerize, forming inclusions that will impede the passage of the cell through the capillaries. Passage is further delayed by an unexplained tendency of cells containing hemoglobin S to stick to the endothelium. The continued transfer of oxygen from the retarded red cell to the tissues will cause an additional rise in the intracellular deoxyhemoglobin S concentration, resulting in an increase in the size of the inclusions. They may grow to the point where the cell can no longer move through the capillary at all, and the vessel becomes plugged. More red cells pile up behind the obstructing cell, give up their oxygen, and are themselves incorporated into the growing plug. Meanwhile, the oxygen demand of the small volume of tissue that was originally supplied by the plugged vessel must be satisfied by red cells in nearby capillaries and arterioles. These cells are now obliged to unload more oxygen than usual, because they have to supply a greater volume of tissue than under ordinary circumstances. Deoxyhemoglobin inclusions now grow in these cells, and the blockade is extended to adjacent vessels. The ultimate outcome is the complete obliteration of the blood supply to the blockaded region, with necrosis of tissues and symptoms of both an acute and chronic nature.

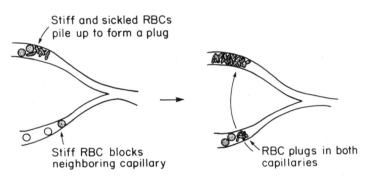

Fig. 11-5. How sickle cells block the microcirculation.

SICKLE CELL DISEASES

Sickle cell diseases occur primarily in blacks. These diseases are common in the equatorial regions of Africa; natives of this region brought the disease with them to North America when they were transported to that continent, primarily during the eighteenth and nineteenth centuries. The diseases are also seen in Arabs and in persons from the Indian subcontinent and are present, although at very low incidence, among Mediterranean Europeans, primarily Greeks, Italians, and Mediterranean islanders (Sicilians and Sardinians).

Sickle Cell Anemia (Homozygous Hemoglobin S Disease)

The worst of the sickle cell diseases is sickle cell anemia. Like other hemoglobinopathies, it is an inherited disease. It is transmitted in an autosomal recessive manner, occurring in persons who have inherited two β^S-globin genes. In these persons, hemoglobin S accounts for more than 90 percent of the hemoglobin in the red cell. Clinical manifestations that are mild or absent in other varieties of sickle cell disease are fully expressed in sickle cell anemia. These clinical manifestations fall into two categories: those caused by the anemia, and those attributable to occlusions of the microvasculature.

Anemia and Its Consequences

A moderate to severe anemia is characteristic of sickle cell anemia. It results primarily from hemolysis, but folate deficiency may occasionally play a part, because folate requirements are increased in sickle cell anemia. In acute infection, particularly with parvovirus, suppression of erythropoiesis may lead to an abrupt fall in the hematocrit owing to the now

<hr>

Anemia of Sickle Cell Disease

Causes
    Extravascular hemolysis
    Aplastic crisis with infections
    Folate deficiency (occasional)
Consequences
    Slowed growth and development
    Chronic congestive heart failure
    Gallstones

<hr>

uncompensated hemolytic process; this situation, known as an *aplastic crisis*, is exactly analogous to what happens under similar circumstances in patients with other hemolytic anemias.

Manifestations of hemolysis are also seen. Serum lactate dehydrogenase and indirect bilirubin are elevated. The spleen is initially enlarged, but in four patients out of five it begins to shrink again after a few years, eventually becoming reduced to an atrophic vestige by repeated microinfarction and scarring; splenic atrophy is so routine that splenomegaly in sickle cell patients over the age of 8 or 10 years is an indication to search carefully for another variety of sickle cell disease. Whether enlarged or atrophied, the spleen loses its function by the time the patient is just a few months of age. Gallstones are exceptionally common in sickle cell anemia, leading to diagnostic complications (see below).

As in thalassemia major, signs and symptoms of cardiac overload are important consequences of the anemia in this condition. The cardiac output is chronically high, leading to hypertrophy, cardiac enlargement, and eventually chronic congestive heart failure. The effects of the anemia on the function of the heart are aggravated by the fact that this organ, like others in sickle cell anemia, is subject to microvascular occlusive disease, with microinfarctions and fibrosis.

Another similarity with thalassemia major is the effect of the anemia on growth and development. Growth may be retarded in patients with severe sickle cell anemia, and resistance to other diseases, particularly infections, is diminished. The high mortality rate in children with sickle cell anemia is largely the result of this impaired ability to resist infection.

The hematocrit in patients with sickle cell anemia is invariably low. The red cells tend to be normal in size, but examination of the smear shows that they are grossly abnormal in shape. Targets, distorted shapes, and the characteristically deformed sickle cells are easily detected (Fig. 11-6). Reticulocytes are substantially increased (on routine smears these appear as polychromatophilic cells), and signs of splenic hypofunction such as basophilic stippling, nucleated red cells, Howell-Jolly bodies, and Cabot rings are seen in the smears of almost all patients of sufficient age, even in those in whom the spleen remains enlarged to palpation. The marrow shows marked red cell hyperplasia, and marrow iron is increased. Megaloblastic changes may occasionally be seen in the red and white cell precursors because of a deficiency in folate superimposed on the underlying disease.

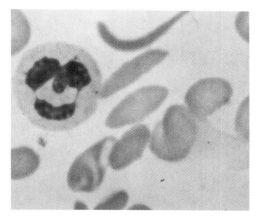

Fig. 11-6. Blood smear in sickle cell anemia. Irreversibly sickled cells are the most characteristic finding. Target cells are also present. The smear may also show nucleated red cells, basophilic stippling, and nuclear remnants (Howell-Jolly bodies and Cabot rings), all of which are indications that the spleen has lost its function. (From Wintrobe, M.M. et al. (1974) Clinical Hematology. 7th ed. Lea & Febiger, Philadelphia, with permission.)

Microvascular Occlusions

Microvascular occlusions are thought to be responsible for most of the clinical manifestations of sickle cell anemia. They may involve most of the organ systems of the body and are frequently characterized by pain as well as by various signs and symptoms of organ dysfunction (Fig. 11-7).

Sickle Cell Crisis

Perhaps the most characteristic manifestation of sickle cell anemia, and certainly one of the most distressing, is the sickle cell crisis. It consists of an episode of severe pain of 1 to 2 weeks' duration, often accompanied by a relatively low-grade fever and leukocytosis. A crisis may be precipitated by infection, dehydration, or acidosis, but it frequently comes out of the clear blue sky. The pain can involve the extremities, the chest, and either the abdomen or the back, or both; it can be so severe as to mimic an acute surgical emergency. Notable

Features of a Sickle Cell Crisis

Precipitated by
    Infection
    Dehydration
    Acidosis
    No special event

Signs and symptoms
    Severe pain
    Modest fever and leukocytosis in
      some cases

No change in hematocrit or in the number
  of sickle cells in the blood smear

by its absence is any change in the red cell status in sickle cell crisis; the hematocrit holds steady (unless there is a simultaneous aplastic crisis, which may coincide with a sickle cell crisis in infected patients), and the number of irreversibly sickled cells in the blood smear remains unchanged. The crisis will subside spon-

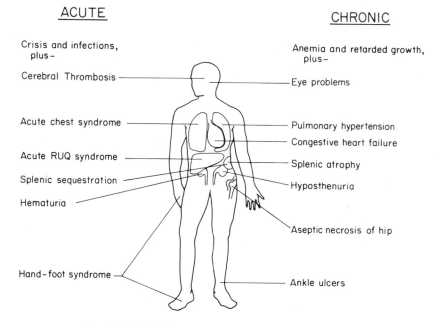

ACUTE

Crisis and infections, plus –

Cerebral Thrombosis

Acute chest syndrome

Acute RUQ syndrome

Splenic sequestration

Hematuria

Hand-foot syndrome

CHRONIC

Anemia and retarded growth, plus –

Eye problems

Pulmonary hypertension

Congestive heart failure

Splenic atrophy

Hyposthenuria

Aseptic necrosis of hip

Ankle ulcers

Fig. 11-7. Clinical manifestations of sickle cell anemia.

taneously, only to recur after a few weeks or months to afflict the patient once again. Because the pain is severe enough to require narcotics for adequate analgesia, drug addiction is not uncommon in patients with sickle cell anemia.

Cardiopulmonary

The cardiac complications of sickle cell disease have been discussed above. Pulmonary problems may be acute or chronic. The acute chest syndrome of sickle cell disease consists of chest pain, fever, cough, and a pulmonary infiltrate, all of relatively abrupt onset. This may be caused by bacterial pneumonia or by a pulmonary infarct resulting from a sickle cell crisis involving the pulmonary circulation; these may be impossible to tell apart, especially because they may occur together, and decisions as to specific treatment may have to be made more or less empirically. In a few patients, pulmonary hypertension with cor pulmonale may develop, the result of recurrent occlusive episodes over many years involving the pulmonary circulation.

Abdominal Organs

The liver is often involved in sickle cell disease. It is usually enlarged, and gallstones are common. Acute right upper quadrant pain is most frequently attributable to a sickle cell crisis, which, if it involves the liver directly, may lead to rapid enlargement of that organ. It may also be attributable to cholelithiasis or to hepatitis of other etiologies. As with the acute chest syndrome, the cause of acute right upper quadrant pain in patients with sickle cell anemia may be exceedingly difficult to determine.

The other abdominal organ routinely involved in sickle cell disease is the spleen. Changes in spleen size and function in sickle cell disease have been discussed above. In children, the spleen can become involved in a very serious complication known as the splenic

sequestration syndrome, in which sudden massive intrasplenic sickling leads to acute severe left upper quadrant pain, a rapid increase in the size of the spleen, and hypovolemia with an abrupt fall in the hematocrit, rapidly leading to shock. The splenic sequestration syndrome constitutes a medical emergency that can cause death if not quickly treated.

Genitourinary System

Genitourinary manifestations of sickle cell anemia include (1) the excretion of a dilute urine (hyposthenuria), a common problem that appears to result from infarction of the inner portion of the renal medulla, a region of tissue in which the oxygen tension is ordinarily quite low; and (2) hematuria, a rare problem arising from the same cause. There is an increase in the incidence of pyelonephritis in sickle cell anemia. Priapism is a rare but characteristic complication.

Bones, Joints, and Extremities

The bones and joints are often affected in sickle cell disease. Bone films may show sclerotic areas that denote regions of prior bony infarction. On a larger scale, aseptic necrosis of the hip frequently occurs. An acute arthritis can result from a vascular occlusion involving the synovium. The incidence of osteomyelitis is increased.

The hand–foot syndrome is an arthritis-like condition seen in children younger than 3 years of age with sickle cell anemia. Often the first clinical manifestation of the disorder, it is characterized by transient painful swelling of the hands and feet lasting about 2 weeks and associated with such signs of inflammation as fever and leukocytosis. It may be confused with a number of other diseases affecting the hands and feet of children, especially rheumatic fever. Chronic nonhealing ankle ulcers are common in sickle cell anemia. They respond poorly to treatment and can be very hard to deal with.

Central Nervous System and Eyes

In sickle cell anemia, strokes may occur at a young age as a result of thrombosis of the cerebral arteries. Recurrent occlusions of retinal arterioles and capillaries may cause blinding eye disease.

Pregnancy

Placental infarctions occur in pregnant women with sickle cell disease, leading to an increase in the incidence of fetal loss and toxemia. Congestive heart failure and thrombophlebitis are more common than usual, and the acute chest syndrome often occurs in the third trimester of pregnancy. In addition, the frequency of crisis is increased throughout the course of the pregnancy. It is evident that the hazards of pregnancy for both the mother and the fetus are substantially increased by sickle cell anemia.

Course of the Disease

The foregoing litany of clinical manifestations shows that sickle cell anemia is a highly generalized disease with acute and chronic effects involving virtually every organ system in the body. Accordingly, it would seem logical to conclude that a short life filled with pain and debility is the fate of patients afflicted with this disease. This is true in many cases, but some patients with sickle cell anemia have surprisingly little trouble with their condition. Crisis are mild and infrequent, and complications develop very slowly.

A number of reasons have been offered to explain why sickle cell anemia varies so widely in severity from patient to patient:

1. *Fetal hemoglobin*. There is a wide variation in hemoglobin F among patients with sickle cell anemia, with levels ranging from 2 to greater than 20 percent (normal 1 to 3 percent). It has been suggested that patients with a mild clinical course have high levels of hemoglobin F, which would diminish the incidence of crisis by impeding deoxyhemoglobin S polymerization through a "Trojan horse" effect.

2. *Total hemoglobin*. The total red cell hemoglobin concentration has been suggested as a factor affecting the course of sickle cell anemia. If the concentration is low, nucleation should be retarded, thereby decreasing the incidence of crises.

3. *Irreversibly sickled cells*. The number of irreversibly sickled cells in the circulation has also been proposed as an index of the severity of the disease, greater numbers predicted a worse course.

All these explanations have some validity, but the correlations only hold at the extremes. The disease is mild in the few patients with very high levels of hemoglobin F or very low red cell hemoglobin concentrations, and severe in the very few patients in whom the numbers of irreversibly sickled cells are exceptionally high. In most patients, however, the severity of the disease cannot be predicted from any measurement.

Whether the course is mild or severe, however, almost all patients with sickle cell anemia sooner or later die of their disease. Some will die in childhood of overwhelming bacterial infections, to which they are unusually susceptible because of their general debility and the fact that their splenic function is gone. Most, however, survive into adulthood, eventually succumbing to the complications of their disease: overwhelming infection, as seen in childhood; renal failure, caused by the accumulation of kidney damage over the course of a lifetime of microinfarctions; and most importantly, cardiac failure, probably the major cause of death in sickle cell anemia.

Other Sickle Cell Diseases

Sickle cell trait
S/β-thalassemia
SC
SD
SO

Other Sickle Cell Diseases

With rare exceptions, patients with sickle cell diseases other than sickle cell anemia are β-globin gene heterozygotes. One of their β-globin genes is the β^S (i.e., sickle) gene, whereas the other is either a normal β-globin gene or a gene with a mutation different from β^S. Because of this genetic makeup, red cells from these patients (except for sickle/β-thalassemia) contain two major hemoglobins. The presence of the second hemoglobin interferes with the ability of the deoxyhemoglobin S to polymerize in the cell. Consequently, these variant forms of sickle cell disease are almost always milder than sickle cell anemia. Depending on the extent to which polymerization is disrupted, the severity of the variant diseases ranges from virtually asymptomatic to almost as bad as homozygous sickle cell anemia.

Sickle Cell Trait

Patients with one normal β-globin gene and one β^S-gene are said to have sickle cell trait. This condition is by far the most common of the sickle cell variants, occurring in nearly one out of every 10 North American blacks.

From a clinical standpoint, sickle cell trait is important principally because patients with trait are carriers of a very serious disease that may appear in their offspring. Statistically, one out of every four children born of parents with sickle cell trait will have sickle cell anemia (autosomal recessive), whereas one out of two will inherit sickle cell trait (autosomal dominant) (Fig. 11-8). Sickle cell trait itself, however, is almost always clinically benign. The hematocrit is normal, blood smears generally shown no abnormalities, and the life expectancy is statistically normal. On the other hand, certain problems, some serious, do arise as a result of sickle cell trait. Most patients with trait eventually develop hyposthenuria because of destruction of the inner portion of the renal medulla, a region so hypoxic and hyperosmolar that even cells with trait will stiffen there and sickle. Splenic infacts have occurred in these patients during flights in planes with unpressurized cabins. Of most concern, patients with sickle cell trait are at increased risk of sudden death under circumstances that combine high tissue oxygen demand with dehydration (e.g., during strenuous military training exercises in hot, muggy climates).

Red cells from patients with sickle cell trait contain major quantities of both hemoglobin S and hemoglobin A, but hemoglobin A exceeds hemoglobin S by a factor of about 1.5:1. This happens at least in part because α-chains combine more rapidly with normal β-chains than with β^S-chains during the formation of hemoglobin tetramers, so that in the competition for the scarce α-chains, the normal β-chains have the edge. In the relatively common combina-

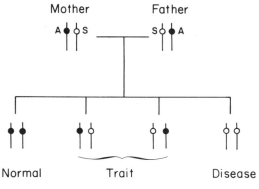

Fig. 11-8. Parents with sickle cell trait can have children with sickle cell anemia.

tion of sickle trait and mild α-thalassemia, the A:S imbalance is exaggerated because the free α-chains are even scarcer than normal; A:S ratios of 3:1 are typical of sickle trait/α-thalassemia minor.

Sickle Cell/β-Thalassemia

Certain patients who are sickle cell heterozygotes also carry a gene for β-thalassemia, a disease in which β-globin chain synthesis is greatly slowed or absent (see Ch. 10). These patients have a form of sickle cell disease the severity of which depends on the degree of production of normal β-chains permitted by their thalassemia gene. Patients whose cells produce relatively large quantities of normal β-chains will have a very mild form of the disease, because their red cells will contain enough hemoglobin A to prevent symptoms by interfering with the polymerization of deoxyhemoglobin S. In contrast, patients whose cells make few or no normal β-chains can have a disease almost as severe as homozygous sickle cell anemia.

In patients with this disease, anemia is the rule. Cells are small rather than normal in size, a point of distinction from homozygous sickle cell anemia, and there are more target cells than in sickle cell anemia (Fig. 11-9). Splenomegaly is common, another clinical difference between S/β-thalassemia and the homozygous

disease. In other respects, the two conditions are clinically identical.

Red cells from patients with S/β-thalassemia may or may not contain hemoglobin A, depending on whether the thalassemic component of the disease is β^+ or β^0. Where hemoglobin A is present, its concentration is always lower than that of hemoglobin S, differentiating S/β-thalassemia from sickle cell trait. When hemoglobin A is absent, differentiating this disease from homozygous sickle cell anemia may be difficult, but it can usually be accomplished by family studies, which will show some form of thalassemia in one parent and some form of sickle cell disease in the other.

Hemoglobin C and SC Disease

Hemoglobin C is a mutant hemoglobin in which the β6 glutamate is replaced by lysine (it will be recalled that in the β^S chain, this glutamate is replaced by valine). The gene for hemoglobin C is found exclusively in blacks, in whom its frequency is about one-fourth that of the sickle gene.

Hemoglobin C trait (one normal β-globin gene and one β^C gene) is an asymptomatic condition. Homozygous hemoglobin C disease causes a mild hemolytic anemia that is entirely similar to other mild extravascular hemolytic anemias (e.g., reticulocytosis, splenomegaly), except for the characteristic appearance of the

Fig. 11-9. Blood smears in S/β-thalassemia (**A**) and sickle cell anemia (**B**). The S/β-thalassemia cells are microcytic. Target cells are more abundant in S/β-thalassemia than in sickle cell anemia. (From Bunn, H.F., Forget, B.G., & Ranney, H.M. (1977) Human hemoglobin variants. Ch. 6. In Human Hemoglobin. W.B. Saunders, Philadelphia, with permission.)

Fig. 11-10. Hemoglobin C disease. Target cells are very prominent. A few deeply stained bricklike rectangular cells are seen; these are characteristic of hemoglobin C disease. (From Bunn, H.F., Forget, B.G., & Ranney, H.M. (1977) Human hemoglobin variants. Ch. 6. In Human Hemoglobin. W.B. Saunders, Philadelphia, with permission.)

red cells on the blood smear. These show a striking degree of targeting (Fig. 11-10), together with an occasional rectangular cell that appears to be formed by intracellular crystallization of the abnormal hemoglobin during the preparation of the smear. Patients with homozygous hemoglobin C disease are not incapacitated in any way by their disease, and their life expectancy is normal.

Problems with hemoglobin C arise in patients who are doubly heterozygous for hemoglobin C and hemoglobin S. These patients have a form of sickle cell disease that in most respects resembles mild homozygous sickle cell anemia. The principal difference between SC disease and the homozygous disease is the mildness of the anemia, hematocrits above 25 ml/dl being the rule in SC disease. As a result, the cardiac problems so prominent in sickle cell anemia are minimal in patients with SC disease, and their life expectancy is only slightly shorter than normal. As in S/β-thalassemia, but in contrast to SS, splenomegaly is common in SC disease.

Routine laboratory tests in SC disease show a mild to moderate anemia, with normal-size red cells. The smear shows many target cells and a few fat sickle forms (Fig. 11-11). Red cells contain hemoglobin S and hemoglobin C, in equal amounts.

SD and SO

Hemoglobin D Punjab ($\beta^{121glu \rightarrow gln}$) and O Arabia ($\beta^{121glu \rightarrow lys}$) are other mutant hemoglobins that cause little disease by themselves, but result in sickle cell disease when present in combination with hemoglobin S. Both are relatively common compared with most mutant hemoglobins, but not nearly as common as hemoglobin S or C. Disease in these double heterozygotes is mild, and splenomegaly is common. The diagnosis is made by demonstrating the presence of the two hemoglobins in the red cells of affected patients. The features of the most important of

Fig. 11-11. **(A)** SC disease. **(B)** Sickle cell disease. In SC disease, target cells are abundant. The sickle forms are shorter and fatter than in sickle cell anemia, a subtle distinction. (From Bunn, H.F., Forget, B.G., & Ranney, H.M. (1977) Human hemoglobin variants. Ch. 6. In Human Hemoglobin. W.B. Saunders, Philadelphia, with permission.)

Table 11-1. Features of the Most Important Heterozygous Sickle Cell Diseases

Disease	Clinical Features	Red Cell Morphology	Hemoglobins
Sickle trait	No crises	Normal	A > S
S/β-thalassemia	Moderate to severe crises Severe anemia Splenomegaly	Small sickle cells Microcytosis 4^+ targets	A absent (β^0) or present but < (β^+); A_2 variably ↑
SC disease	Moderate to severe crises Modest anemia Splenomegaly	Fat sickle cells 4^+ targets	C equals S

the heterozygous sickle cell diseases are listed in Table 11-1.

MANAGEMENT OF SICKLE CELL DISEASES

Diagnosis

Making the diagnosis of a sickle cell disease usually involves two steps: (1) demonstrating that red cells from a patient suspected of having a sickle cell disease actually contain hemoglobin S, and (2) identifying all the hemoglobins present in those red cells by electrophoresis. Evidence for the presence of hemoglobin S is usually obtained by one of two screening tests: the solubility test or the sickle

Fig. 11-12. The sickle cell preparation. (From Castoldi, G.L. (1981) Erythrocytes. Ch. 3. In Zucker-Franklin, D. et al. (eds.) Atlas of Blood Cells: Function and Pathology. Edi. Ermes s.r.l., Milan, with permission.)

cell preparation. Both are based on the principle that when oxygen is removed from a preparation of hemoglobin S, the hemoglobin will polymerize and precipitate. The agent used to remove the oxygen is usually sodium metabisulfite ($Na_2S_2O_5$), a powerful reducing agent.

1. *Solubility test.* The sodium metabisulfite is added to a solution of hemoglobin in concentrated buffer (usually prepared by releasing the hemoglobin from the suspected red cells with distilled water and then adding buffer as needed); if hemoglobin S is present, a dark red precipitate of deoxyhemoglobin S will appear in the solution.

2. *Sickle cell preparation.* The metabisulfite is added to a suspension of whole red cells in saline. Cells containing any quantity of hemoglobin S—even those from patients with sickle cell trait—will sickle under these conditions. The sickling of these cells is readily seen under the microscope (Fig. 11-12).

As a model of the pathogenetic event in sickle cell diseases, the sickle cell preparation has the appeal of relevance and analogy; screening, however, is usually carried out by the solubility test because it is easier.

Identification of the hemoglobins is accomplished by electrophoresis, which is performed by applying a streak of hemolysate to one end of a solid supporting strip that has been dampened with buffer at the desired pH (usually pH 8.6), then passing an electrical current along the strip for a given period of time. The hemoglobin molecules march along the strip at rates that depend mainly on their net charge. The various species of hemoglobin in the normal

Fig. 11-13. Electrophoresis of the hemoglobins from normal red cells. The most prominent band is hemoglobin A. Hemoglobins A and A_2 are well separated on the strip, whereas hemoglobin F runs just behind hemoglobin A. Hemoglobin A is not homogeneous, but actually consists of a group of closely related species that migrate together in the electrical field. These species represent hemoglobin A tetramers ($\alpha_2\beta_2$) variably substituted with sugars or sugar phosphates on the N-terminal amino group of the β-chain. The major constituent of this group is unsubstituted hemoglobin A. Second is hemoglobin A_{1c}, a molecule in which a glucose has become attached to the β-chain by a nonenzymatic process. The concentration of hemoglobin A_{1c} is an excellent indicator of blood sugar control in diabetics.

red cell separate nicely, as shown in Figure 11-13, and can be quantitated by their color.

Abnormal hemoglobins characteristic of sickle cell disease differ from hemoglobin A in their net charge. The two most common of these—hemoglobins S and C—differ from hemoglobin A in the loss of one ($\beta^{S:glu\rightarrow val}$) and two ($\beta^{C:glu\rightarrow lys}$) negative charges, respectively. These losses of negative charge translate directly into losses in electrophoretic mobility, which decrease in the order: Hb A > Hb S > Hb C (Fig. 11-14). Accordingly,

hemoglobins A, S, and C are easily distinguished by their behavior in an electrical field, and hemoglobin electrophoresis becomes a simple and convenient way to demonstrate their presence in patients with sickle cell disease.

A diagnostic monkey wrench is occasionally thrown into the works in the form of the uncommon abnormal hemoglobins D and O-Arab. These forms produce heterozygous sickle cell disease when combined with hemoglobin S. The problem is that each of these hemoglobins moves with one of the more common hemoglobins under the usual conditions of electrophoresis: D migrates with S, and O Arabia migrates with C. SD therefore looks like SS on the electrophoresis strip, and SO Arabia looks like SC. If the problem should arise, it can be settled by electrophoresis at pH 6.2, which separates the confusing pairs.

The hemoglobin electrophoretic patterns corresponding to the various sickle cell diseases are shown in Figure 11-14. It is worth repeating that the following pairs of sickle cell diseases give identical electrophoretic patterns: SS and SD; SC and SO Arabia; and SS and S/β^0-thalassemia (although with S/β^0-thalassemia, increases in A_2 similar to those seen in β-thalassemia trait may provide a clue to the true diagnosis). With such pairs of diseases, the decision to look further in order to make a diagnosis is usually based on clinical clues. For example, mild disease in an adult with

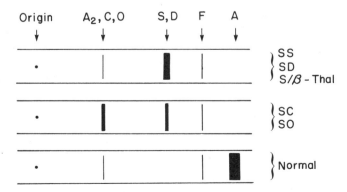

Fig. 11-14. Hemoglobin electrophoresis in the sickle cell diseases.

splenomegaly whose hemoglobin electrophoresis gives an SS pattern is an indication to look for SD, because true homozygous sickle cell anemia is usually a severe disease in which splenomegaly is uncommon. Finally, it should be recalled that hemoglobins A and S are found in both sickle cell trait and S/β^+-thalassemia, but that in sickle cell trait, A > S, whereas in S/β^+-thalassemia, S > A.

Prenatal Diagnosis

Like thalassemia, sickle cell anemia can sometimes be diagnosed prenatally. The diagnosis can be made by demonstrating the presence of the sickle mutation in the fetal β-globin gene through the use of MstI, a restriction endonuclease whose recognition sequence is altered by the $\beta^{A\rightarrow}\beta^S$ mutation. It may be more difficult to know what to do with this information than in the case of prenatally diagnosed thalassemia major, because the course of

---

Treatment of Acute Problems in Sickle Cell Diseases

Treatment of crisis
    Fluids
    Analgesics
    Oxygen and alkali if indicated

Indications for antibiotics
    Infections
    Acute chest syndrome

Indications for partial exchange transfusions
    Acute chest syndrome
    Splenic sequestration syndrome[a]
    General anesthesia
    Acute clinical deterioration in a sickle
      cell patient

---

[a] Splenic sequestration constitutes an *acute emergency*. Shock must be treated immediately. Emergency splenectomy may be necessary.

Long-term Treatment of Sickle Cell Diseases

Folic acid
Prophylactic antibiotics in children under
    age 6
Long-term transfusion therapy
    Children with stroke
    Pregnant women (?)

---

homozygous sickle cell anemia is highly variable, with many patients pursuing a relatively symptom-free course throughout a long and generally healthy life.

Treatment

The treatment of sickle cell diseases generally boils down to the management of the episodes of illness or stress that occur during the course of the disease. The anemia itself generally does not require treatment, although folate supplements should be given routinely to patients with sickle cell disease, just as it is to patients with other forms of chronic hemolytic anemia.

Crisis

Despite thousands of man-years of investigation, nothing has been found as yet that can shorten the duration of a sickle cell crisis. Treatment is therefore restricted to supportive measures: analgesics, plenty of fluids, and alkali and oxygen if necessary to correct acidosis or hypoxia, but not on a routine basis. Patients with abdominal crisis must be watched carefully to make sure they do not have an acute surgical abdomen. The *acute chest syndrome* should be treated empirically with antibiotics; partial exchange transfusions should be carried out to replace sickle cells with normal cells;

and oxygen should be freely administered to maintain tissue oxygenation and prevent further complications. The *splenic sequestration syndrome* requires immediate fluids, oxygen, and partial exchange transfusions to reverse hypovolemia and shock; emergency splenectomy may be necessary. A program of exchange transfusion, or long-term transfusion to hematocrits of approximately 35 ml/dl (a level high enough to reduce levels of hemoglobin S by suppressing endogenous erythropoiesis), is recommended for children with strokes and for pregnant women in the third trimester.

Infections

Bacterial infections are an exceedingly serious problem in patients with sickle cell disease and should be treated aggressively. Pneumococcal infections, which occur frequently in sickle cell disease, can be prevented to some extent by vaccination. Prophylactic antibiotics are recommended for children younger than age 6.

General Anesthesia

General anesthesia is an indication for partial exchange transfusion therapy to decrease the proportion of hemoglobin-S-containing cells in the circulation. This may need to be done on an emergency basis.

SUGGESTED READINGS

Bunn, H.F. (1987) Subunit assembly of hemoglobin: An important determinant of hematologic phenotype. Blood *69*:1.

Bunn, H.F. & Forget, B.D. (1984) Human Hemoglobins, 2nd Ed. W.B. Saunders, Philadelphia.

Charache, S. (1981) Treatment of sickle cell anemia. Annu. Rev. Med. *32*:195.

Dean, J. & Schechter, A.N. (1978) Sickle-cell anemia: Molecular and cellular bases of therapeutic approaches. N. Engl. J. Med. *299*:752, 804, 863.

Steinberg, M.H. & Embury, S.H. (1986) Alpha-thalassemia in blacks: genetic and clinical aspects and interactions with the sickle hemoglobin gene. Blood *68*:985.

Thurn, J. (1988) Human parvovirus B19: historical and clinical review. Rev. Infect. Dis. *10*:1005.

Vichinsky, E.P. & Lubin, B.H. (1980) Sickle cell anemia and related hemoglobinopathies. Pediatr. Clin. North. Am. *27*:429.

Polycythemia

Contrasting with the anemias are the polycythemias, a group of disorders in which the total volume of red cells in the patient is abnormally high. Most forms of polycythemia are caused by the overproduction of erythropoietin, which leads to excessive red cell formation. One variety, however, known as *polycythemia vera*, is caused by an intrinsic abnormality of the stem cell. There is in addition a condition known as *stress erythrocytosis* that closely resembles the polycythemias but in which the patient's total red cell volume is often in the normal range.

The hallmark of all these conditions is an elevation of the hemoglobin level. A high hemoglobin level generally means that the patient has polycythemia, though further testing is sometimes necessary to confirm this impression. Once the existence of polycythemia has been established, its cause must be determined. This determination is based on further clinical and laboratory findings that vary among the different forms of polycythemia (Table 12-1).

THE SECONDARY POLYCYTHEMIAS

The secondary polycythemias are those forms of polycythemia that result from the overproduction of erythropoietin. Erythropoietin increases red cell formation by specifically stimulating the growth of the late-committed stem cells of the erythrocyte series (see Ch. 2). Erythropoietin production is ordinarily regulated by the rate of oxygen delivery to the kidney, a figure that is tied closely to the amount of hemoglobin in the blood. Secondary polycythemia develops when the production of erythropoietin is inappropriately high for the blood hemoglobin level.

Causes

Polycythemia due to inappropriately high erythropoietin production is caused by one of two factors: chronically low tissue oxygenation or an abnormal cell population that produces erythropoietin autonomously.

Chronically Inadequate Tissue Oxygenation

As mentioned above, the level of erythropoietin in the blood is normally regulated by the delivery of oxygen to the kidneys. With normal renal oxygen delivery, the kidneys manufacture only small quantities of erythropoietin and the hematocrit and hemoglobin remain in the normal range. Impaired renal oxygen delivery, however, signals the kidneys to secrete increased amounts of erythropoietin, which in turn stimulates the bone marrow to increase red cell production in order to correct renal oxygen delivery by providing the blood

Table 12-1. The Differential Diagnosis of Polycythemia

Finding	Secondary polycythemia	Polycythemia vera	Stress erythrocytosis
Arterial oxygen tension	Normal or low	Normal	Normal
Splenomegaly	Absent	Present	Absent
White blood count and platelet count	Normal	Usually high	Normal
Uric acid	Normal	Often high	Normal
Red cell mass	High	High	High normal

with additional oxygen-delivering capacity. Polycythemia occurs when even at a normal hemoglobin concentration the blood cannot deliver oxygen to the kidneys rapidly enough to hold erythropoietin secretion to normal levels. This is seen most commonly in conditions associated with a chronic reduction in arterial oxygen saturation (chronic hypoxemia). Much less frequently, it arises through a failure of fully oxygenated hemoglobin to release its oxygen to the tissues.

The cause of *polycythemia due to chronic hypoxemia* are listed below. The most frequent cause is chronic lung disease, in which hypoxemia occurs because of the mixing of well-oxygenated blood draining from relatively normal regions of the lung with poorly oxygenated blood draining from more diseased regions of the lung, regions that are well-perfused but poorly aerated. Another cause of this form of polycythemia, one that may be subtle and difficult to diagnose, is sleep apnea.

Causes of Polycythemia Due to Chronically Inadequate Tissue Oxygenation

Low arterial oxygen saturation
   Chronic lung disease
   Right-to-left shunts
   High altitude

Normal arterial oxygen saturation
   Sleep apnea
   High affinity hemoglobin
   Abnormal 2,3-DPG metabolism

In this condition, intermittent obstruction of the upper airway during sleep causes episodes of low arterial oxygen saturation that may be frequent enough to lead to secondary polycythemia. Less common causes include right-to-left shunts secondary to congenital heart disease or other vascular anomalies and oxygen-poor living environments such as high mountains.

Polycythemia due to impaired oxygen release occurs in patients with high-affinity hemoglobins and with certain rare abnormalities of 2,3-disphosphoglyceric acid (2,3-DPG) metabolism. These have been discussed in Chapter 3.

Autonomous Erythropoietin Production

Erythropoietin may be secreted autonomously from certain kinds of tumors, and occasionally from tissues involved with other diseases. Polycythemia due to autonomous erythropoietin production is seen most commonly in patients with renal cell carcinoma, 5 percent of whom develop this problem. This form of polycythemia is also seen occasionally in patients with hepatomas, and invariably in patients with the cerebellar hemangioblastomas of von Hippel-Lindau disease. Secondary polycythemia may also be caused by certain benign renal lesions such as polycystic kidney and hydroneophrosis, which probably act by interfering with the renal circulation so that critical regions of the organ are underperfused and begin to secrete excess erythropoietin. In patients with autonomous erythropoietin production, polycythemia occurs because

> ## Causes of Polycythemia Due to Inappropriate Erythropoietin Secretion
>
> Renal
> >   Renal cell carcinoma
> >   Renal cysts
> >   Hydronephrosis
> >   Renal graft rejection
>
> Extrarenal
> >   Hepatoma
> >   Pheochromocytoma
> >   Cerebellar hemangioblastoma (von Hippel-Lindau disease)

the secretion of the hormone by the abnormal tissue is unregulated and fails to shut down even in response to the abnormally large amounts of oxygen that are delivered to the secreting tissue by the hemoglobin-rich polycythemic blood.

Manifestations

General

The characteristic sign of polycythemia of any kind is an elevation in the hemoglobin (and hematocrit). This is usually detected in the laboratory, though the patient's flushed, ruddy complexion often furnishes an early clue to its presence. The degree of elevation of the hemoglobin and hematocrit varies from patient to patient, ranging from just above normal to twice the normal value or even higher. If the hemoglobin level is sufficiently high, symptoms can result from the associated increase in blood volume and blood viscosity (Fig. 12-1). These symptoms may include fatigue, headaches, a feeling of engorgement in the head, and shortness of breath, as well as aggravation of congestive heart failure. The blood pressure may be elevated, and the veins in the eyegrounds engorged.

Certain features are especially important in helping to make the very important distinction between secondary polycythemia and polycythemia vera (see box). The spleen is almost never felt on physical examination in a patient with uncomplicated secondary polycythemia, but is palpable in the majority of patients with polycythemia vera. The white blood count, platelet count, and uric acid levels are generally normal in secondary polycythemia, but are likely to be high in polycythemia vera. For a fuller discussion of polycythemia vera, see the chapter on myeloproliferative disorders (see Ch. 28).

Decreased versus Normal Arterial Oxygen Saturation

One of the most useful tests for evaluating patients with polycythemia is the measurement of the hemoglobin oxygen saturation in their arterial blood. From the results of this test, patients with polycythemia can be divided into two groups: those who show a decrease in arterial oxygen saturation and those who do not. The diseases responsible for the polycythemia are very different in these two groups.

Decreased Arterial Oxygen Saturation

If the oxygen saturation of the arterial hemoglobin is 89 percent or less, then the polycythemia is probably due to one of the conditions that cause chronic hypoxemia (see p. 172). In persons living at very high altitudes and in patients with congenital heart disease with a right-to-left shunt, the hematocrit and hemoglobin can rise to remarkably high levels; hematocrits of 80 ml/dl or more may be seen in such persons. In contrast, hematocrits rarely exceed the high 50s in patients with chronic lung disease, probably because the smoldering pulmonary infection present in most of these patients gives rise to an anemia of chronic dis-

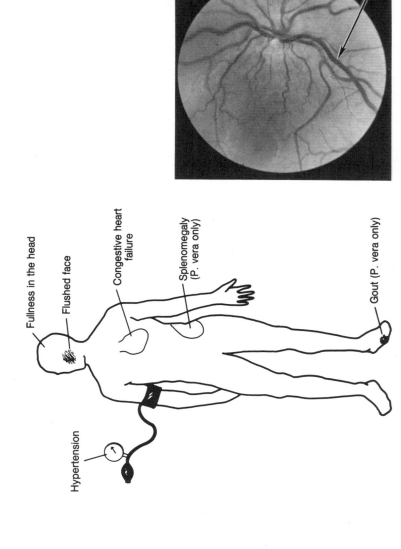

Fig. 12-1. Signs and symptoms of polycythemia. Most of the signs and symptoms are caused by the combination of increased total blood volume and increased blood viscosity. Splenomegaly occurs only in polycythemia vera.

Findings Seen in Polycythemia Vera But Not in Secondary Polycythemia

Splenomegaly

High white cell count

High platelet count

Elevated uric acid

ease that partly offsets their hypoxia-driven increase in red cell production.

Normal Arterial Oxygen Saturation

Polycythemia combined with a normal arterial oxygen saturation is most frequently due to "stress erythrocytosis" (see below) or to polycythemia vera (see Ch. 28). On occasion, however, this combination may betray the presence of certain forms of secondary polycythemia. These include polycythemias caused by erythropoietin-producing lesions (e.g., a renal cell carcinoma) and the rare cases of polycythemia due to a high-affinity hemoglobin or an abnormality in 2,3-DPG metabolism.

Among the causes of secondary polycythemia, sleep apnea is unique because, even though polycythemia in this disorder results from chronic hypoxemia, random arterial oxygen saturations are almost always normal. This is because random arterial oxygen saturations are usually drawn during the day, when the patient's breathing is normal and his blood is fully oxygenated, whereas desaturation occurs only in sleep, during episodes of apnea, which in severe cases may number hundreds in the course of a night. The diagnosis of sleep apnea is generally made in a sleep laboratory, although its presence is suggested by overwhelming daytime drowsiness and a history of violent snoring (the latter elicited, of course,

from the patient's spouse or other nocturnal companion).

Borderline Arterial Oxygen Saturation

Arterial oxygen saturations of 89 to 92 percent are on the borderline between normal and decreased. This oxygen saturation, though low enough to give rise to polycythemia as a secondary response, also occurs in forms of polycythemia more typically associated with a normal arterial oxygen saturation (e.g., polycythemia vera). A borderline oxygen saturation is seen with exasperating frequency in polycythemias of all kinds and offers little help in diagnosis.

Polycythemia versus High Hematocrit

In thinking about diseases characterized by overproduction of red cells, it is important to keep in mind the distinction between polycythemia and high hematocrit. Polycythemia refers to the elevation of red cell mass that is the hallmark of these diseases, whereas a high hematocrit refers only to an abnormally high red cell mass/plasma volume ratio. (The term "red cell mass" refers to the total quantity of red cells in the patient. Despite this terminology, the red cell "mass" is always expressed as a volume—usually as milliliters of red cells.) An elevated hematocrit, although highly suggestive of polycythemia, may not be enough to make the diagnosis, because there are circumstances under which the hematocrit can be as high as 60 ml/dl in the face of a normal red cell mass. To diagnose polycythemia, it is often necessary to measure the red cell mass directly. This is accomplished by labeling a known quantity of the patient's red cells with ^{51}Cr, reinjecting them, and, after allowing sufficient time for complete mixing, determining by what factor the tagged cells were diluted by the patient's own circulating red cells.

Fig. 12-2. Determination of the red cell mass helps establish whether a patient with a moderately elevated hematocrit has true polycythemia or not. (**Left**) The normal situation: The hematocrit, red cell mass, and plasma volume are all normal. (**Center**) An elevated hematocrit but no polycythemia; the red cell mass is normal and the plasma volume is low. (**Right**) An elevated hematocrit with true polycythemia; the red cell mass and the plasma volume are both high.

Patients with clinically significant secondary polycythemia will almost invariably show an increase in the red cell mass (Fig. 12-2).

Management

The secondary polycythemias are ideally managed by treating the underlying disease. This may not be possible, however, or even if possible may yield only a partial response. The question then remains as to what to do about the elevated hemoglobin. Often, the answer to this question is "Nothing." If, however, the hemoglobin level is sufficiently high, symptoms may occur because the high viscosity of the polycythemic blood reduces tissue oxygen delivery and imposes a strain on the heart (see Ch. 2). In this situation, phlebotomy can be used to lower the hemoglobin and relieve symptoms.

In patients whose polycythemia is due to chronic hypoxemia, treatment by phlebotomy appears contrary to logic, because the elevation in red cell volume would seem to be needed to compensate for the reduction in arterial oxygen saturation. In severe chronic lung disease, however, it has been found that patients do best when their hemoglobins are in the range of 18 g/100ml. Thus even in chronic hypoxemia, more hemoglobin is not necessarily better, and a symptomatic patient with a very high hemoglobin will often benefit from phlebotomy.

POLYCYTHEMIA VERA

In polycythemia vera, normal marrow stem cells are replaced by an abnormal stem cell population whose response to growth regulators (e.g., erythropoietin) is disturbed. As discussed above, the high hemoglobin in polycythemia vera is usually accompanied by findings that are very unusual in the secondary polycythemias, including splenomegaly and high white cell and platelet counts. Polycythemia vera is covered in more detail in Chapter 23.

STRESS ERYTHROCYTOSIS

The combination of a modest elevation in the hematocrit and a normal red cell mass is common. Known as Gaisböck's syndrome or stress erythrocytosis, this combination is typically seen in hard-driving middle-aged men, usually smokers, who in addition tend to be overweight and hypertensive. The red cell mass in these patients is generally on the high side of normal, whereas plasma volumes are in the low-normal range, leading to a high hemoglobin without an increase in red cell mass.

Fig. 12-3. The effect of carbon monoxide on the oxygen saturation curve of whole blood. When some of the four oxygen-binding sites on a hemoglobin molecule are occupied by CO, the remaining oxygen-binding sites lose much of their cooperativity. The result is a high-affinity hemoglobin that carries fewer oxygens than normal and is reluctant to release any of its oxygen to the tissues.

Stress erythrocytosis is important to diagnose, because patients with this condition are at risk for heart attacks and other vascular occlusive disease.

In the pathogenesis of stress erythrocytosis, the carbon monoxide (CO) inhaled with the tobacco smoke plays a special role. When a CO molecule is taken up by hemoglobin, the CO both prevents the binding of oxygen to the occupied site and eliminates cooperativity in the binding of oxygen to the remaining three sites (see Ch. 3), so that a hemoglobin one of

whose four binding sites is occupied by CO, behaves like a high affinity hemoglobin (Fig. 12-3). Furthermore, CO inhalation causes an abrupt drop in plasma volume, for reasons that are not clear. It is easy to see how CO, producing both a "high affinity"-like hemoglobin and a low plasma volume, can give rise to the syndrome of stress erythrocytosis.

SUGGESTED READINGS

Doll D.C. & Weiss, R.B. (1985) Neoplasia and the erythron. J. Clin. Oncol. *3*:429.

Erslev, A.J. & Caro, J. (1983) Pathophysiology and classification of polycythaemia. Scand. J. Haematol. *31*:287.

Flenley, D.C. (1982) Oxygen transport in chronic hypoxic lung disease. J. Clin. Pathol. *35*:797.

Golde, D.W., Hocking, W.G., Koeffler, H.P. & Adamson, J.W. (1981) Polycythemia: mechanisms and management. Ann. Intern. Med. *95*:71.

Harrison, B.D. & Stokes, T.C. (1982) Secondary polycythaemia: its causes, effects and treatment. Br. J. Dis. Chest *76*:313.

Typical Patient with Stress Erythrocytosis

Middle-aged man

Intense personality

Smoker

Overweight

Hypertensive

Hocking, W.G. (1987) Hematologic abnormalities in patients with renal diseases. Hematol. Oncol. Clin. North. Am. *1*:229.

Perloff, J.K., Rosove, M.H., Child. J.S. & Wright, G.B. (1988) Adults with cyanotic congenital heart disease: hematologic management. Ann. Intern. Med. *109*:406.

Stradling, J.R. & Lane, D.J. (1981) Development of secondary polycythaemia in chronic airways obstruction. Thorax *36*:321.

SECTION II

Coagulation

Blood clotting involves two components of the circulation: the clotting factors, a group of circulating proteins most of which are made in the liver; and the platelets, which are manufactured in the bone marrow. These are the elements of a highly complex system that is elaborately regulated so as to permit clotting to take place only at precisely defined times and locations. Clotting disorders occur when the function of one or more of these elements is disturbed. Patients with clotting disorders usually present with abnormal bleeding; occasionally, they may present because of the occurrence of spontaneous coagulation under inappropriate circumstances.

13

The Clotting Cascade and Its Regulation: Congenital and Acquired Clotting Factor Disorders

At the simplest level, the formation of a clot involves the gelation of a protein known as fibrin. This protein is not normally present as such in the circulation, but is produced in large quantities at the site of coagulation from a circulating precursor, fibrinogen. The production of fibrin from fibrinogen involves a sequence of reactions the effect of which is to amplify the tiny biochemical signal produced by a damaged blood vessel into a fibrin-generating reaction vigorous enough to form a clot capable of stopping the bleeding from the damaged vessel. Because this process of amplification occurs in a series of stages, the sequence of reactions by which the initial signal is transmuted into a fibrin clot is known as the clotting cascade.

THE CLOTTING CASCADE

The proteins involved in the formation of a clot are all present in the plasma, but they circulate as precursors with little or no activity. When blood vessels and surrounding tissues are damaged, two of these clotting factors, factor VII and factor XII (contact or Hageman

factor), are converted from an inactive to an active form. In their active form, these two clotting factors activate the next factors down the line. These in turn activate the succeeding factors, the final outcome being the production of a fibrin clot. In every case, the inactive clotting factor is converted to the active form by the cleavage of one or two particular peptide bonds, a process known as *activation by limited proteolysis*.

Stages and Factors

The clotting cascade can be divided into three stages: the initial stage, the intermediate stage, and the stage of clot formation. These stages and the clotting factor activated during each are listed in Table 13–1.

Initial Stage

The initial stage consists of two distinct events: the so-called contact phase of coagulation and the activation of factor VII.

Table 13-1. Stages of the Clotting Cascade

Stage	Factors Activated
Initial	XII, prekallikrein, XI, VII
Intermediate	IX, X, prothrombin
Clot formation	Fibrinogen, XIII

The Contact Phase and the Activation of Factor XI

The contact phase and the activation of factor XI is a set of mutually reinforcing reactions, the end result of which is the production of activated factor XI (usually designated factor XIa) (Fig. 13-1). The contact phase begins when blood is exposed to a negatively charged surface (in vivo, a site of blood vessel injury; in vitro, glass or clay). The negative surface charge attracts from the bloodstream the four proteins of the contact phase: *factor XII* and *high molecular weight kininogen*, which attach directly to the negatively charged surface, and *factor XI* and *prekallikrein*, which are bound to high molecular weight kininogen and travel with it to the surface.

On the negatively charged surface, factor XII, acquiring a weak but highly specific proteolytic activity, begins to convert prekallikrein to kallikrein. Reinforcement results from the prekallikrein → kallikrein conversion: the kallikrein, itself a very specific protease, con-

verts circulating XII into XIIa (i.e., activated XII); the newly formed XIIa generates more kallikrein from prekallikrein. By activating XII, kallikrein accelerates its own formation and vice versa, a clear case of positive feedback.

Meanwhile, the principal goal of the contact phase—namely, the production of XIa—is rapidly accomplished, because both kallikrein and XIIa can catalyze the activation of factor XI:

$$XI \rightarrow XIa$$

The self-amplifying character of the contact phase makes it a highly efficient mechanism for generating XIa.

Activation of Factor VII

Most cells contain tissue factor, a membrane-associated protein that binds VII. When these cells are damaged, their tissue factor is exposed to the VII in the blood, and the tissue factor–VII complex forms. This complex is a feeble protease that slowly converts X, the next clotting factor down the line, to its active form Xa. Positive feedback now enters the picture as the Xa transforms the tissue factor–VII complex to the much more potent tissue factor–VIIa complex, which now converts X to Xa much faster than it did before activation

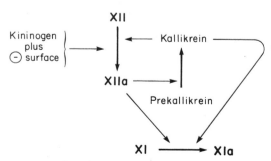

Fig. 13-1. The contact phase.

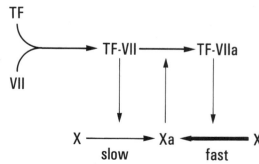

Fig. 13-2. Activation of factor VII. TF, tissue factor.

(Fig. 13–2). In this way VIIa production, like XIa production, becomes a self-amplifying process.

Intermediate Stage

In the intermediate stage, factor IX, factor X, and factor II (prothrombin) are activated, Activated factor II (thrombin) is the enzyme that converts fibrinogen to fibrin, initiating the formation of the clot per se. Its production is the final step in the intermediate stage.

Activation of Factor IX

Both products of the initial stage—XIa and VIIa—are able to activate factor IX (Fig. 13–3). Activation is accomplished as usual by limited proteolysis. Calcium is necessary for activation by XIa; calcium and phospholipid are both required for VIIa-mediated activation.

Factor IXa can do nothing further by itself. In association with Ca^{2+}, phospholipid, and factor VIII, however, it becomes a potent activator of factor X, the next factor in line. This complex of factor IXa, factor VIII, Ca^{2+}, and phospholipid is known as the "factor X converting complex." In this complex, factor IXa functions as a protease, while factor VIII plays a purely accessory role as an accelerator of the reaction, having no proteolytic activity of its own. The importance of this accessory role must not be underestimated, however; one of the most severe coagulation disorders in clinical medicine is attributable to the deficiency of factor VIII.

Activation of Factor X

Like factor IX, factor X can be activated in two ways (Fig. 13-4). It can be activated by the factor X converting complex, the factor IXa- and VIII-containing species described in the preceding section, or it can be activated by factor VIIa in the presence of Ca^{2+} and phospholipid. Activation again involves limited proteolysis.

Activated factor X (factor Xa) now associates with factor V plus Ca^{2+} and phospholipid to form the, *prothrombin-converting complex*, the species that catalyzes the activation of prothrombin to thrombin. Factor Xa is the protease, carrying out the peptide-splitting reactions by which the prothrombin activation reaction is accomplished, while factor V serves as accelerator. The resemblance between this prothrombin converting complex and the factor X converting complex is evident.

Activation of Prothrombin (Factor II)

The conversion of prothrombin to thrombin is carried out solely by the prothrombin-converting complex. No other activated clotting

Fig. 13-3. Activation of factor IX. Factor IX can be activated by either of the two complexes shown in brackets. PL stands for phospholipid.

Fig. 13-4. Activation of factor X. Factor X can be activated by either of the two complexes shown in brackets. PL stands for phospholipid.

Fig. 13-5. Conversion of prothrombin to thrombin. Prothrombin is converted to thrombin by limited proteolysis—that is, by the cleavage of a few specific peptide bonds (*arrows*). When a prothrombin molecule binds to the prothrombin converting complex, these bonds are exposed to the action of factor Xa, the proteolytic component of the converting complex. The factor Xa converts prothrombin to thrombin by (1) splitting off the activation peptide and (2) cutting the loop made by the disulfide bridge.

factor or clotting factor complex is able to carry out this reaction. Limited proteolysis is aonce again the mechanism of activation. Figure 13-5 shows that active thrombin is generated from prothrombin by two proteolytic cleavages: one that removes the amino-terminal half of the prothrombin molecule, and one that splits the remaining peptide chain into two pieces held together by a disulfide bridge. Because the removal of the large amino-terminal fragment is necessary for the activation of prothrombin to thrombin, this fragment is called the activation peptide. The activation of

factors VII, IX, and X follows a very similar pattern.

Thrombin too is a protease, the final one produced in the clotting cascade. It has several actions. It can convert factors V and VIII into forms that are much more potent than the native circulating factors, thereby promoting its own production—another example of positive feedback in the clotting cascade. It converts plasminogen to plasmin, an effect that helps control the coagulation process. The way in which thrombin acts on platelets is discussed in Chapter 14. Its most obvious effect, however, is to convert fibrinogen into a clot.

Actions of Thrombin

Fibrinogen → fibrin

Activation of factors V and VIII

XIII → XIIIa

Plasminogen → plasmin

Activation of protein C

Effects on platelets

Final Stage: Clot Formation

Clot formation begins with the thrombin-catalyzed conversion of fibrinogen to monomeric fibrin (Fig. 13-6). This conversion transforms a molecule of solitary habits into one that is driven to polymerize. The rapid spontaneously polymerization of these fibrin monomers is what forms the clot, a gelatinous mass consisting of tangled strands of polymer-

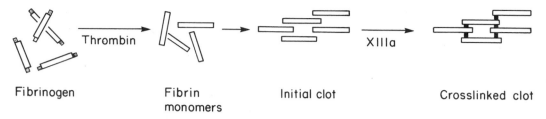

Fibrinogen   Fibrin   Initial clot   Crosslinked clot
              monomers

Fig. 13-6. Formation of the fibrin clot.

ized fibrin molecules. Initially, the clot is held together by the weak noncovalent forces responsible for the polymerization of the fibrin monomers. Within minutes, however, the strands are joined covalently through the action of a cross-linking enzyme, factor XIIIa. This cross-linking causes the clot to reach maturity and achieve its maximum strength.

The conversion of fibrinogen to fibrin monomer occurs by limited proteolysis, the recurrent theme of coagulation. Fibrinogen is a long, thin molecule composed of three pairs of chains—Aα, Bβ, and γ—tied together at their C-terminal ends by a group of disulfide bonds known as the *disulfide knot*. Thrombin acts on fibrinogen by splitting pieces off the N-terminal ends of the Aα- and Bβ-chains (Fig. 13-7). With the release of these pieces, known as *fibrinopeptide A* and *fibrinopeptide B*, the fibrinogen is converted to fibrin monomer,

which polymerizes spontaneously to form the initial clot.

The cross-linking enzyme also circulates as an inactive precursor. This precursor, factor XIII, is converted to factor XIIIa by thrombin. factor XIIIa forms cross-links between the outer ends of the fibrin molecules by replacing the —NH$_2$ of a glutamine in one of its constituents chains with the ε-amino group of a lysine in an adjacent chain (Fig. 13-8). The γ-chains are cross-linked first, then later the α-chains. The exchange of glutamine amino groups is known as *transglutamination*; factor XIIIa is referred to as a *tranglutaminase*.

The Clotting Cascade in Summary

The clotting cascade is clearly a complex subject that may be hard to grasp in toto on the first or even second reading. The process can

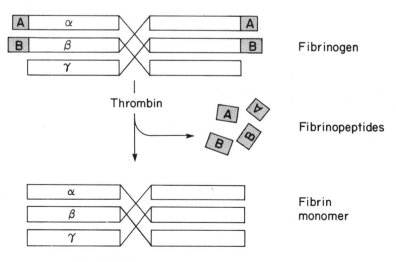

Fig. 13-7. Cleavage of fibrinogen by thrombin.

Fig. 13-8. Transglutamination.

be summarized, however, by the following two statements, which may serve as guides through the maze and may assist in explaining the basis for the various tests used in evaluating the clotting cascade:

1. Up through the activation of factor X, the clotting cascade actually consists of a pair of activation sequences that run in parallel. One comprises the sequence

$$(XIIa, kallikrein) \rightarrow XIa \rightarrow IXa \rightarrow Xa$$

This sequence is called the intrinsic pathway, because it is triggered by factors intrinsic to (i.e., present in) the plasma. The other consists of the sequence

$$Tissue factor \rightarrow VIIa \rightarrow Xa$$

This sequence is referred to as the extrinsic pathway, because it is triggered by tissue factor, which is extrinsic to the plasma. Apart from the single crossover reaction

$$VIIa \rightarrow IXa$$

the intrinsic and extrinsic pathways represent completely separate activating tracks. From factor X on, of course, there is only the single common track:

$$Xa \rightarrow IIa \rightarrow clot$$

These sequences are summarized in Figure 13-9.

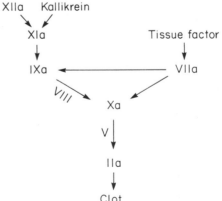

Fig. 13-9. Clotting cascade. The cascade consists of two separate activating pathways—the intrinsic pathway and the extrinsic pathway—which converge to a common pathway at factor X. Except for factors V and VIII, all the clotting factors named in this diagram are proteases.

2. Calcium and phospholipid are necessary for almost all the steps in the initial and intermediate stages. The only exceptions are the activation of factor IX by XIa, which requires only Ca^{2v}, and the reactions of the contact phase, which require neither.

Testing the Cascade

The methods for testing the cascade are summarized in Table 13-2.

Screening Tests

Screening tests for the clotting cascade are carried out on plasma in which clotting has been prevented by a calcium-sequestering agent—citrate or oxalate. The cascade is initiated by adding calcium plus an activating agent, and the time required for the formation of a clot is measured. There are three such tests, each using a different activating agent and each examining a different portion of the cascade: partial thromboplastin time (PTT), prothrombin time (PT), and thrombin time (TT).

Partial Thromboplastin Time

For the PTT test, activation is accomplished by a negatively charged surface: the glass wall of a test tube or (for the so-called activated PTT) a contact activator such as finely divided kaolin, a form of clay. Phospholipid is also added. This test measures the intrinsic system and the common track.

Prothrombin Time

For the PT test, tissue thromboplastin, which contains phospholipid plus tissue factor, is used as the activating agent. This test measures factor VII and the common track.

Thrombin Time

In the TT test, thrombin is the activating agent. This test measures the sequence: fibrinogen→fibrin monomer→initial clot.

The end point for each of these tests is the production of the initial clot. Therefore, none of these tests measures factor XIII, although among them they measure all the other factors in the clotting cascade.

Specific Factors

Fibrinogen

Fibrinogen is usually measured as thrombin-clottable protein. Enough thrombin is added to convert all the fibrinogen to fibrin, and the amount of protein in the resulting fibrin clot is determined by one of a variety of techniques.

Table 13-2. Testing the Clotting Cascade

Method	Component Tested	Test
Screening tests	Intrinsic and common pathways VII and the common pathway Fibrinogen → clot	Partial thromboplastin time Prothrombin time Thrombin time
Specific factors	Fibrinogen XIII Other factors	Thrombin-clottable protein Solubility of clot in urea or $ClCH_2\,COOH$ PT or PTT of test plasma mixed with plasmas deficient in known factors Immunoassay
Inhibitors		PT or PTT of test plasma mixed with normal plasma

Fibrinogen can also be determined by immunological and precipitation methods; these measure the factor by its structure, not its function.

Factor XIII

The initial clot, held together only by weak noncovalent forces, is soluble in mild denaturing agents, whereas a clot cross-linked by factor XIIIa is not. The solubility of a clot in a solution of a mild denaturant (urea or monochloroacetic acid) is therefore used to measure factor XIII.

Other Factors

A PT or PTT may be prolonged because of a deficiency in a specific clotting factor. Such a test would be fully corrected by mixing the deficient plasma with an equal volume of normal plasma, or of a second plasma lacking a different clotting factor, but would remain uncorrected if the second plasma were lacking the same clotting factor that was missing from the first. A clotting factor deficiency can therefore be diagnosed by showing that an abnormal PT or PTT is corrected by all but one of a panel of plasmas with known deficiencies: The unknown plasma and the plasma that fails to correct the test are missing the same clotting factor.

The concentration of the deficient clotting factor, an important consideration in the treatment of clotting factor deficiencies, can be determined from the PT or PTT using a standard curve obtained with mixtures of normal plasma and plasma with a known deficiency. The concentration of a clotting factor can also be determined by immunological testing. Clotting factor concentrations as measured by immunological testing often agree with concentrations as measured functionally (i.e., by the PT or PTT), but sometimes there is a discrepancy, with the immunological concentration exceeding the functional concentration. Such a dis-crepancy indicates the presence of an abnormal clotting factor that is antigenically close to normal but functionally defective.

Inhibitors

When an abnormal screening test fails to be corrected by mixing the defective plasma with an equal volume of normal plasma, the presence of an inhibitor is indicated. The potency of the inhibitor can be determined by measuring the effect of various concentrations of the inhibitor-containing plasma on the clotting properties of normal plasma. Identifying which factor(s) the inhibitor acts against may be difficult, however, because both the PT and the PTT depend on the activation of many factors, and an inhibitor acting against any one of them will prolong the test. Fortunately, identification of the inhibited factor can usually be accomplished through special assay techniques.

Bleeding Time

The bleeding time, a crude but valuable screening test, is performed by measuring how long it takes for bleeding to stop from a fresh cut of defined size. The cut is ordinarily made on the inner surface of the forearm, its length and depth being fixed by means of a template. A prolonged bleeding time usually indicates a platelet disorder (qualitative or quantitative); very occasionally, it may be caused by an abnormality of small blood vessels (e.g., scurvy). In pure disorders of the clotting cascade, the bleeding time is almost invariably normal.

BIOSYNTHESIS OF CLOTTING FACTORS

The liver is the site of biosynthesis of most clotting factors. Factor VIII is synthesized in parts, one portion coming from endothelium and megakaryocytes and the rest being pro-

Clotting Factors Made in the Liver

Fibrinogen

II (Prothrombin)[a]

V

VII[a]

VIII

IX[a]

X[a]

XIII

---

[a] Require vitamin K for their production

Fig. 13-11. Formation of gla from a glutamic acid residue.

quires vitamin K. It will be seen that the drugs most commonly used for long-term therapeutic anticoagulation act by interfering with this reaction.

Vitamin K is also required for the production of two anticoagulant proteins: protein C and protein S.

REGULATION OF CLOTTING

The clotting process is regulated by two general mechanisms: the elimination of activated clotting factors and the destruction of the fibrin clot.

Elimination of Activated Clotting Factors

Activated clotting factors are rapidly removed from the circulation by the liver. They may also be directly inactivated in the plasma

duced in many kinds of cells. (For a full explanation of the makeup of factor VIII, see the discussion of von Willebrand's disease in Ch. 14). It is not known where the remaining clotting factors are made.

A lipid-soluble vitamin, vitamin K (Fig. 13-10), is required for the production of four of the clotting factors made in the liver: factors II (prothrombin), VII, IX, and X. The N-terminal (activation peptide) portions of all four of these clotting factors contain a series of γ-carboxyglutamyl (gla) residues that appear to function in calcium binding. The gla residues are not incorporated into the proteins during translation, but rather are produced by the post-translational addition of CO_2 to selected glutamate residues in the protein chain (Fig. 13-11). It is this carboxylation reaction that re-

Fig. 13-10. Vitamin K. R, a long hydrocarbon side

Elimination of Clotting Factors from the Blood

Clearance by the liver

Inactivation by
Antithrombin III (proteases except VIIa)
Protein C (thrombin-activated V and VIII)

by two circulating anticoagulant systems: the antithrombin III (AT III)/proteoglycan system and the protein C/protein S system.

AT III

A protease inhibitor, AT III works by combining with the clotting factor to form an extremely stable, inactive 1:1 complex (Fig. 13-12). It acts against all the proteolytic clotting factors except VIIa (Fig. 13-9). Its importance in vivo is shown by the fact that persons with an inherited deficiency of AT III are highly susceptible to thrombosis on the venous side of the circulation.

The action of AT III is greatly potentiated by binding to certain proteoglycans. These include *endothelial cell proteoglycans*, which bind AT III to line the inner surfaces of blood vessels with a layer of anticoagulant, and *heparin*, an anticoagulant drug that works through its interaction with AT III.

Protein C and Protein S

Protein C is a vitamin-K-dependent protein that neutralizes factors V and VIII by limited proteolysis. Like the clotting factors, protein C circulates as an inert precursor and must itself be activated before it can function as an anticoagulant. Activation is accomplished by a limited proteolytic reaction in which thrombin

is the active protease. Before it can act on protein C, however, thrombin has to be modulated in a such a way as to alter its substrate specificity. Modulation is accomplished by thrombomodulin, an endothelial cell protein that forms a complex with thrombin, eliminating its coagulant activity and at the same time endowing it with a protein C-converting activity that it lacks when free. Because protein C can only function after being activated by thrombin, its effect tends to be limited to regions where active clotting is taking place.

Activated protein C then destroys the activity of factors V and VIII. To carry out this task, the activated protein C combines with Ca^{2+}, phospholipid, and another vitamin-K-dependent protein known as protein S to form what might be termed a "factor V/VIII inactivating complex" (Fig. 13-13). This complex, containing a protease (activated protein C) and an accelerator (protein S), plus Ca^{2+} and phospholipid, is completely analogous to the factor X- and prothrombin-converting complexes described above. The "factor V/VIII inactivating complex" inactivates these factors by limited proteolysis.

Protein C is complementary to AT III, working on nonproteolytic clotting factors against which AT III has no effect. Patients deficient in either protein C or protein S have a greatly increased risk of venous thrombosis. In infants homozygous for protein C or protein S deficiency, this is expressed as *purpura fulminans*, a rapidly spreading hemorrhagic ne-

Fig. 13-12. The mechanism of action of antithrombin III.

Fig. 13-13. Inactivation of factors V and VIII by protein C. Thrombin liberated in the vicinity of a clot attaches to thrombomodulin on the surface of an endothelial cell. When it binds to thrombomodulin, thrombin acquires the ability to activate protein C. The activated protein C combines with protein S, Ca^{2+} and phospholipid to form a "factor V/VIII inactivating complex" that destroys the activities of factors V and VIII by proteolysis.

crosis of the skin that is often fatal. This indicates that, like AT III, protein C and protein S have important roles in the prevention of coagulation in vivo.

Fibrinolysis

As important as the formation of a clot at a site of injury is its removal when its usefulness is over. The clot is removed by enzymatic digestion, a process referred to as *fibrinolysis*.

Plasmin and Fibrin-Split Products

Fibrinolysis is accomplished by a fibrin-splitting protease called *plasmin*. This enzyme is produced in the vicinity of a clot by limited proteolysis of plasminogen, its circulating precursor. Plasminogen is converted to plasmin by two activators: tissue plasminogen activator, which initiates clot lysis by activating plasminogen bound to the fibrin in the clot (it has little effect on circulating plasminogen); and urokinase, which keeps hollow organs (e.g., the ureter) free from clots. Both are secreted in active form by appropriately stimulated endothelial cells and mononuclear phago-

cytes, and urokinase is secreted by epithelial cells as well. The route of plasmin formation is shown in Figure 13-14.

The activities of both tissue plasminogen activator and plasmin itself are regulated by specific inhibitors: tissue plasminogen activator inhibitor and α_2-antiplasmin, respectively. The physiological importance of α_2-antiplasmin is demonstrated by the very severe bleeding disorder that occurs in patients lacking this protein.

The digestion by plasmin of an individual fibrin molecule takes place in an orderly manner (Fig. 13-15). Plasmin first releases the outer portions of the α-chains, producing the so-called X fragment. This fragment is then split on one side of the disulfide knot into a D (small) and a Y (large) fragment. A similar cleavage on the other side of the disulfide knot releases a second D fragment, leaving behind a small piece known as the E fragment.

When digesting a clot, plasmin cuts the covalently linked fibrin polymers in the same places: at the outer portions of the α-chains and next to the disulfide knots. The fragments of polymer cut away by the plasmin are released from the clot as fibrin-degradation products (FDPs) [or fibrin-split products (FSPs)]. Some of these fragments are identical to those

Fig. 13-14. Formation of plasmin.

produced by the digestion of an individual fibrin molecule. Many, however, are larger, containing portions of two or more fibrin molecules. These are produced when fragments are released from the polymer by cuts in two separate fibrin units (Fig. 13–15).

Fig. 13-15. Digestion of fibrin by plasmin. (**Top**) Digestion of a single molecule. (**Bottom**) Digestion of a cross-linked clot.

Fibrin-split products are potent inhibitors of clotting. They impair coagulation through two mechanisms, both based on their close similarity to fibrin and fibrinogen:

1. They interfere with the action of thrombin by binding to thrombin at its fibrinogen-binding site.

2. They interfere with the polymerization of fibrin monomers by forming monomer-split product complexes. Some of these complexes remain in solution; others bind abnormally to the growing clot, weakening its structure.

Normally, the quantities of fibrin-split products in the blood are too small to affect coagulation. In certain conditions, however, they can increase sufficiently to cause clinical bleeding through their anticoagulant action.

Plasmin also degrades other proteins of the clotting cascade. The most important of these is fibrinogen, but plasmin also acts to destroy factors V and VIII.

Measuring Fibrinolysis

Although fibrinolysis in the normal person is so slow as to be undetectable, there are diseases in which it is greatly accelerated. Accelerated fibrinolysis can be diagnosed by demonstrating the presence of fibrin-split products in the serum or by finding increased plasminogen activation in the circulation.

Fibrin-Split Products

Like other anticoagulants, fibrin-split products cause abnormalities in the screening assays (PT, PTT, and especially TT); their presence may be suspected on that basis. To confirm their presence, two types of tests are used: paracoagulation, and direct measurements.

Paracoagulation. Ethanol or protamine gelation paracoagulation tests depend on the fact that fibrin-split products can form soluble complexes with fibrin monomers, preventing the bound monomers from polymerizing into a fibrin clot. When ethanol or protamine is added to serum containing such complexes, the complexes fall apart, releasing their fibrin monomers. The liberated monomers polymerize in a normal fashion, forming a visible clot. This is known as paracoagulation. It is a quick but indirect way of demonstrating that fibrin-split products are present in a serum sample.

Direct Measurements. There are several ways to measure the levels of fibrin-split products in serum directly. The most widely used are the Staphylococcus clumping assay, which is based on the ability of fibrin-split products to agglutinate *Staphylococcus aureus*, and an immunological assay, which uses an antibody against the split products.

Euglobulin Lysis Time

This test determines whether the plasma contains any circulating activators of the fibrinolytic system (i.e., plasminogen activators) (Fig. 13–16). It takes advantage of the fact that when plasma is treated with dilute acid, fibrinogen precipitates out, carrying with it (1) other clotting factors, and (2) the components of the fibrinolytic system (plasmin, plasminogen, and any circulating plasminogen activators), but leaving behind circulating inhibitors of the fibrinolytic system. This precipitate, known as the *euglobulin fraction*, can be isolated and redissolved in neutral buffer containing a calcium-binding anticoagulant. When excess calcium is added to this solution of euglobulin fraction, the clotting factors act on fibrinogen to produce a fibrin clot. This clot will dissolve over the next few hours if plasminogen activators are present, because of the unopposed action of the plasmin newly generated by the activators during the period of incubation. The rate at which the clot dissolves is closely related to the quantity of circulating plasminogen activators present in the original

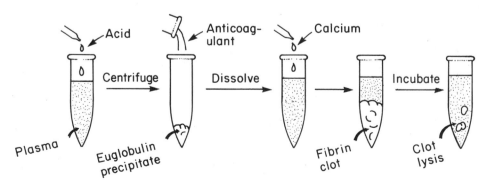

Fig. 13-16. Euglobulin lysis time.

plasma. The time required for the euglobulin precipitate to dissolve, a period referred to as the *euglobulin lysis time*, is thus a measure of the fibrinolytic activity of the plasma; the shorter the euglobulin lysis time, the greater the fibrinolytic activity.

DISORDERS OF THE CLOTTING CASCADE

Inherited Disorders

Hemophilia

Hemophilia A (hereinafter referred to as hemophilia) is a clotting disorder caused by an inherited deficiency of factor VIII. In some instances, the factor VIII deficiency is caused by an absolute reduction in the amount of circulating factor VIII; in others it is caused by the production of normal quantities of a defective clotting factor. hemophilia is both the most common and the most serious of the inherited disorders of the clotting cascade.

Hemophilia is transmitted in an X-linked manner. This means that the disease is seen almost exclusively in males, although it is transmitted by both carrier mothers and affected fathers. The pattern of transmission (Fig. 13-17) guarantees that the sons of a carrier mother have a 50:50 chance of having hemophilia. A hemophiliac male can only transmit the condition to his daughers, all of whom will be carriers. Carriers of hemophilia are usually recognized by virtue of the fact that they have had a hemophiliac child, but it is sometimes possible to identify them before this occurs.

Clinical Manifestations

Intractable bleeding is the problem in hemophilia. It is seen after injury, of course, but it can occur spontaneously in otherwise healthy patients. The sites affected by spontaneous bleeding are characteristic (Fig. 13-18):

Joints. The large joints—especially the hip, knee, and ankle—are the sites most commonly involved in a spontaneous bleed. The affected joint swells and becomes extremely painful over the course of a few hours. Because the joint is a closed space, the bleeding eventually stops, so signs and symptoms regress over several days. Recurrent bleeding is the rule, however, eventually leading to a crippling arthritis caused by repeated joint injury.

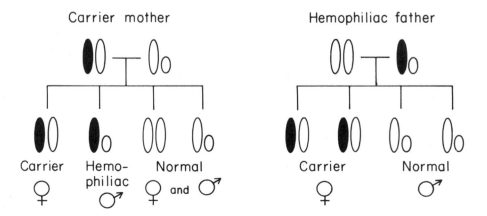

Fig. 13-17. Transmission of hemophilia. X and Y chromosomes of the parents and children are shown. Defective X chromosomes are black.

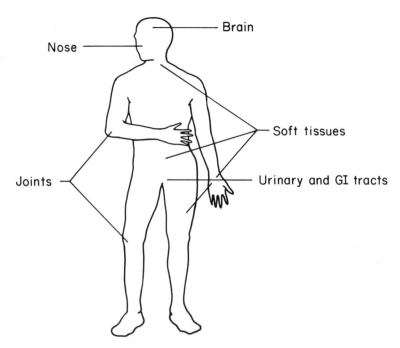

Fig. 13-18. Sites of spontaneous bleeding in hemophilia.

Soft Tissues. Spontaneous bleeding into soft tissues may take place. Seepage of blood may continue for hours or days, with the gradual development of a massive hematoma. The diagnosis is made on the basis of the presence of a growing mass (demonstrated by physical examination or scan) along with signs of blood loss (falling hematocrit and shock). Symptoms of compression may also occur, depending on the site of the bleed. Hemorrhage into the iliopsoas muscle, for example, can cause an entrapment syndrome affecting the nerves of the lumbar plexus. One of the most dangerous places for a soft-tissue bleed is the base of the tongue, because of the possibility of death from asphyxia owing to closure of the pharynx.

Other Problems. Nosebleeds and urinary bleeding are common, although not especially dangerous, in patients with hemophilia. Gastrointestinal (GI) bleeding, either spontaneous or from a lesion in the GI tract, is a moderately frequent complication. A particularly dangerous problem is bleeding into the brain, a frequent cause of death in hemophilia. *Headaches and head injuries, however mild they may seem, have to be taken extremely seriously in these patients.*

Bleeding after trauma is also a problem. A major injury such as that resulting from an automobile accident causes massive bleeding that must be stopped to prevent death from exsanguination. Minor injuries, however, may also result in extensive blood loss. For example, a small cut in a hemophiliac will typically stop bleeding after a few minutes as a result of arteriolar constriction and the formation of a platelet plug, but will then begin to bleed again a few hours later and continue to leak blood in a slow, steady trickle for days. The amount of blood that can be lost from a slow leak should not be underestimated; unstanched bleeding at the seemingly trivial rate of 0.5 ml/min represents a loss of 3 units/day.

The clinical severity of the disease varies from patient to patient depending on the factor VIII level, which tends to remain constant in a given hemophiliac. Patients whose factor VIII level is greater than 5 percent of normal have few problems with spontaneous bleeds or minor injuries. As the factor VIII level drops, the severity of the disease increases. The worst problems are seen in patients whose factor VIII level is less than 1 percent of normal.

A complication that poses great difficulties for the management of the disease is the appearance of a so-called inducible inhibitor. Inhibitors are factor VIII-neutralizing antibodies that develop in about 10 percent of patients with hemophilia. One-half of these are "stable" inhibitors whose levels remain constant over time. The other half are referred to as "inducible" inhibitors because their levels respond anamnestically to factor VIII treatment, rising sharply within a few days after replacement therapy is started and remaining at elevated levels for weeks or months thereafter. The problems of treating hemophiliacs with inducible inhibitors are discussed below.

Management

Hemophilia is suspected in a patient with a history of bleeding, especially spontaneous bleeding and most especially spontaneous bleeding into a joint. Male sex and a family history are of course highly suggestive, although hemophilia is seen from time to time in females and will occasionally occur sporadically, the result, it is thought, of a spontaneous mutation.

In the laboratory, the only abnormal screening test is a prolonged PTT. The bleeding time is normal, but bleeding from the cut is likely to resume after an hour or so. The diagnosis is made by showing that factor VIII is decreased. In making the diagnosis, it is important not simply to demonstrate the deficiency, but to determine the level of the clotting factor as well, because the severity of the disease depends critically on the degree of the deficiency. Laboratory data can also help identify carriers. Molecular genetic techniques (see Ch. 10) for carrier identification and prenatal diag-

---

Diagnosing Hemophilia in the Laboratory

Patient
> PTT prolonged
> VIII activity greatly reduced

Carrier
> Normal clotting screen
> VIII activity moderately reduced
> VIII activity/VIII antigen about half normal
> Diagnostic restriction fragment length polymorphisms

---

nosis are under development, but are not yet available to practicing physicians. It is sometimes possible to identify a carrier, not absolutely, but with a high probability, by demonstrating intermediate levels of factor VIII activity in a female relative of a hemophiliac. An even more reliable way of diagnosing the carrier state depends on measuring the "factor VIII antigen" as well as the factor VIII clotting activity. Unfortunately, the term "factor VIII antigen" does not refer to the factor VIII coagulant protein. It refers instead to another circulating protein, the von Willebrand factor, one of whose functions seems to be to stabilize the real factor VIII in the blood (which is how it got the name "factor VIII antigen"). This confusing state of affairs is discussed more fully in Chapter 14. With respect to the detection of the carrier state, the important point is that the factor VIII clotting activity: factor VIII antigen ratio is much more constant from person to person than is the absolute level of factor VIII clotting activity. This ratio is therefore a much more reliable indicator of carrier status than the factor VIII level; as a result, a carrier can sometimes be identified from her activity:antigen ratio (usually about half-normal) even when her factor VIII activity is in the ambiguous "low-normal" range. When the measurements are made with care, the activity:antigen ratio can detect five carriers out of six.

The treatment of hemophilia involves replacement therapy with factor VIII concentrates; it is generally based on the principle that factor VIII is given when, and only when, bleeding occurs. Two types of concentrates are currently in use: cryoprecipitate, which in addition to factor VIII contains fibrinogen and von Willebrand factor, and purified factor VIII, which contains little of either. Minor bleeds may be treated at home by the patient, who has been taught how to administer the concentrate and keeps a supply in his refrigerator. Home therapy has resulted in much better control of minor bleeds, because patients are instructed to treat themselves at the first sign of bleeding. As a result, severe hemarthroses are much less common than they used to be and crippling arthritis is no longer an inevitable outcome of hemophilia. In patients with mild hemophilia, minor bleeds can also be treated with desmopressin (DDAVP), a vasopressin analogue that increases plasma factor VIII levels by stimulating the secretion of "Factor VIII antigen" (see above) by the endothelium.

Major bleeds usually require hospitalization. The approach to therapy is to administer enough factor VIII concentrate so that the plasma factor VIII always remains above a fixed level, the exact value of which depends on the severity of the bleed. To do this it is necessary to know how rapidly factor VIII disappears from the circulation. The half-life of factor VIII averages about 12 hours, but it is generally a good idea to measure the half-life in the patient by giving him an infusion of concentrate and measuring factor VIII levels before and at various times after the infusion is administered. From this measured half-life and the patient's plasma volume (estimated at 40 ml/kg) the dose of factor VIII can be calculated. The dose is checked and adjusted if necessary by measuring factor VIII levels during the course of therapy. Factor VIII is generally given two or three times a day; treatment for a major bleed may need to be continued for 10 days to 2 weeks. These same principles apply to factor VIII coverage for surgery.

A recent complication of replacement therapy is the occurrence of acquired immune deficiency syndrome (AIDS) in patients with hemophilia. With the spread of AIDS (which became epidemic in the middle 1970s), the factor VIII supply, produced from thousands of units of pooled plasma, became widely contaminated with HIV (human immunodeficiency virus, the cause of AIDS). As a result, most patients with hemophilia are now infected with HIV, and the majority will probably die of AIDS. The factor VIII supply is now much safer than before, because ways have been developed to eliminate HIV from factor VIII preparations without destroying the clotting factor, but the years of HIV contamination have left a tragic legacy.

Certain strict caveats apply to the management of hemophilia. Drugs that inhibit platelet function (e.g., aspirin) are strictly contraindicated. Venipuncture is usually not a problem, but biopsies, including bone marrow aspiration, must not be performed without factor VIII coverage.

What about the patient who has an inhibitor? If the inhibitor is stable, treatment is the same, except that the dose of concentrate must be high enough to overcome the inhibitor and provide therapeutic levels of factor VIII. If the inhibitor is inducible, the whole approach to treatment changes. With a high level of inhibitor, the best chance for hemostasis is offered by preparations containing activated clotting factors, although these carry with them the hazards of hepatitis and venous thromboembolism, and they are exceedingly expensive (treatment can cost thousands of dollars a day). If such a preparation is not available, very large doses of factor VIII concentrate may be used; neutralization of factor VIII by the antibody requires a certain amount of time, so the rapid administration of large doses of concentrate may permit a small amount of active factor VIII to reach the bleeding site and exert its effect. If the inhibitor level is low, treatment with more or less standard doses of concentrate is likely to be effective, at least until the inhibitor level begins to rise, at which time treatment will have to be changed unless the bleeding has stopped. Hemarthrosis is treated by immobilization, ice packs, and analgesics. Factor VIII is avoided if at all possible, because the induction of the inhibitor poses worse problems than does a blood-filled joint. The ideal treatment, of course, would be the elimination of the inhibitor. This has not been possible by plasmapheresis or immunosuppressive therapy; one current approach, still experimental, is to attempt to eliminate the antibody by inducing tolerance through the long-term administration of factor VIII. The treatment of hemophilia is summarized below.

Factor IX Deficiency (Hemophilia B; Christmas Disease)

Factor IX deficiency is about one-fifth as common as factor VIII deficiency. Clinically, the two diseases are virtually identical; both

---

Treatment of Hemophilia

No inhibitor
  Cryoprecipitate or purified factor VIII
  Home therapy for minor bleeds
  DDAVP for mild hemophilia

Inhibitor present
  Stable
    Replacement at doses sufficient to overcome the inhibitor
  Inducible
    Low level: standard doses of purified factor VIII
    High level (initial, or after induction): Activated clotting factors, or very high doses of purified factor VIII
    Hemarthrosis: no replacement; immobilization and local measures

Contraindicated
  Aspirin and other antiplatelet drugs
  Biopsy or other invasive procedures without factor VIII coverage

---

are X-linked, and both show the same patterns of bleeding. Treatment is with a concentrate (prothrombin concentrate) that contains the vitamin-K-dependent clotting factors: II, VII, IX, and X.

Contact Factor Deficiencies

The contact factors are Hageman factor (XII), prekallikrein, and high-molecular-weight kininogen. Deficiencies of each of these factors have been described; XII deficiency is the most common. These deficiencies are laboratory diseases, presenting as an isolated prolongation of the PTT and a reduction in the level of the deficient factor. There is no clinical bleeding tendency whatsoever. Indeed, Mr. Hageman, the patient who lent his name to the clotting factor that was missing from his blood, died of pulmonary embolism at a ripe old age.

Dysfibrinogenemias

The hereditary dysfibrinogenemias are diseases in which normal quantities of a defective fibrinogen circulate in the bloodstream. The defect is expressed functionally as an abnormality involving one or another of the steps leading from circulating fibrinogen to the cross-linked fibrin clot. Patients with a dysfibrinogenemia may be clinically normal, or they may show a mild tendency toward either bleeding or venous thrombosis. The typical laboratory findings are a prolonged thrombin time and a disparity between the fibrinogen levels as determined by different techniques, those measuring thrombin-clottable protein giving lower values than those measuring fibrinogen itself (immunological or precipitation methods).

Others

The inherited clotting factor deficiencies are listed in Table 13-3. The mode of transmission and features unique to each disorder are also

Table 13-3. Inherited Clotting Factor Disorders

Deficiency	Transmission[a]	Special Features	Treatment
Fibrinogen	A	Bleeding from umbilical stump; poor wound healing	Cryoprecipitate or purified fibrinogen
Prothrombin	A	Screening tests may be normal	Plasma or prothrombin concentrate
Factor V	A	Bleeding time may be prolonged	Fresh frozen plasma
Factor VII	A	PTT normal, PT prolonged	Plasma or prothrombin concentrate
Factor VIII	X		Cryoprecipitate or purified Factor VIII
Factor IX	X		Prothrombin concentrate
Factor XI	A	Usually mild	Plasma
Contact factors	A	No clinical manifestations	None needed
Factor XIII	A	Bleeding from umbilical stump; poor wound healing. Screening tests always normal	Plasma

a A, Autosomal recessive, X, X-linked.

given. A point worth noting is that the screening tests (PTT, PT, TT, and bleeding time) are invariably normal in factor XIII deficiency and are sometimes normal in prothrombin deficiency.

ACQUIRED DISORDERS

Vitamin K Deficiency

Vitamin K deficiency causes a bleeding disorder that results from impaired production of the vitamin-K-dependent clotting factors: II (prothrombin), VII, IX, and X. The causes of vitamin K deficiency are listed below. The deficiency is most often seen in conditions associated with the malabsorption of fat (e.g., chronic pancreatitis, biliary cirrhosis, sprue), but it may occasionally result from malnutrition, especially in the elderly or in patients receiving oral antibiotics whose alternative source of the vitamin (intestinal bacteria, which provide small amount of vitamin K to all of us) has been destroyed. In the newborn, vitamin K levels are marginal, and any factors that impose an additional stress on vitamin K metabolism (e.g., postpartum malnutrition or hypoxia during delivery with damage to an already immature liver) can lead to frank vitamin K deficiency and hemorrhagic disease of the newborn. Finally, certain anticoagulants are antagonists of vitamin K and give rise to a clotting disorder identical to that of vitamin K deficiency.

The outstanding abnormality on laboratory testing is a prolonged PT. The PTT may also be prolonged, although it is generally not as abnormal as the prothrombin time. Other tests are normal except for decreased levels of the vitamin-K-dependent clotting factors. It is usually not necessary to measure these, however; a PT that corrects within 2 days after vitamin K treatment confirms the diagnosis.

The deficiency is treated by giving vitamin K. Oral treatment is usually good enough, but parenteral therapy is occasionally necessary

---

Causes of Vitamin K Deficiency

Malabsorption of fat

Malnutrition
  In the elderly
  In patients receiving oral antibiotics

Newborn

Anticoagulation with vitamin K antagonists

in patients with malabsorption. Hemorrhagic disease of the newborn is prevented by the routine administration of the vitamin to all newborns. The response to treatment is exceedingly rapid; in the absence of other diseases, the clotting defect will be fully corrected within 2 days. Management of vitamin K deficiency is summarized below.

Liver Disease

Liver disease causes a very complex acquired coagulopathy affecting virtually every segment of the clotting cascade. The coagulopathy results mainly from a failure of clotting factor production by the diseased liver, but it also reflects the release of an abnormal clotting factor, as well as the failure of the liver to clear certain coagulation-related proteins from the blood. Specifically:

1. Failure of clotting factor production leads to falls in factor II (prothrombin), V, VII, IX, and X, as well as a fall in prekallikrein. Fibrinogen falls as well, but this appears to be caused primarily by increased fibrinolysis (see point 3).

2. A functionally abnormal fibrinogen is produced that contains insufficient quantities of sialic acid. This amounts to an acquired dysfibrinogenemia.

3. Clearance of activated clotting factors (IXa, Xa, and XIa) is impaired, as is the clearance of plasminogen activator. The latter is the

cause of the increased fibrinolysis that is so typical of liver disease. In addition to these, platelets are decreased, mainly because of the splenomegaly that is a common concomitant of liver disease.

Because of the comprehensive nature of the clotting disorder, virtually every test of coagulation is abnormal. The specific abnormalities and their probable causes are listed in Table 13-4. It will be seen that these abnormalities are virtually indistinguishable from those caused by disseminated intravascular coagulation (DIC), a condition common in seriously ill patients. Attempts to make the diagnosis of DIC in the presence of severe liver disease are usually in vain.

As to treatment, any patient with liver disease should be given a single large dose of vitamin K on the change that vitamin K deficiency is a contributing factor, but improvement after a dose of vitamin K is rare. The mainstay of treatment is replacement therapy. This is only used in patients who are actively bleeding. Fresh frozen plasma is given (fresh frozen plasma contains all the clotting factors deficient in liver disease), along with platelets if the patient is sufficiently thrombocytopenic. Replacement is only a stopgap measure; improvement, although frequent, is transient, often lasting only a few hours before additional replacement is needed. The only definitive treatment of the coagulopathy is cure of the underlying liver disease.

Acquired Anticoagulants (Circulating Inhibitors)

The acquired anticoagulants of clinical significance are listed in the box on the next page. Their presence is suspected from mixing studies.

The lupus anticoagulant is an antibody that recognizes certain phospholipids. This anticoagulant is sometimes seen in patients with lupus erythematosus, the prototypical auto-immune disease. It also appears from time to

---

Management of Vitamin K Deficiency

Diagnosis
Prolonged prothrombin time corrected by vitamin K

Treatment
Replacement with vitamin K

Table 13-4. Clotting Disorder in Liver Failure

Abnormality	Explanation
Long prothrombin time	Deficiency of vitamin K-dependent clotting factors; presence of fibrin-split products
Long partial thromboplastin time	Deficiency of II, V, IX, prekallikrein; presence of fibrin-split products
Long thrombin time	Presence of fibrin-split products; abnormal fibrinogen
Long bleeding time	Decreased platelets
Low fibrinogen	
Increased fibrin-split products	Increased fibrinolysis
Shortened euglobulin lysis time	

Acquired Anticoagulants

Lupus anticoagulant

Fibrin-split products

Anti-factor VIII in hemophilia

Abnormal immunoglobulins in multiple myeloma and related diseases

Anticoagulant drugs

time in the elderly, and occasionally in pregnant women, in whom it can cause repeated spontaneous abortions. The lupus anticoagulant rarely causes clinical problems, and those it causes are related to thrombosis, not hemorrhage. Most often it is solely a laboratory disease, presenting as a prolonged PTT not corrected by normal plasma. An inhibitor found by accident in a patient with no clinical bleeding disorder is usually the lupus anticoagulant.

Other acquired anticoagulants are discussed in Chapters 15 and 16.

SUGGESTED READINGS

Antonarakis, S.E. The molecular genetics of hemophilia A and B in man. Factor VIII and factor IX deficiency. Adv. Hum. Genet. *17*:27.

Clouse, L.H. & Comp. P.C. (1986) The regulation of hemostasis: The protein C system. New Engl. J. Med. *314*:1298.

Furie, B. & Furie, B.C. (1988) The molecular basis of blood coagulation. Cell *53*:505.

Hoyer, L.W. (1981) The factor VIII complex: Structure and function. Blood *58*:1.

Jackson, C.M. & Nemerson, Y. (1980) Blood coagulation. Annu. Rev. Biochem. *49*:767.

Jones, P. (1977) Developments and problems in the management of hemophilia. Semin. Hematol. *14*:375.

Kane, W.H. & Davie, E.W. (1988) Blood coagulation factors V and VIII: Structural and functional similarities and their relationship to hemorrhagic and thrombotic disorders. Blood *71*:539.

Kaplan, A.P. (1978) Initiation of the intrinsic coagulation and fibrinolytic pathways of man. Prog. Hemost. Thromb. *4*:127.

Kaplan, A.P. & Silverberg, M. (1987) The coagulation-kinin pathway of human plasma. Blood *70*:1.

Kasper, C.K. (1989) Treatment of factor VIII inhibitors. Prog. Hemost. Thromb. *9*:57.

Mann, K.G. (1987) The assembly of blood clotting complexes on membranes. Trends Biochem. Sci. *12*:229.

Nemerson, Y. (1988) Tissue factor and hemostasis. Blood *71*:1.

Shapiro, S.S. & Thiagarajan, P. 1982) Lupus anticoagulants. Prog. Hemost. Thromb. 6:263–285.

White, G.C. & Shoemaker, C.B. (1989) Factor VIII gene and hemophilia A. Blood *73*:1.

Platelets

Platelets are small cell fragments that circulate in the bloodstream. They are produced by the disintegration of megakaryocytes, the large precursor cells found in the bone marrow. Platelets play an indispensable role in coagulation, plugging breaches in small blood vessels and helping initiate the processes of repair in injured tissues.

NORMAL PLATELETS

Platelet Structure

Platelets in the circulation are disc-shaped objects about one-fifth the diameter of a red cell (Fig. 14-1). Their shape is maintained by a ring of microtubules at the margin of the disc. Of special importance to their hemostatic function are the plasma membrane, granules, and the canalicular system.

The Plasma Membrane

The plasma membrane contains a number of glycoproteins that function in the interactions of platelets with external surfaces as well as receptors for exogenous activators (including thrombin) and for the von Willebrand factor. On stimulation of the platelet, receptors for fibrinogen and factor V appear in the membrane; a stimulated platelet moves in a cloud of clotting factors.

Granules

The platelet contains three types of granules: the α-granules, the dense granules, and the lysosomes. Each granule consists of a packet of materials wrapped within a single layer of membrane. The contents differ by granule class. On activation of the platelet, the α- and dense granules release their contents into the external environment. This degranulation event is of great importance with respect to damage control by platelets.

The Canalicular System

The canalicular system of tubules extends inward from the outer surface of the platelet and ramifies through its cytoplasm. Granule contents are thought to be discharged into the system, from which they make their way into the external environment.

Platelet Production

Platelets are produced from distinctive cells called megakaryocytes (*mega-*, "large"; *karyo-*, "nucleus"). These very large cells with multiform nuclei are easily seen in the marrow even under low power (Fig. 14-2). They arise from stem cells that commit themselves to the megakaryocyte line. These committed stem

Fig. 14-1. Platelet viewed through an electron microscope. A bullseye-like dense granule and a uniformly gray α-granule are indicated by the *arrows*. Small empty spaces representing sections through the canalicular tubules can be seen, and the marginal ring of microtubules is clearly apparent. (From White, J.G. (1974) Electron microscopic studies of platelet secretion. Progr. Hemost. 2:49–98, with permission.)

Contents of the Platelet Granules

Dense granules
    ADP
    Serotonin
    Calcium
α-Granules
    Clotting factors (fibrinogen and factor V)
    von Willebrand factor
    Thrombospondin
    Platelet factor 4
    β-Thromboglobulin
    Platelet-derived growth factor
Lysosomes
    Hydrolytic enzymes active at low pH

cells grow into megakaryocytes by a unique process known as *endomitosis*. In this process, the DNA of the cell is repeatedly duplicated, but the nucleus does not divide. Instead, it grows bigger and more bizarre in shape, its DNA content doubling with each cycle of

Fig. 14-2. Megakaryocytes. (**A**) Viewed under low power. (**B**) Electron micrograph, showing demarcation membranes (*arrows*) and granules. (**A:** From Lessin, L.F. & Bessis, M. (1972) Morphology of the erythron. In Williams, W.J. et al.: Hematology. McGraw-Hill, New York. © 1972. The McGraw-Hill Book Co., with permission. **B:** From Zucker-Franklin, D. (1981) Megakaryocytes and platelets. Ch. 10. In Zucker-Franklin, D. et al. (eds.) Atlas of Blood Cells: Function and Pathology. Edi. Ermes s.r.l., Milan, with permission.)

DNA replication. At the same time, the cytoplasm grows, roughly doubling its mass each time the DNA is replicated. As the cell grows, it differentiates, acquiring the structures and functions of mature platelets—for example, the three classes of granules and the ability to secrete von Willebrand factor. The cell also acquires an intricate network of internal channels, the demarcation membranes, that divide it into platelet-size domains. Finally, after two to five cycles of DNA replication, the cell disintegrates: its cytoplasm folds into pseudopods that work their way through the wall of a marrow sinusoid into the stream of flowing blood, then break apart along the demarcation membranes into individual platelets, while its huge shapeless nucleus remains behind to be destroyed by the mononuclear phagocytes. The production of platelets is summarized in Figure 14-3.

It takes roughly 5 days for a committed stem cell to give birth to a mass of new platelets. The new platelets then circulate for about 10 days before disappearing from the bloodstream. Aging as they circulate, the platelets shrink in size and steadily lose functional capacity, until they finally become senile and are swept from the blood. What finally happens to these outdated, expendable fragments is not known.

Platelet production is stimulated by interleukin-3 (IL-3) and granulocyte-macrophage colony stimulating factor (GM-CSF), two of the five known hematopoietic growth factors. It also appears to be under the influence of a hormone called *thrombopoietin*, about which almost nothing is known except that it can be detected in the blood of patients with thrombocytopenia. In response to these growth factors (and perhaps others yet to be discovered), the

Fig. 14-3. How platelets are made. The megakaryocyte grows by endomitosis (DNA replication without nuclear division), doubling in size with each endomitotic cycle. After 2 to 4 cycles (ploidy z 8N to 32N, where 2N is the amount of DNA in a normal diploid cell), the cell stops growing and begins to differentiate, acquiring platelet-specific granules and a network of demarcation membranes as it matures. Maturation reaches completion with the disintegration of the megakaryocyte, which breaks apart along the demarcation membrane network into thousands of platelets. (Based on the work of Odell, T.T., & Anderson, H.R. (1959) Production and life span of platelets. In Stohlman, F. (ed.) The Kinetics of Cellular Proliferation. Grune & Stratton, Orlando FL, and Odell, T.T., & McDonald, T.P. (1961) Life span of mouse blood platelets. Proc. Soc. Exp. Biol. Med. *106*:107. Modified from Hirsh, J., & Doery, J.C.G. (1972) Platelet function in health and disease. Prog. Hematol. *7*:185. In Wintrobe, M.M. (1981) Platelets and megakaryocytes. Ch. 15 in Clinical Hematology. 8th ed. Lea & Febiger, Philadelphia, with permission.)

marrow can increase platelet production by as much as six- or sevenfold. Increased production results from increase in (1) the number of megakaryocytes in the marrow and (2) the number of platelets per megakaryocyte as each cell doubles its size by an extra cycle of DNA replication before it breaks up.

Platelet Function

In the circulation, platelets normally travel separately, showing little tendency to interact with each other or with the endothelial cells that form the capillaries and line the walls of larger blood vessels. When tissues are damaged, however, the platelets are exposed to activating agents that are released at the site of injury. This contact with activating agents initiates an integrated series of events, the final outcome of which is the formation of a hemostatic plug composed of thousands of platelets fused into a single mass.

Activation of the Platelet

The encounter of a platelet with an activating agent provokes major changes in the platelet's shape and properties (Fig. 14-4). A disc at rest, the stimulated platelet rapidly assumes the shape of a sphere. Its granules retreat to the center, and from its surface sprout a number of long hairlike projections known as *filipodia*. It then undergoes the *release reaction*, a complicated series of events during which (1) the α- and dense granules discharge their contents to the outside; (2) an exceedingly potent lipid mediator is secreted; and (3) the ability of the platelet to promote the activation of the clotting cascade is greatly augmented.

During activation, platelets grow very sticky and begin to adhere to each other in a process known as *aggregation*. Simultaneously, the release reaction of the freshly activated platelets liberates substances that are able to activate other platelets. Like the first crop of activated platelets, these newly activated platelets become sticky, adhering to each other as well as to the original platelet aggregate. The newly activated platelets also undergo the release reaction, activating still more platelets and recruiting them into the growing aggregate. It can be seen how this sequence of events will lead to the formation of a large platelet mass at a site of tissue injury. Eventually, this mass will grow large enough to plug the injured vessel and bleeding will stop. (Obviously, this

Disc   Sphere

Aggregation   Coalescence

Fig. 14-4. Activation of platelet. (From Barnhart, M.I., Walsh, R.T., & Robinson, J.A. (1972) A three-dimensional view of platelet responses to chemical stimuli. Ann N.Y. Acad. Sci. *201*: 360–390, with permission.)

mechanism will only work for vessels below a certain size; there is no way that bleeding from a major vessel can be stopped by a platelet plug.) It appears that the platelet plug is responsible for initial hemostasis in minor injuries, the fibrin clot forming later to reinforce the hemostatic occlusion. During the course of a few hours, the platelets in this mass coalesce and lose their identity. The final plug is a homogeneous, featureless gel, nearly indistinguishable from the fibrin clot in which it will have become enmeshed.

Products Liberated in the Release Reaction

Granule contents
    α-Granules
    Dense granules

Thromboxane A_2

Platelet surface procoagulant

The Release Reaction

In the release reaction, a stimulated platelet makes available various substances that affect clotting, inflammation, and repair at a site of injury. The substances made available in the release reaction include the α- and dense granule contents, the lipid mediator thromboxane A_2, and a procoagulant on the platelet surface that stimulates the formation of a fibrin clot.

Degranulation

The release of α- and dense granule contents occurs within a few seconds after an encounter between platelets and an activating agent. The dense granule contents discharged during the release are low molecular weight substances, whereas the α-granule contents are proteins

(see Platelet Structure, above). Functions for several of these substances are recognized.

With respect to the dense granule contents, the only substance having a clearly defined role is adenosine diphosphate (ADP). This is one of the two endogenous platelet activators liberated during the release reaction (the other is thromboxane A_2). Precise functions for the serotonin and Ca^{2+} liberated during the release reaction are still unknown.

As to the α-granules, roles have been proposed for a number of the proteins liberated from these granules during the release reaction, as summarized in Table 14-1. Factor V promotes the formation of a fibrin clot at sites of platelet release. The α-granule fibrinogen, however, probably has little to do with fibrin clot formation, as it is released in such small quantities; this fibrinogen may have a role in platelet aggregation. The von Willebrand factor helps the platelet adhere to surfaces, and

Table 14-1. Functions of the α-Granule Contents

Component	Function
Factor V	Promotes formation of fibrin clot
Fibrinogen	Required for platelet aggregation
von Willebrand factor	Required for platelet adherence
Thrombospondin	Aggregates platelets
Platelet factor 4	Neutralizes heparin; ?acts against a heparinlike molecule in blood vessels or tissues
β-Thromboglobulin	?
Platelet-derived growth factor	Stimulates growth of fibroblasts and smooth muscle cells; probably promotes tissue repair; may promote atherosclerosis

thrombospondin promotes platelet aggregation by binding simultaneously to fibrinogen and the platelet surface. Platelet factor 4 neutralizes the anticoagulant heparin in vitro and possibly exerts a similar effect in vivo, perhaps counteracting AT III activation by endothelial proteoglycans (see Ch. 13). Platelet-derived growth factor stimulates the growth of fibrinoblasts and smooth muscle cells in culture; it has been postulated to function in the repair of damaged tissue (as well as in the formation of the atherosclerotic plaque, perhaps an example of overrepair).

Lipid Mediators

Lipid mediators are low molecular weight lipid-soluble compounds that exert potent biological effects on a wide variety of cell types at very low concentrations. These mediators can be classified according to their structures into several groups. Among these groups are the phospholipid mediators, which are closely related to phosphatidylcholine; the leukotrienes, which are straight-chain compounds derived from arachidonic acid; and the prostaglandin/thromboxane group, also derived from arachidonic acid but containing a ring.

Of these, the group most directly involved with platelets is the prostaglandin/thromboxane group. The members of this group can be divided into two categories: stable (prostaglandins of the E and F classes), and unstable (thromboxane A_2 and prostacyclin). The unstable members play the major role in platelet function.

The first of these, thromboxane A_2, is an exceedingly potent platelet activator that is produced by the platelets themselves during the release reaction. Its route of metabolism is shown in Figure 14-5. This can be divided into three steps:

1. *Production of arachidonic acid.* Arachidonic acid is produced in platelets by the hydrolysis of membrane phospholipids. Phosphatidylinositol in particular is a major source.

This phospholipid contains almost 100 percent arachidonic acid at its 2- (i.e., middle) position. When platelets are stimulated, a phospholipase is activated that is highly specific for this phosphatidylinositol, splitting it into inositol phosphate and diglyceride. Arachidonic acid is then released from this diglyceride by the action of another enzyme, diglyceride lipase. Arachidonic acid can also be released in a one-step reaction. Release by this direct route results from the activation of a second phospholipase, one that splits the fatty acid from the 2-position of several classes of phospholipids. The products of this reaction are arachidonic acid and a lysophospholipid (Fig. 14-5).

2. *Production of thromboxane* A_2. Arachidonic acid is converted to thromboxane A_2 by an oxidation reaction followed by rearrangement. The oxidation is catalyzed by cyclooxygenase and takes arachidonic acid to an intermediate product known as *prostaglandin* H_2. This is coverted by thromboxane A_2 by a rearrangement of the ring, which is catalyzed by thromboxane synthetase.

3. *Destruction of thromboxane* A_2. The duration of action of thromboxane A_2 is very brief because it is extremely unstable, hydrolyzing in seconds to the stable but biologically inert thromboxane B_2. Because of its stability, thromboxane B_2 is a useful footprint of its precursor, its presence indicating that thromboxane A_2 was produced at some earlier time.

Prostacyclin, the other unstable member of the prostaglandin/thromboxane group, is a powerful antagonist of platelet activation. It is produced by the vascular endothelium and is thought to aid in preventing activation of platelets in the bloodstream. Like thromboxane A_2, it is made from arachidonic acid via the cyclooxygenase product, prostaglandin H_2. In the endothelial cell, however, the rearrangement of prostaglandin H_2 is catalyzed by prostacyclin synthetase, not thromboxane synthetase, and the product is prostacyclin (Fig. 14-5). The life span of prostacyclin is as short as that of thromboxane A_2; it is hydrolyzed in sec-

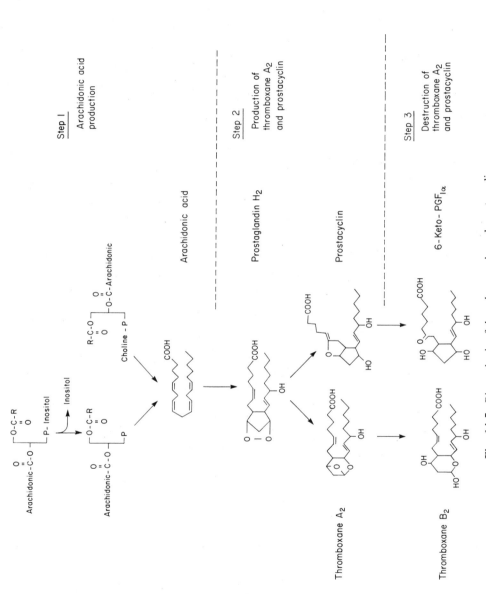

Fig. 14-5. Biosynthesis of thromboxane A$_2$ and prostacyclin.

onds to 6-keto $PGF_{1\alpha}$, a stable, inert compound whose presence signifies the prior release of prostacyclin.

Surface Procoagulant

Platelets participate directly in the clotting cascade by serving as constituents of the factor X- and prothrombin-converting complexes (see Ch. 13). Their effectiveness as clotting cascade participants depends on their history: platelets that have undergone the release reaction are much more potent in this regard than are resting platelets. This increase in potency is thought to be due to the appearance of new clotting factor receptors on the platelet surface during the release reaction. Two receptors are known to appear during release: the fibrinogen receptor and the factor V receptor. The fibrinogen receptor probably participates in platelet aggregation, rather than the clotting cascade. The factor V receptor, however, could well be involved in the clotting cascade. In particular, it is not unreasonable to imagine that the prothrombin converting complex is put together by the Ca^{2+} -dependent binding of a factor Xa molecule to a factor Va molecule sitting in its receptor on the surface of an activated platelet.* Such an event would explain the increased effectiveness of activated platelets as promoters of fibrin clot formation.

Aggregation

Platelet aggregation is easily seen when an activating agent is added to a well-stirred suspension of resting platelets (Fig. 14-6). It begins about 30 seconds after the stimulus is added and normally reaches completion in 5 to 10 minutes. Fibrinogen must be present in the medium or the platelets will not aggregate; this

---

*Similarly, an as yet unidentified factor VIIIa receptor on the platelet surface could explain how platelets stimulate factor X activation.

has clinical ramifications, notably in Glanzmann's thrombasthenia.

From the way they elicit aggregation, platelet-activating agents can be divided into two categories: (1) *direct activators*, which cause platelets to aggregate as a primary effect of the platelet-activator interaction; and (2) *indirect activators*, which work entirely through platelet release, the platelets aggregating solely because of the endogenous aggregating agents (ADP and thromboxane A_2) liberated during the release reaction. With indirect activators, aggregation is a straightforward one-phase event (Fig. 14-6A). With direct activators, however, aggregation often occurs in two phases (Fig. 14-6B). The first phase, known as the primary wave, results directly from the interaction between the activator and the platelets. The second phase, or secondary wave, is caused by further stimulation of the platelets by the endogenous aggregating agents liberated in the associated release reaction.

Platelet aggregation during a primary wave is imperfect; complete aggregation is achieved only during the secondary wave. In certain platelet disorders, or with very low concentrations of stimulus, platelets exposed to a direct stimulus will fail to undergo a secondary wave because the release reaction is inadequate. Under these circumstances, the weak aggregates formed during the primary wave will disperse. Conversely, platelets exposed to very high concentrations of a direct stimulus will aggregate in a one-phase manner.

Platelet Activators

At sites of tissue injury, the principal platelet activators are thrombin and collagen. Activation of the clotting cascade steeps the platelets in thrombin, whereas damage to blood vessels and underlying tissues brings the platelets into contact with collagen, a ubiquitous tissue component from which they are ordinarily separated by the thin vascular endothelium. Thrombin is a direct aggregating agent, causing platelets to aggregate and release in

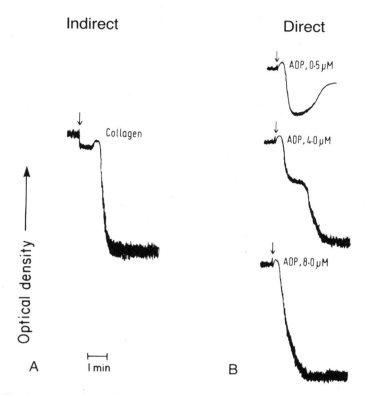

Fig. 14-6. Platelet aggregation. Platelet aggregation is measured by following the change in light transmission after adding an aggregating agent to a stirred sample of platelet-rich plasma, prepared by centrifuging heparinized blood at low speed to remove red cells and white cells. Before aggregation, the platelets form turbid suspension through which light passes with difficulty. The suspension clears up as platelets cluster into aggregates, increasing light transmission. The magnitude of change in light transmission gives a rough indication of the degree to which platelets have aggregated in response to the stimulus. (**A**) One-phase aggregation: response to indirect aggregating agent. (**B**) Two-phase aggregation: response to direct aggregating agent. (Modified from Holmsen, H., Salganicoff, L. & Fukami, M.H. (1977) Platelet behavior in biochemistry. In Ogston, D. & Bennett: Hemostasis: Biochemistry, Physiology, Pathology. John Wiley & Sons Ltd., Chichester, England, with permission.)

the circulation. Collagen, however, brings the platelets to the injured surface. On encountering the exposed collagen, platelets attach tightly to a collagen fibril in a process known as *adhesion*. Stimulated by the collagen, an indirect activating agent, the attached platelets undergo the release reaction, attracting additional platelets to form an aggregate in response to released ADP and thromboxane A_2.

Other platelet activators include epinephrine, ADP, and thromboxane A_2. As discussed above, the last two are platelet constituents that are secreted during the release reaction. Epinephrine and (at low concentrations) ADP are direct activators that cause platelets to aggregate in a classic biphasic manner. The platelet activating agents are classified into direct and indirect activators as shown below.

Platelets are also agglutinated by the antibiotic ristocetin. Unlike the agents discussed above, ristocetin acts on dead (formalin-fixed) as well as live platelets. It is therefore clear that the response of platelets to ristocetin can have little physiological significance. Never-

---

Platelet Activating Agents

Indirect
    Collagen

Direct
    Thrombin
    Epinephrine
    ADP
    Thromboxane A_2

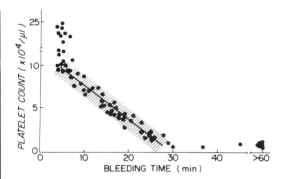

Fig. 14-7. Relationship between platelet count and bleeding time. (From Malpass, T.W. & Harker, L.A. (1980) Acquired disorders of platelet function. Semin, Hematol. *17*:243, with permission.)

theless, ristocetin-mediated platelet agglutination has proved extremely useful in diagnosing platelet function disorders.

Testing Platelet Function

Bleeding Time

The bleeding time is the most general test of platelet function (Table 14-2). It is usually performed by making a 1 cm × 1 mm incision in the skin of the inner forearm, then blotting every 30 seconds until the bleeding stops. The time required for the bleeding to stop is the bleeding time.

Any disorder affecting the platelets will pro-

long the bleeding time, if sufficiently severe. In milder forms of such disorders the bleeding time is often normal, but it may be brought into the abnormal range by an aspirin taken a few hours before the test. This is true for both quantitative and qualitative disorders. In conditions associated with reduced numbers of platelets (e.g., thrombocytopenia), there is a nice correlation between platelet count and bleeding time (Fig. 14-7). In conditions associated with defective platelet function, the bleeding time will be prolonged regardless of the platelet count. Because it is so general a test, the bleeding time is exceedingly useful as a screen for platelet function disorders. By the same token, however, it provides little information beyond the fact that a platelet function disorder exists.

Platelet Adhesion

Platelet adhesion used to be measured directly by pouring platelet-rich plasma through a column of glass beads and counting the number of platelets retained by the beads. It is now known that the same information can be obtained by measuring platelet agglutination in response to ristocetin. Ristocetin agglutination has supplanted the glass bead column as the

Table 14-2. Platelet Function Tests

Test	Function Tested
Bleeding time	General
Aggregation	
Indirect stimuli	Aggregation
Direct stimuli	Aggregation; release of ADP and thromboxane
Ristocetin	Adhesion
Granule content release	
Serotonin	Discharge of dense granules
Platelet factor 4 and β-thromboglobulin	Discharge of α-granules
Thromboxane B_2	Thromboxane secretion

means of diagnosing disorders of platelet adhesion.

Ristocetin agglutination is defective in von Willebrand's disease and Bernard-Soulier disease, two inherited disorders in which platelet adhesion is impaired. It is generally normal in other platelet diseases.

Aggregation and the Release Reaction

Plate aggregation is measured by an optical method using platelet-rich plasma. The technique is described in Figure 14-6, which presents examples of typical aggregation patterns in response to direct and indirect activators.

Defects in platelet aggregation fall into two classes: those in which the entire aggregation response is affected, and those in which only the secondary wave is missing. The latter always result from an impairment in the release reaction; endogenous aggregation agents fail to be secreted from the platelets, and the secondary wave does not occur.

The release reaction can be evaluated more completely by directly measuring degranulation and thromboxane production. These can be determined by assaying the quantities of granule components and thromboxane secreted into the medium by stimulated platelets. For this purpose, serotonin is generally used as the dense granule marker, platelet factor 4 and β-thromboglobulin as the α-granule markers, and thromboxane B_2 as the index of thromboxane production. These measurements are seldom needed in the workup of a platelet function disorder, because release can be assessed well enough for most purposes just by examining the secondary wave of aggregation. Their primary use is for research.

By far the most common cause of a defective release reaction is aspirin ingestion. Other nonsteroidal anti-inflammatory agents cause a defect in platelet release as well. Inherited disorders of platelet function are less frequent causes of defective release.

PLATELET FUNCTION DISORDERS

Platelet function is disturbed in a number of conditions, both inherited and acquired. Most of these conditions show a bleeding tendency, but this tendency is surprisingly mild except in a few rare platelet diseases (notably Bernard-Soulier disease and some cases of von Willebrand's disease). The absence of bleeding problems in patients with platelet function defects should be contrasted with their frequency and gravity in patients with severe thrombocytopenia, in whom death from exsanguination or intracranial hemorrhage is a real hazard.

As a rule, bleeding patterns in platelet disorders are distinctly different from bleeding patterns in disorders involving soluble clotting factors (Table 14-3). Patients with clotting factor disorders tend to bleed into joints and soft tissues, sites that are seldom involved in thrombocytopenia or qualitative platelet function defects. The most frequent site of bleeding in platelet disorders is the skin. Patients with severe platelet function disorders or thrombocytopenia will often develop multiple tiny hemorrhagic spots known as *petechiae*; these are not seen in clotting factor disorders. Larger confluent hemorrhagic areas (purpura) also appear in the skin in platelet function disorders, but these are seen in clotting factor disorders as well. Other sites of bleeding common to both clotting factor and platelet disorders include the orifices (nose, upper and lower GI, urinary, and vaginal) and the brain.

Inherited Defects of Platelet Adhesion

There are two inherited disorders of platelet adhesion: von Willebrand's disease and Bernard-Soulier disease (Table 14–4). Both are

Table 14-3. Bleeding Sites: Platelet Disorders versus Clotting Factor Disorders

Platelets	Clotting Factors	Both
Petechiae	Joints	Purpura
	Soft tissues	Orifices
		Brain

Table 14-4. Distinguishing among von Willebrand's Disease, Bernard-Soulier Disease, and Glanzmann's Thrombasthenia

	von Willebrand's Disease	Bernard-Soulier Disease	Glanzmann's Thrombasthenia
Defect	Adhesion	Adhesion	Primary aggregation
Cause	Low plasma vWF[a]	Absent vWF[a] receptors	Absent fibrinogen receptors
Poor aggregation in response to	Ristocetin	Ristocetin, thrombin	Everything except ristocetin (ristocetin aggregation is normal)
Other	Low plasma vWF[a]	Huge platelets	No clot retraction
	Low plasma factor VIII	Absence of GP Ib[b]	Absence of GP IIb and GP IIIa[b]

[a] von Willebrand factor.
[b] Glycoprotein Ib, IIb, IIIa.

characterized by a defect in the attachment of platelets to collagen. Excessive bleeding occurs because the platelets are unable to adhere normally to the collagen to which they are exposed when blood vessels are torn at sites of injury.

von Willebrand's Disease

von Willebrand's disease is by far the most common inherited abnormality of platelet function. It is transmitted as an autosomal dominant trait. The bleeding disorder tends to be mild in the heterozygote, but is exceedingly severe in the rare homozygote.

von Willebrand Factor

The hallmark of von Willebrand's disease is defective platelet function. The platelets themselves are perfectly normal, however. The actual cause of the platelet function defect is a deficiency of a plasma constituent known as the von Willebrand factor.

The von Willebrand factor is a group of multimeric proteins secreted by megakaryocytes and endothelial cells. All are made up of a single monomer of MW of approximately 250,000. This monomer polymerizes to form a series of huge complexes of regularly increasingly molecular weight, some as large as 15 to 20 million (Fig. 14-8). These very large complexes must be present in order for platelets to (1) adhere to surfaces (e.g., collagen or glass) and (2) aggregate in response to ristocetin. Promotion of adherence is probably the major

Fig. 14-8. Multimers of von Willebrand factor. (Modified from Ruggeri, Z.M. et al. (1982) Multimeric composition of Factor VIII/von Willebrand factor following administration of DDAVP: Implications for pathophysiology and therapy of von Willebrand's disease subtypes. Blood 59:1271–1278, with permission.)

in vivo function of the von Willebrand factor.

A second function of the von Willebrand factor has to do with its long-recognized relationship to factor VIII, the clotting factor of hemophilia.* This relationship is clearly evident in von Willebrand's disease. In most patients with this condition, levels of both factor

---

*A set of three symbols derived from the factor VIII–von Willebrand factor relationship is sometimes used in discussions of von Willebrand's disease. These symbols contain the numeral VIII (for factor VIII) followed by a letter that specifies one or another of the associated activities. The symbols are VIII:C, for factor VIII coagulant activity (that which is missing in hemophilia); VIII:R, for ristocetin cofactor activity (that which promotes platelet aggregation by ristocetin); and VIII:A, for the von Willebrand antigen (that which is detected by an antibody against the von Willebrand factor). In this chapter, von Willebrand factor is named in full, and the term factor VIII always refers to the clotting factor that is missing in hemophilia.

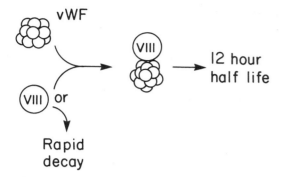

Fig. 14-9. Relationship between factor VIII and von Willebrand factor.

VIII and von Willebrand factor are reduced to a similar extent (when expressed as percent of normal). By contrast, patients with hemophilia have normal levels of von Willebrand factor, even though their factor VIII levels may be close to zero.

The reason for this relationship between factor VIII and von Willebrand factor is that the von Willebrand factor acts to stabilize factor VIII by forming a complex with it in the circulation (Fig. 14-9). In von Willebrand's disease, the factor VIII level is low because of a deficiency in von Willebrand factor, the factor VIII-stabilizing protein. In hemophilia, though, the factor VIII level is low because factor VIII itself is defective, whereas the von Willebrand factor is completely normal.

Diagnosis of von Willebrand's Disease

All patients with inherited platelet disorders have the same clinical picture: a family history of bleeding of a greater or lesser degree of severity. Laboratory investigations are required to make the diagnosis.

Classic von Willebrand's disease is caused by a deficiency of von Willebrand factor. This deficiency can be demonstrated directly in the laboratory by an assay that uses an antibody against the von Willebrand factor. In addition, there is a characteristic combination of other laboratory abnormalities: (1) the bleeding time is prolonged as expected in any platelet disorder; (2) platelet function is disturbed in a particular way: adhesion is impaired and the platelets fail to agglutinate with ristocetin, although they aggregate and release in a completely normal fashion with any other aggregating agent; and (3) factor VIII activity is reduced, a consequence of the relationship between this clotting factor and the von Willebrand factor.

Variant forms of von Willebrand's disease also occur (Table 14-5). In some variants, levels of factor VIII and von Willebrand antigen are normal. Two of the variant forms are caused by a functionally defective von Willebrand factor that is unable to form large polymers; another is due to an intrinsic platelet defect. They are uncommon, but are important to recognize because they are managed somewhat differently than classic von Willebrand's disease.

Management

Like other plasma clotting factor deficiencies, von Willebrand's disease is managed by replacement therapy. Patients can be given either fresh frozen plasma or cryoprecipitate (the same preparation used to treat hemophilia). Purified factor VIII should not be used, however, because it contains little active von Willebrand factor. DDAVP is useful in mild type I and type IIA von Willebrand's disease, but should not be given in type IIb or pseudo-von Willebrand's disease, because it worsens the thrombocytopenia. The effect of treatment should be evaluated by the clinical response and the bleeding time. Other tests are not helpful in managing von Willebrand's disease, because they can show improvement after re-

---

Making the Diagnosis of von Willebrand's Disease

Bleeding time prolonged

Ristocetin aggregation decreased or absent

Factor VIII decreased

von Willebrand antigen decreased

Table 14-5. Classification of von Willebrand's Disease

Type	Defect	Platelet count	Ristocetin aggregation	Response to DDAVP
I	All vWF multimers decreased	Normal	Absent	+
IIa	Large vWF multimers decreased	Normal	Absent	+
IIb	Large vWF multimers decreased, intermediate multimers increased	Low	Increased	Contraindicated
Pseudo-	Like type IIb; platelets show abnormally high affinity for largest vWF multimers	Low	Increased	Contraindicated
III	vWF multimers absent	Normal	Absent	No effect

placement therapy without any improvement in the patient's bleeding tendency.

Levels of factor VIII behave in a curious way after a patient with von Willebrand's disease is given a dose of plasma or cryoprecipitate. Factor VIII rises quickly to greater-than-normal levels, then stays high for 2 to 3 days before dropping off again. This reaction contrasts with that found in hemophiliacs, whose factor VIII levels begin to fall rapidly immediately after therapy. This behavior is undoubtedly another consequence of the relationship between factor VIII and the von Willebrand factor.

Bernard-Soulier Disease

Bernard-Soulier disease can be looked at as the platelet counterpart of von Willebrand's disease. In von Willebrand's disease, the problem is with the plasma, which lacks the von Willebrand factor. In Bernard-Soulier disease, the problem is with the platelets, which lack the ability to interact with the von Willebrand factor.

The bleeding problem in Bernard-Soulier disease is extremely severe, although it tends to improve with age. Diagnosis depends on the laboratory results. The platelet count is low, but the individual platelets are huge—the size of the red cells (Fig. 14-10). Platelet function studies are by and large the same as von Wil-

Fig. 14-10. Platelets in Bernard-Soulier disease. (Modified from Bithell, T.C., Parekh, S.S., & Strong, R.R. (1972) Platelet function in the Bernard-Soulier syndrome. Ann. N.Y. Acad. Sci. *201*:145–160, with permission).

Management of von Willebrand's Disease

Replacement therapy: Fresh frozen plasma or cryoprecipitate (not purified factor VIII)

Stimulate vWF production: DDAVP

Follow: Clinical effect and bleeding time studies

Bernard-
Soulier

Glanz-
mann's

Fig. 14-11. Platelet glycoproteins. (**Left**) Bernard-Soulier disease. (Modified from Nurden, A.T. et al. (1981) Analysis of the glycoprotein and protein composition of Bernard-Soulier platelets by single- and two-dimensional sodium dodecyl sulfate-polyacrylamide gel electrophoresis. J. Clin. Invest. *67*:1431–1440, with permission.) (**Right**) Glanzmann's thrombasthenia. (Modified from Phillips, D.R. & Agin, P.P. (1977) Platelet membrane defects in Glanzmann's thrombasthenia. J. Clin. Invest. *60*:535–545, with permission.)

lebrand's disease, showing faulty adhesion and ristocetin agglutination, but a normal response to other aggregating agents (except thrombin; see Table 14-4). The critical defect in Bernard-Soulier disease is the absence of the glycoprotein designated GP Ib from the membrane of the platelet (Fig. 14–11). This glycoprotein appears to be the platelet receptor for the von Willebrand factor. It is the lack of this receptor protein that accounts for the abnormalities in hemostasis and platelet function in Bernard-Soulier disease.

Inherited Defect of Aggregation

Glanzmann's Thrombasthenia

Glanzmann's thrombasthenia (Table 14–4) appears to result from a defect in the interaction between platelets and fibrinogen. When normal platelets are activated, fibrinogen binding sites appear on their surface. Presumably,

these binding sites have something to do with the need for fibrinogen in platelet aggregation. Thrombasthenic platelets lack these fibrinogen binding sites and show a general defect in aggregation.

Thrombasthenics have a moderately severe bleeding disorder. Unlike Bernard-Soulier disease, platelets are normal in number and size and adhesion is intact in Glanzmann's thrombasthenia. The aggregation defect is precisely complementary to the von Willebrand defect: These platelets aggregate only in response to ristocetin, and to nothing else. A characteristic feature, somehow related to the platelet defect, is the failure of the thrombasthenic clot to retract (i.e., to shrink and squeeze out serum over the course of a few hours) the way normal clots do.

Like Bernard-Soulier disease, Glanzmann's thrombasthenia is caused by a membrane glycoprotein deficiency. Two glycoproteins are missing in thrombasthenia: GP IIb and GP IIIa (Fig. 14-11). Together, these two glycoproteins form the fibrinogen receptor. Their absence explains the fibrinogen binding defect and other abnormalities in Glanzmann's thrombasthenia.

Disorders of Release

In these disorders, platelets fail to complete the release reaction. In some instances, this is because of a defect in thromboxane production. In other cases, a deficiency of dense granule ADP is at fault.

Defective thromboxane production almost always results from the administration of anti-inflammatory drugs. Many of these drugs work by blocking the production of prostaglandins and thromboxanes. Such drugs will interfere will the release reaction by preventing the formation of thromboxane A_2. The best example is aspirin, which inactivates cyclooxygenase, the first enzyme of the thromboxane A_2 synthetic pathway. One aspirin tablet will completely destroy all the cyclooxygenase in whatever megakaryocytes and platelets are present

Disorders of Release

Defective thromboxane production
    Inherited
    Acquired (anti-inflammatory drugs)

Storage pool deficiency

Release
disorder

Normal

Optical density

⊢——⊣
1 min

Fig. 14-12. Aggregation defect in release disorders. (From Holmsen, H., Salganicoff, L. & Fukami, M.H. (1977) Platelet behavior in biochemistry. In Ogston, D. & Bennett,: Hemostasis: Biochemistry, Physiology, Pathology. John Wiley & Sons Ltd., Chichester, England, with permission.)

at the time of ingestion. This leads to a defect in platelet release that is corrected only when fresh platelets made from newly differentiated megakaryocytes appear in the bloodstream. Other drugs also interfere with thromboxane formation; unlike aspirin, these agents inhibit thromboxane production reversibly, so their effects lasts only as long as they are present in the body. In addition to drugs, some inherited abnormalities in thromboxane production cause defective platelet release. Such conditions are very rare.

Steroids, the most potent of the anti-inflammatory drugs, have little effect on normal platelets.

A few patients are found whose platelets contain abnormal dense granules, or lack these granules altogether. Such patients are said to have *storage pool deficiency*. In their platelets, dense granule ADP, referred to as "storage pool" ADP to distinguish it from the ADP in the platelet cytoplasm, is greatly decreased. These platelets cannot discharge ADP during the release reaction because they have no storage pool ADP to discharge; release is therefore incomplete.

All release defects produce the same clinical picture. There is usually little in the way of abnormal bleeding, unless the defect is superimposed on some other clotting disorder (e.g., thrombocytopenia or hemophilia). The bleeding time may be normal or prolonged. Platelet function studies show an absence of the secondary wave of aggregation (Fig. 14-12); this is the most characteristic finding in platelet release defects and occurs because the abnormal platelets are unable to release their own aggregating agents when exposed to platelet activators. The diagnosis of a release defect can be confirmed by measuring the levels of released products (e.g., thromboxane or ADP), but such studies are ordinarily done only for research purposes.

Drugs That Interfere with Thromboxane Formation

Aspirin

Indomethacin

Phenylbutazone

Ibuprofen and related drugs

Sulfinpyrazone

Acquired Platelet Function Disorders

A number of diseases show disturbances of platelet function. These disturbances may be caused by the disease itself, or they may result from drugs or procedures used in therapy.

Clinical bleeding is fairly common in acquired platelet function disorders and occasionally can be severe. The diagnosis is suspected in any patient who (1) has one of the associated diseases or (2) has received a form of treatment known to interfere with platelet function. The laboratory results usually include a long bleeding time and a variety of abnormalities in platelet aggregation and platelet factor III release.

Uremia

An acquired platelet function defect is the rule in uremia. The defect is caused by the accumulation in uremic plasma of waste products of unknown identity that interfere with platelet function.

The platelet function defect can be severe, with a very long bleeding time and grossly abnormal platelet function studies. The defect is thought to have a major role in the bleeding associated with uremia: cutaneous, gastrointestinal, and pericardial. It responds to dialysis or kidney transplantation. It has also rather surprisingly been reported to respond to cryoprecipitate, the same material used to treat hemophilia and von Willebrand's disease, as well as to DDAVP. Platelet transfusions are useless, however, because the underlying problem has to do with the plasma, not the platelets.

Drugs

Several classes of drugs cause platelet function defects. Those of clinical importance are certain anti-inflammatory drugs, the β-lactam antibiotics (e.g., penicillins and cephalothins), and alcohol. The anti-inflammatory drugs have been discussed above. The β-lactam antibiotics cause platelet function disorders when given in high doses; they act by interfering with the binding of stimuli to platelet receptors. The way in which alcohol impairs platelet function is not known.

Drug-induced platelet dysfunction usually requires no treatment. When treatment is necessary, it is generally best to withdraw the drug causing the problem or to cut its dose. Platelet transfusions can be helpful in an emergency.

Postcardiopulmonary Bypass

Patients undergoing cardiopulmonary bypass surgery may bleed postoperatively because of an acquired platelet function defect. The platelets acquire the defect as they pass through the pump. The defect is characterized by the discharge of the α-granules and the development of an exceedingly long bleeding time. The long bleeding time does not seem to be related to the loss of α-granules, however, because bleeding time returns to normal within a few hours, even though the α-granules are lost permanently. If bleeding occurs as a result of this defect, it may be treated with platelet transfusions.

The second important cause of post-pump bleeding is inadequate ligation of bleeding vessels at the operative site. Other problems include a low platelet count resulting from dilution by transfusions, activation of the clotting cascade within the blood vessels because of disseminated intravascular coagulation (Ch. 15), and underneutralization of the heparin used during surgery to prevent clotting in the pump.

Other Disorders

Other causes of acquired platelet dysfunction include stem cell disorders and the presence of abnormal circulating proteins (see box on preceding page).

REFERENCES

Bellucci, S. & Caen, J.P. (1988) Congenital platelet disorders. Blood Rev. 2:16–26.

Deranleau, D.A. (1987) Blood platelet shape change ABCs. Trends Biochem. Sci. *12*:439.

Malmsten, C. (1979) Prostaglandins, thromboxanes and platelets. Br. J. Haematol. *41*:453.

Malpass, T.W. & Harker, L.A. (1980) Acquired disorders of platelet function. Semin. Hematol. *17*:242.

Marcus, A.J. (1979) The role of prostaglandins in platelet function. Progr. Hematol. *11*:147.

McDonald, T.P. (1987) Regulation of megakaryocytopoiesis by thrombopoietin. Ann. N. Y. Acad. Sci. *509*:1–24.

Nurden, A.T. & Caen, J.P. (1978) Membrane glycoproteins and human platelet function. Br. J. Haematol. *38*:155.

Oates, J.A., Fitzgerald, G.A., Branch, R.A., et al. (1988) Clinical implications of prostaglandin and thromboxane A_2 formation (first of two parts). N. Engl. J. Med. *319*:689.

Remuzzi, G. (1988) Bleeding in renal failure. Lancet *1*:1205–1208.

Ruggeri, Z.M. & Zimmerman, T.S. (1987) von Willebrand factor and von Willebrand disease. Blood *70*:895.

Schick, P. & Stormoken, H. (eds.) (1985) Platelets and megakaryocytes. Semin. Hematol. *22*:123.

Schick, P. & Stormorken, H. (eds.) (1986) Platelets and megakaryocytes. Semin. Hematol. *23*:1.

Tavassoli, M. (1980) Megakaryocyte-platelet axis and the process of platelet formation and release. Blood *55*:537.

Vainchenker, W. & Kieffer, N. (1988) Human megakaryocytopoiesis: in vitro regulation and characterization of megakaryocytic precursor cells by differentiation markers. Blood Rev. *2*:102–107.

Weiss, H.J. (1980) Congenital disorders of platelet function. Semin. Hematol. *17*:228.

Weksler, B.B. & Nachman, R.L. (1981) Platelets and atherosclerosis. Am. J. Med. *71*:331.

Disseminated Intravascular Coagulation and Thrombotic Thrombocytopenic Purpura

Disseminated intravascular coagulation (DIC) and thrombotic thrombocytopenic purpura (TTP) are highly complex clotting disorders that occur in a setting of serious illness. These disorders are conveniently discussed together because they have certain clinical features in common: complexity, abrupt onset, and a rapid fall in the platelet count. It will be seen, however, that these are two totally different diseases having two entirely different mechanisms.

DISSEMINATED INTRAVASCULAR COAGULATION

DIC is the condition that results when the clotting system is activated in all or a substantial part of the vascular tree. Despite widespread fibrin production, the major problem is usually bleeding, not thrombosis.

Pathogenesis

DIC is caused by the presence in the bloodstream of thromboplastic substances—substances that can trip off the clotting cascade (Fig. 15-1). Small amounts of these substances normally leak into the bloodstream every day—for example, gram-negative bacteria, whose endotoxin coats can activate clotting through several mechanisms, are constantly entering the portal circulation from the intestine—but the usual defenses against runaway coagulation (i.e., antithrombin III, protein C, and clearance by the mononuclear phagocyte system) are more than adequate to handle this small thromboplastic load. In certain diseases, however, large quantities of thromboplastic substances are discharged into the circulation. The defenses are swamped, and DIC ensues.

The thromboplastic material thought to be responsible for most cases of DIC is tissue

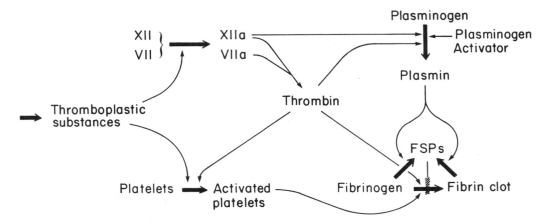

Fig. 15-1. Pathogenesis of DIC. DIC begins when thromboplastic substances are released into the bloodstream in large amounts. These thromboplastic substances activate factors VII and XII, triggering clotting cascade through both extrinsic and intrinsic pathways. Thrombin generated via this cascade then activates circulating platelets (also activated by thromboplastic substances). The combination of thrombin plus activated platelets causes fibrinogen to be converted to fibrin, resulting in formation of clots within the circulatory system. At the same time, plasminogen is converted to plasmin through actions of thrombin, factor XIIa, and plasminogen activator (released from endothelial cells and mononuclear phagocytes during the course of the intravascular clotting process). Plasmin digests both fibrinogen and clotted fibrin, dissolving clots while also releasing fibrin-split products (FSPs), potent anticoagulants that interfere with further conversion of fibrinogen to a fibrin clot. Net effect: Consumption of fibrinogen, platelets, and certain clotting factors and establishment of a confused state in which fibrin clots are perpetually formed and destroyed in circulation, while coagulation at sites of injury is impeded because of depleted platelets and clotting factors and anticoagulant effects of FSPs.

thromboplastin. This is an ill-defined group of substances that have the following two properties: (1) they are released from damaged cells, and (2) they cause blood to clot. Tissue thromboplastin probably includes the factor-VII-activating protein, tissue factor.

Another thromboplastic material thought to have a role in many cases of DIC is endotoxin. This complex lipid forms the outermost layer of gram-negative organisms and appears in large quantities in the circulation of patients who have serious gram-negative infections. Endotoxin activates factor VII by inducing the release of tissue factor from phagocytes; it also activates factor XII and platelets.

Other substances are also believed capable of triggering DIC. Antigen–antibody complexes are one example, and snake venoms, especially those of the pit vipers, are another.

Aiding the thromboplastic materials in their

work are certain factors that affect the properties of the blood itself in patients with DIC. Tissue acidosis, common in these patients, promotes the activation of the clotting cascade by reducing the local pH of the blood. Stasis of the circulation permits activated clotting factors to accumulate in one region, making it easier for a little thromboplastin to push the clotting system past the point of control and into a state of DIC.

Acting on factor XII, factor VII, and sometimes the platelets, thromboplastic substances trigger every component of the coagulation system. Fibrin is generated through the action of the clotting cascade. Plasmin is generated from plasminogen by factor XIIa, thrombin, and plasminogen activator, which is manufactured in increased amounts by mononuclear phagocytes and endothelial cells under conditions of stress. The plasmin splits both fibrinogen and the newly generated fibrin, releasing fibrin-split products with their anticoagulant properties. Platelets are activated by newly formed thrombin, by exposed collagen, and sometimes by the thromboplastic substances themselves. Activation exposes the platelet factor Va binding site, which feeds back to accelerate the clotting cascade. The activated platelets are consumed as they aggregate and adhere to damaged tissues. The net effects of all these events are as follows:

1. Loss of plasma fibrinogen as it is consumed by the clotting process and by the action of plasmin.
2. Loss of other clotting factors, notably V, VIII, and XIII, as they are used up during the operation of the clotting cascade.
3. Fall in the platelet count, as the platelets aggregate and leave the circulation.
4. Appearance of fibrin-split products, as plasmin acts on its substrates.

The end result is DIC, a complex bleeding disorder caused by these platelet and clotting factor deficiencies and the anticoagulant effects of the fibrin-split products.

Clinical Manifestations

DIC has two forms: acute and chronic. The acute form occurs in a setting of serious illness and is characterized mainly by bleeding. In the chronic form, both bleeding and thrombosis occur.

Acute DIC

Acute DIC occurs when a mass of thromboplastic material is introduced into the bloodstream. This occurs in several clinical situations.

Causes

Obstetrical Complications. The fetus, the placenta, and the amniotic fluid are filled with thromboplastic substances. Acute DIC caused by the entry of these thromboplastic substances into the maternal circulation is typical of certain complications of pregnancy: abruptio placenta, in which a portion of the placenta tears away from the uterus; missed abortion, in which a dead fetus is retained in the uterus; and amniotic fluid embolism.

Infections. Infections provide many sources of thromboplastic material. Tissue thromboplastins are liberated and collagen is exposed to the bloodstream at sites of infection. Endotoxin is also produced if the infection is caused by a gram-negative organism. It is not surprising that acute DIC is a common complication of serious infections, both bacterial and viral.

Injuries and Burns. Acute DIC is often seen with serious injuries and burns, caused by the release of thromboplastic material from damaged tissues into the bloodstream.

Antigen–Antibody Complexes in the Circulation. Antigen–antibody complexes can trigger DIC, most likely through a primary effect on the platelets. This may account for the DIC sometimes seen in hemolytic transfusion reactions.

Shock and Acidosis. Shock and acidosis are general features of many illnesses once they become sufficiently severe. Illnesses this severe are frequently complicated by acute DIC. Whether the shock and acidosis have an initiating (i.e., thromboplastinlike) role in this DIC is not clear. It is clear, however, that both aggravate the clotting abnormality through stasis and a lowered blood pH, and perhaps through impaired clearance of activated clotting factors by the mononuclear phagocyte system as well.

Symptoms

Bleeding. The prime symptom of acute DIC is bleeding. The bleeding starts all at once and may be very severe. Bleeding from venipuncture sites is highly characteristic and is often the first sign of acute DIC. Areas of purpura, sometimes very large, appear on the skin. The nose, gums, and the gastrointestinal and urinary tract are common sites of bleeding. In fact, in acute DIC bleeding can occur from any site.

Traumatic Hemolytic Anemia. Problems are sometimes caused by the fibrin deposited in the small blood vessels. A traumatic anemia often occurs as circulating red cells are sliced apart by fibrin strands stretched across their path ("clotheslining").

Bilateral Necrosis of the Renal Cortex. A rare manifestation of DIC involves the deposition of fibrin in the glomeruli of the kidney. This cuts off the blood supply to the renal cortex, causing bilateral cortical necrosis and severe acute renal failure.

The clue to the diagnosis of acute DIC is the abrupt onset of bleeding in a sick patient who does not have a prior history of underlying clotting defect. In any such patient, acute DIC should be high on the list of possibilities.

Chronic DIC

Chronic DIC occurs when thromboplastic material is delivered into the bloodstream in a slow, steady trickle. It is less commonly diagnosed than acute DIC, but because it is a subtle condition, many cases perhaps go unrecognized.

Causes

Cancer. Malignant tumors are constantly discharging small amounts of thromboplastic material into the circulation. This material may be derived from cells that die within the tumor. It is responsible for the state of chronic DIC seen in many patients with cancer. Occasionally, it contributes to episodes of acute DIC in these patients. Acute DIC is a particu-

lar problem in patients with acute promyelocytic leukemia of the hypergranular variety (see Ch. 23).

Missed Abortion. In some patients with missed abortion, thromboplastic substances leak only slowly from the dead fetus into the circulation. Such patients will develop a chronic rather than an acute form of DIC.

Giant Hemangioma (Kasabach-Merritt Syndrome). Giant hemangiomas can cause a state of chronic DIC. The mechanism is unclear, but it is thought that stasis of blood in the hemangioma may somehow contribute to the condition.

Antigen–Antibody Complexes. Chronic DIC can occur in diseases in which antigen–antibody complexes circulate on a long-term basis. Systemic lupus erythematosus is the best example of such a disease.

Symptoms

Thrombosis. The most frequent symptom of chronic DIC is thrombosis. The thrombi usually form in the veins (recurrent thrombophlebitis is the most typical manifestation of chronic DIC), but they sometimes form on the valves of the heart. The real hazard of thrombosis is the danger of pulmonary or arterial embolism, in which fragments of the thrombi are torn away and carried downstream by the circulation, plugging distant vessels.

Bleeding. Also common in chronic DIC, bleeding is less common than thrombosis. In contrast to acute DIC, the bleeding in chronic DIC is usually not widespread.

Laboratory Findings

DIC is associated with a characteristic pattern of abnormalities in the clotting function tests. These are listed in Table 15-1, together

Table 15-1. Clotting Studies in DIC: Classic Pattern

Abnormality	Cause
Prolonged screening tests: PTT, PT, TT[a]	Decreased plasma clotting factor levels; elevated fibrin-split products
Low platelets	Consumption of platelets
Low fibrinogen	Consumption by the clotting cascade; destruction by plasmin
Elevated fibrin-split products	Destruction of fibrinogen by plasmin
Normal euglobulin lysis time	? Removal of plasminogen activator and plasmin from the circulation through binding to intravascular fibrin clots

[a] Partial thromboplastin time, prothrombin time, thrombin time.

with their underlying mechanisms. The pattern given in the table is classic, but not invariable:

1. The fibrinogen level may be normal. This is because fibrinogen is an acute-phase reactant whose rate of production increases during illness. Sometimes this increase in production is enough to offset the increase in consumption caused by the DIC, so fibrinogen remains within the normal range.

2. In chronic DIC, it often happens that the increase in the production of the platelets and clotting factors that occur in response to the clotting disorder are enough to prevent the expected drop in their blood levels. For this reason, many of the clotting tests may be normal in chronic DIC. Fibrin-split products, however, are usually elevated.

Measurements of clotting factors other than fibrinogen are of little help in diagnosing DIC. The levels of these clotting factors are supposed to behave in a predictable way when clotting takes place, but they actually vary widely in DIC and are only occasionally in agreement with what would be expected on theoretical grounds.

In addition to the clotting abnormalities, DIC shows the laboratory features of a traumatic hemolytic anemia. The hematocrit level may be low, broken cells (schistocytes) are seen on the blood smear, and haptoglobin is reduced or absent. These and other manifestations of this type of anemia are discussed more fully in Chapter 9.

Treatment

There are three aspects to the management of DIC: the treatment of the underlying condition, the replacement of deficient clotting components, and the administration of heparin.

Treatment of the Underlying Condition. This is by far the most important aspect of management. DIC can sometimes be held in check by replacement therapy and heparin, but it can only be cured by eliminating the underlying disease.

Replacement of Deficient Clotting Components. If bleeding in DIC is accompanied by low blood fibrinogen or platelets, these should be restored by transfusion: cryoprecipitate for fibrinogen deficiency, fresh frozen plasma to correct for possible deficiencies of other clotting factors, and platelets for thrombocytopenia. It may seem that this treatment is adding fuel to the fire by supplying more clotting components to a patient whose clotting system is already too active, but, in fact, bleeding patients do better, not worse, when their clotting deficiencies are corrected in this way.

Heparin Therapy. The treatment of DIC with heparin is a controversial matter. Theoretically, it should be possible to cure acute DIC by blocking ongoing coagulation with heparin, but in practice this mode of treatment has been far from an overwhelming success. The problems with use of heparin in acute DIC have been that bleeding can be aggravated by heparinizing patients who already have severe bleeding problems and that the death rate in large groups of patients with acute DIC have not been improved by heparin. On the other hand, there have been numerous instances in which heparin appears to have saved the lives of individual patients with acute, severe DIC.

What is the current consensus among the experts with regard to the use of heparin in acute DIC? There is none. Some experts believe that heparin should be used in all patients with DIC. Others advise against its use under any circumstances. The middle view, perhaps the most widespread, holds that heparin need not be used routinely in DIC, but should be given as a life-saving measure to patients with truly severe DIC, to tide them over until other forms of treatment have had a chance to take effect. Patients with DIC who are given heparin must be monitored very carefully; bleeding must be watched for, and the status of the DIC should be followed by the fibrinogen level and the platelet count.

The use of anticoagulants may be of help in chronic DIC, when the problem is thrombosis rather than bleeding. Vitamin K antagonists are generally tried first, but they tend not to work in these patients. Low-dose heparin has proved effective in some patients. A full discussion of anticoagulants is given in Chapter 16.

PRIMARY FIBRINOGENOLYSIS

Primary fibrinogenolysis occurs when active plasmin is generated in the circulation at a time when the clotting cascade is not in operation. It is an occasional feature of certain diseases—most commonly severe liver disease —but once in a great while it is seen in cancer of the lung or prostate or in heat stroke. It is very rare.

The symptom of this disease is bleeding, which can be very severe. Bleeding occurs for two reasons: (1) because of depleted fibrinogen as it is split by the plasmin, and (2) because of the accumulation of "fibrin" (actually, fibrinogen)-split products, with their anticoagulant properties.

The condition that must be ruled out in order to make the diagnosis of primary fibrinogenolysis is DIC. At first glance this may appear difficult, because the laboratory findings in these two disorders have a number of similarities. The clotting factor screening tests— partial thromboplastin time (PTT), prothrombin time (PT), and thrombin time (TT)—are prolonged in both disorders, fibrinogen levels are reduced, and fibrin-split products are found in the plasma. A traumatic anemia is also present. There are, however, some distinct differences between the two (Table 15-2):

1. The platelet count is normal, not low, in primary fibrinogenolysis.

2. The euglobulin lysis time, a crude but useful measure of circulating plasmin, is shortened in primary fibrinogenolysis, but normal in DIC. The normality of the euglobulin lysis time in DIC is somewhat unexpected, because a great deal of active plasmin is generated in that condition. It may be that in DIC most of the components of the plasmin system are associated with intravascular fibrin clots (both plasminogen activator and plasmin itself are known to bind avidly to polymerized fibrin)

Table 15-2. Differences Between Primary Fibrinogenolysis and DIC

Parameters	Primary Fibrinogenolysis	DIC
Laboratory findings		
Platelet count	Normal	Low
Euglobulin lysis	Shortened	Normal
Fibrin-split products		
By structural assays	+	+
By paracoagulation tests	0	+
Treatment with ε-aminocaproic acid	Useful	Dangerous

and are therefore left behind when blood is drawn for laboratory analysis.

3. The results of tests for fibrin-split products are different in the two conditions. Tests that detect split products by their structure (immunological or staphylococcal clumping assays) are positive in both conditions, whereas tests that depend on paracoagulation (ethanol or protamine gelation) are positive in DIC but negative in primary fibrinogenolysis. The reason is as follows. In DIC, the plasma contains fibrin monomers that are unable to form a fibrin gel because they are complexed to split products. When ethanol or protamine is added to this plasma, these complexes fall apart, and the liberated fibrin monomers polymerize to form the telltale gel. In fibrinogenolysis, the split products are there, but the fibrin monomers are not, so a gel does not form on the addition of ethanol or protamine.

Making the distinction between DIC and fibrinogenolysis is important for therapeutic reasons. Fibrinogenolysis can be treated with ε-aminocaproic acid (or its structural cousin, tranexamic acid), which corrects the condition by inhibiting both plasmin and plasminogen activator. In DIC, however, this drug can be very dangerous, because that condition requires active plasmin to keep the blood vessels from filling with fibrin clot, and the administration of ε-aminocaproic acid can lead to a diffuse thrombotic disorder far worse than the bleeding for which the drug was given.

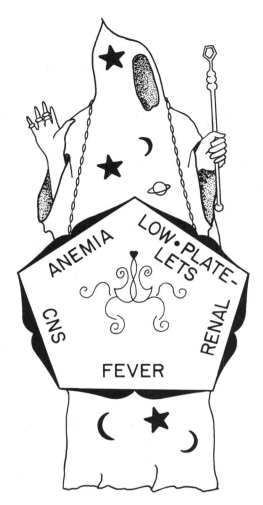

Fig. 15-2. Pentad of TTP.

THROMBOTIC THROMBOCYTOPENIC PURPURA

Thrombotic thrombocytopenic purpura (TTP) is a mysterious and deadly disease in which fibrin plugs appear in small blood vessels throughout the body, with little apparent activation of the clotting cascade or the fibrinolytic system. It is frequently preceded by a minor viral illness, but the connection between this minor illness and the catastrophe that follows is completely obscure.

The disease has a rapid onset, with widespread manifestations appearing over the

The Manifestations of
Thrombotic Thrombocytopenic
Purpura

Fever
Thrombocytopenia with bleeding
Traumatic hemolytic anemia
Acute renal failure
Severe central nervous system (CNS)
disturbances: fluctuating focal signs,
seizures, coma

course of a day or two. In the classic case, these manifestations form what is referred to cabalistically as "the pentad" (Fig. 15-2).

The anemia, kidney failure, and CNS disturbances are probably attributable to the presence of fibrin in the blood vessels. The thrombocytopenia is presently unexplained, though some believe it is due to the appearance of an abnormal circulating protein that precipitates the disease by causing platelets to aggregate within the blood vessels.

A milder form of what may be the same disease is seen in the young—especially infants and young children—and in pregnant women. It is frequently, but not invariably, heralded by an infection. This disorder features all the manifestations of TTP except for the CNS disturbances—a "tetrad" of symptoms—and is known by the descriptive name *hemolytic-uremic syndrome*. Mortality in the hemolytic-uremic syndrome is significant, but is much lower than in TTP.

Laboratory findings are very helpful in making the diagnosis, and especially in making the sometimes difficult distinction between TTP

Laboratory Evidence of TTP

Clotting abnormalities
    Low platelets
    Increased megakaryocytes
    Clotting tests otherwise normal

Traumatic hemolytic anemia
    Low hematocrit and hemoglobin
    Red cell fragments on smear
    Bilirubinemia
    Sometimes hemoglobinuria

---

and DIC (see box). The changes of traumatic hemolytic anemia are present, including a low hematocrit, fragmented red cells on the blood smear, and the other findings described in Chapter 9. The platelet count is low, but there are many megakaryocytes in the marrow, indicating that the reduction in platelets is attributable to increased consumption, rather than to decreased production. Other clotting studies are usually normal, an important distinction

Fig. 15-3. Fibrin-plugged arteriole in gum biopsy from a patient with TTP. Note the absence of an inflammatory response around the arteriole. (From Pisciotta, A.V. & Gottschall, J. (1980) Clinical features of thrombotic thrombocytic purpura. Semin. Thromb. Hemostasis 6:330–340, with permission.)

from DIC; screening tests are normal, fibrinogen levels are normal or increased, and split products are absent.

The diagnosis often has to be made on clinical grounds, but it can sometimes be made by biopsy, usually of the gum. The diagnostic finding is an arteriole that contains a mass of fibrin (Fig. 15-3). There is no evidence of inflammation (i.e., no cellular infiltrate surrounds the fibrin-filled arteriole), and there is no immunoglobulin or complement to be found. The finding of an arteriole filled with a bland fibrin plug is pathognomonic of TTP in this clinical setting.

TTP is usually treated by large-volume plasma exchanges, usually in combination with steroids. This form of therapy has decreased the mortality rate of TTP from 90 precent to something under 50 percent; no one knows why. In patients with TTP who have failed plasma exchange, a combination of steroids, antiplatelet agents, and emergency splenectomy has been used with some success.

REFERENCES

Colman, R.W., Robboy, S.J. & Minna, J.D. (1979) Disseminated intravascular coagulation: A reappraisal. Annu. Rev. Med. *30*:319.

Fong, J.S., de Chadarevian, J.P. & Kaplan, B.S. (1982) Hemolytic-uremic syndrome. Current concepts and management. Pediatr. Clin. North. Am. *29*:835-856.

Murgo, A.J. (1987) Thrombotic microangiopathy in the cancer patient including those induced by chemotherapeutic agents. Semin. Hematol. *24*:161–177.

Ridolfi, R.L. & Bell, W.R. (1981) Thrombotic thrombocytopenic purpura. Medicine *60*:413.

Sills, R.H. (1984) Thrombotic thrombocytopenic purpura. I. Pathophysiology and clinical manifestations. Am. J. Pediatr. Hematol. Oncol. *6*:425–430.

16

Antithrombotic Therapy: Anticoagulants, Antiplatelet Drugs, and Fibrinolytic Agents

Diseases associated with thrombosis—heart attacks, strokes, pulmonary emboli, and so forth—are the most common causes of death in the developed countries. Current treatment of many of these diseases involves the use of drugs that counteract intravascular coagulation. These drugs fall into three categories; anticoagulants, which impede clotting through effects on the soluble clotting factors; fibrinolytic agents, which dissolve clots that have already formed; and the antiplatelet agents.

ANTICOAGULANTS

Anticoagulants are used for the treatment of conditions in which clotting occurs in the heart or blood vessels. They do not work equally well in all such conditions, however, and even when they do work, anticoagulants are hazardous to use because they can increase the risk of bleeding. The decision to use anticoagulants is therefore a serious matter, and the management of anticoagulated patients requires the utmost care and vigilance.

The two major types of anticoagulants are heparin and the vitamin K antagonists. Heparin is used to treat acute thrombosis; vitamin K antagonists are used for long-term anticoagulation.

Heparin

Heparin is a complex polymer of sugars and amino sugars containing a large number of acidic groups [carboxyl ($-COO^-$) and sulfate] that give it very high negative charge at biological pH (Fig. 16-1). Heparin is a member of a general class of acidic sugar polymers known as *mucopolysaccharides*. These mucopolysaccharides are abundant on cell surfaces and in the ground substance of connective tissues. Mucopolysaccharides similar to heparin are thought to be partly responsible for the anticoagulant properties of the endothelial surface (see Ch. 13).

Heparin interferes with clot formation by causing the inactivation of all the clotting factors that work through proteolysis, with the exception of factor VIIa. It accomplishes this by a mechanism involving the plasma protein antithrombin III (Fig. 16-2). Antithrombin III has the ability to bind to proteolytic clotting factors in such a way as to block their active sites irreversibly. This reaction is slow, so that activated clotting factors may be able to do their job before antithrombin III has a chance to interfere with their effects. What heparin does is to combine with antithrombin III to form a complex of greatly enhanced reactivity. In contrast to the slow action of free antithrombin

Fig. 16-1. Portion of the heparin molecule.

III, this complex is able to combine with clotting factors and block their effects almost as fast as the factors appear in the circulation.

The coagulation screening tests in heparinized patients are as expected from the action of the heparin–antithrombin III complex. The partial thromboplastin time (PTT) and thrombin time (TT) are sharply altered. The prothrombin time (PT) is much less affected, because factor VIIa is resistant to the heparin–antithrombin complex. The bleeding time is not affected at all, as long as the platelet count is normal.

Clinical Use

Because of its chemical nature, heparin cannot be absorbed from the intestine, so it must be given parenterally. The best way to administer heparin is continuously by vein. It is sometimes given by intermittent injections (intravenous or subcutaneous), but the risk of bleeding with intermittent therapy is higher than with continuous therapy, undoubtedly because adequate round-the-clock anticoagulation

---

Effect of Heparin on Coagulation Screening Tests

Substantially prolonged: Partial thromboplastin time and thrombin time

Slightly prolonged: Prothrombin time

Unchanged: Bleeding time

---

with intermittent therapy requires a dose of heparin large enough to cause a dangerous paralysis of clotting function for the first hour or two after administration. Heparin is cleared rapidly by the liver, having a half-life in the blood of about 1 hour, so intermittent therapy has to be given fairly often (every 4 to 6 hours is the rule).

It is generally necessary to give large doses of heparin at the start of treatment, because extensive clotting is going on and large amounts of activated clotting factors have to be neutralized in the circulation. Once clotting is under control and the production of active clotting

Fig. 16-2. How heparin works.

Clinical Use of Heparin

Conventional dose
    Best given continuously by vein
    Started with relatively high doses, but
        dose lowered carefully as clotting
        comes under control
    Dose adjusted to give PTT[a] of 1.5 to
        2.0 times control, at arbitrary times
        (continuous therapy) or 1 hour be-
        fore the next dose (intermittent
        therapy)
Low dose
    Given subcutaneously every 8 to 12
        hours
    Not necessary to follow PTT

---

[a] Partial thromboplastin time.

---

factors has fallen back toward normal, the heparin dose must be cut back to avoid overanticoagulation and bleeding.

The degree of anticoagulation is usually determined by the PTT. The heparin dose is adjusted to give a PTT of 1.5 to 2 times control an hour before the next dose (intermittent therapy) or any time at all (continuous therapy). At these levels, heparin has little effect on the PT.

Heparin in very low doses can be used to prevent venous thrombosis in certain high-risk patients (e.g., patients about to undergo abdominal or chest surgery, or patients restricted to bed rest for congestive heart failure). Because the release of only a tiny amount of activated clotting factor in a vein is enough to trigger thrombophlebitis, a low dose of heparin is all that is needed to neutralize that tiny pulse of activated clotting factor and prevent formation of a clot. Once a clot does begin to form, however, major amounts of clotting factors are activated, and large doses of heparin are required to bring the ongoing clotting process under control. Low-dose heparin is given subcutaneously every 8 to 12 hours. It is not nec-

essary to follow treatment with the PTT, as the doses given are too low to affect this test.

Complications

Bleeding

As with all anticoagulants, the major side effect of heparin is bleeding. This problem generally occurs when the patient is overanticoagulated, but it can also take place when the level of anticoagulation is in the therapeutic range as indicated by the PTT. Platelets are particularly important for clot formation in a patient whose soluble clotting system is partly paralyzed by heparin; to reduce the likelihood of bleeding in such a patient, antiplatelet agents must be avoided if possible.

Diagnosis of heparin toxicity is generally simple: Bleeding in a patient receiving heparin therapy who is found to have a long PTT can be considered to be a side effect of heparin, unless proved otherwise. Occasionally the diagnosis presents a problem, generally in patients in whom postoperative bleeding develops after cardiopulmonary bypass surgery. Patients on bypass are always given heparin during surgery to keep their blood from clotting in the pump. At the end of the operation, the heparin is neutralized with protamine, a group of positively charged proteins that form tight complexes with the negatively charged heparin molecules, preventing them from interacting with antithrombin III. These patients sometimes bleed after surgery has been com-

---

Complications of Heparin Treatment

Bleeding

Thrombocytopenia (with paradoxical arterial thrombosis)

Osteoporosis (rare)

pleted and the protamine has been given. Although there are a number of reasons why such bleeding may occur, the situation often boils down to the question: Does the patient have DIC, or has the heparin been incompletely neutralized? Routine testing may not answer this question: Levels of fibrin-split products may be ambiguous, the split products themselves can mimic the anticoagulant activity of heparin, and the platelet count will be low in any postoperative patient who has received many units of blood. Fortunately, there is a test that can distinguish between these two possibilities (Fig. 16-3). This test, known as the *reptilase time*, is carried out by measuring how long it takes for plasma to clot after adding reptilase, the venom from the South American pit viper (*Bothrops jararaca*). Reptilase causes clot formation by splitting off fibrinopeptide A from fibrinogen, acting much like thrombin; in fact, the reptilase time is very similar in principle to the thrombin time. Reptilase, however, is not affected by the heparin–antithrombin III complex. Consequently, the reptilase time will be perfectly normal in heparin toxicity even though the thrombin time may be infinite. Both times will be prolonged in DIC, however, because fibrin-split products will retard the assembly of fibrin monomers into a clot regardless of whether the monomers are produced by thrombin or reptilase.

As to treatment, mild bleeding caused by heparin toxicity can be managed by watchful waiting, as heparin is rapidly cleared from the bloodstream. For serious bleeding, heparin should be neutralized by protamine. Overneutralization should be avoided, however, because there is some indication that protamine itself may interfere with clotting. Transfusions should be used for blood replacement as necessary, but it should be borne in mind that *transfusions will not correct the clotting defect caused by heparin* and should therefore not be administered for that purpose.

Thrombocytopenia and Arterial Thrombosis; Osteoporosis

Some patients receiving heparin will develop a low platelet count, probably because of the development of a heparin-dependent antiplatelet antibody (see Ch. 14). This can be a serious problem, because the reduction in platelets combines with the anticoagulant effect of the heparin to produce a high bleeding hazard, while at the same time the patient mysteriously becomes subject to arterial thrombosis. If unexplained thrombocytopenia should develop in a patient receiving heparin, the heparin should generally be stopped and the patient switched to oral anticoagulants.

Patients on long-term heparin may develop osteoporosis (i.e., washed-out bones). This very rare complication has only been seen in patients who have been on high dose heparin for 6 months or longer.

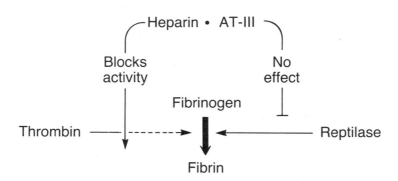

Fig. 16-3. Reptilase time versus thrombin time. AT-III, antithrombin III.

Vitamin K Antagonists

Vitamin K is necessary for the conversion of certain glutamate (glu) residues to γ-carboxyglutamate (gla) residues in factors II (prothrombin), VII, IX, and X. In the course of the glu→gla reaction, the vitamin undergoes oxidation and has to be converted back to the reduced form before it can take part in the formation of another gla residue (Fig. 16-4). Vitamin K antagonists act by blocking the reduction of the oxidized vitamin, leading to a deficiency of reduced vitamin K. As a result, the glu→gla reaction is retarded so the vitamin K-dependent clotting factors are unable to acquire their essential γ-carboxyglutamate residues. Without their γ-carboxyglutamates, these clotting factors cannot bind Ca^{2+}, making them unable to function. The result is a state of impaired coagulation caused by an acquired deficiency of these four clotting factors. The clotting factors do not fall simultaneously, but are lost sequentially: factor VII first, because it turns over in the blood faster than any other

clotting factor (its half-life in the blood is only 6 hours, as compared with the next shortest half-life, that of factor VIII, which is twice as long); factors IX and X next; and finally prothrombin, which requires 3 to 4 days to fall. The anticoagulated state is achieved only when all four clotting factors have reached their final levels.

As the active clotting factors decline, their gla-free precursors accumulate (1) in the liver, where they are manufactured; and (2) in the blood, where they are released from the liver and act as weak anticoagulants.

All the effects of the vitamin K antagonists are reversed by a single dose of vitamin K, provided it is large enough. Carboxylation of glutamates begins as soon as the vitamin reaches the liver, and the clotting factor deficiency is completely corrected within 1 or 2 days. There is some evidence, in fact, for a transient overshoot as the accumulated precursors are rapidly carboxylated and released into the plasma as active clotting factors. This may be the basis for the rebound hypercoagulability

Fig. 16-4. The vitamin K cycle and the mechanism of action of vitamin K antagonists. Vitamin K in its reduced (hydroquinone) form is an essential cofactor for the carboxylation of glutamate (glu) to γ-carboxyglutamate (gla). During the course of this reaction, the vitamin is oxidized to the quinone epoxide and must be reconverted to the hydroquinone before it can participate again in the glu→gla reaction. Reconversion involves two sequential reductions: quinone epoxide→quinone, and quinone→hydroquinone. Vitamin K antagonists block the first of these reductions, thereby retarding the glu→gla conversion by depriving the reaction of its cofactor.

Fig. 16-5. Warfarin and hydroxycoumarin.

that reportedly occurs after a dose of vitamin K is given to correct an anticoagulated state.

All the vitamin K antagonists in current use are derivatives of a compound known as *hydroxycoumarin* (Fig. 16-5). They differ principally in their durations of action. At present, warfarin (Fig. 16-5) appears to be the vitamin K antagonist enjoying the widest use. The popularity of warfarin stems from the fact that its duration of action (5 to 7 days) offers the best compromise between the need for a stable level of anticoagulation and the conflicting need for a rapid response when the dose of the drug is changed.

Clinical Use

Vitamin K antagonists have a very different role in anticoagulant therapy from that of heparin (Table 16-1). The latter is generally used to treat acute episodes of intravascular clotting, and the course of treatment is generally short (10 days or so). It is always given parenterally. In contrast, the vitamin K antagonists are used more to prevent future clotting than to treat immediate episodes of thrombosis. The course of treatment is long, lasting months to years. The vitamin K antagonists are always given by mouth.

Clinical Use of Vitamin K Antagonists

Start at the estimated maintenance dose

Follow prothrombin time daily. Adjust dose to achieve a prothrombin time of 1.2 to 2.0 times normal

Continue heparin until the anticoagulant effect of the vitamin K antagonist is established (generally 5 days)

Once maintenance dose is determined, prothrombin time may be followed less frequently (eventually, every 2 to 3 weeks)

Patients are started on vitamin K antagonists at the dose considered necessary to maintain them at an adequate level of anticoagulation. A loading dose is not needed. The level of anticoagulation is evaluated by following the prothrombin time, which measures all the vitamin K-dependent clotting factors except perhaps factor IX. The aim is to lengthen the PT to 1.2 to 2.0 times normal, the exact value depending on the condition being treated. This generally requires 3 to 4 days. If the patient is on heparin, the vitamin K antagonist is given with the heparin for 5 days, after which the heparin is stopped. Initially, it is generally necessary to measure the prothrombin time daily and to adjust the dose of anticoagulant frequently. Eventually, it is possible in most cases to find a maintenance dose on which the patient will stay properly anticoagulated. Once this dose is discovered, the prothrombin time can be followed less frequently.

Table 16-1. Heparin and the Fibrinolytic Agents versus the Vitamin K Antagonists

	Heparin and the Fibrinolytic Agents	Vitamin K Antagonists
Purpose	Treatment of intravascular clotting	Prevention of future thrombosis
Route of administration	Parenteral	Oral
Duration of treatment	Days	Months to years

Cause of Poor Control

Even under the best of circumstances, anticoagulation therapy is a haphazard affair. The range of therapeutic anticoagulation is narrow, and patients will frequently move in and out of this range even on a constant dose of anticoagulant. In many cases, no reason can be found for those fluctuations in control. Nevertheless, certain possibilities should be considered whenever control lapses in a patient on vitamin K antagonists. These include drug interactions, liver disease, change in diet, and noncompliance.

Drug Interactions

More than any other type of drug, the vitamin K antagonists are affected by other drugs that the patient may be taking. The four mechanisms by which these drug interactions take place are as follows.

Accelerated Destruction of the Vitamin K Antagonist. Vitamin K antagonists are inactivated largely by the cytochrome P-450 system in the liver. The cytochrome P-450 system is an enzyme system (more accurately, a group of closely related enzyme systems) whose function is to oxidize drugs and other foreign chemicals so as to speed their elimination from the body. A property of this enzyme system is that it is induced by certain of the drugs it oxidizes, increasing in quantity whenever these drugs are present. This increase in the quantity of the cytochrome P-450 system naturally leads to an increase in the rate at which its substrates are metabolized. Specifically, it leads to accelerated destruction of the vitamin K antagonists. The result is an abrupt increase in the dose of anticoagulant required to maintain a given level of anticoagulation. Consequently, whenever a patient receiving anticoagulants takes a P-450-inducing drug, he escapes anticoagulation unless the dose is increased. Conversely, if an anticoagulated patient stops taking such a drug without adjusting the anticoagulant dose downward, he will become overanticoagulated as the P-450 level falls to its uninduced value, and is at increased risk of bleeding.

Decreased Destruction of the Vitamin K Antagonist. Certain drugs act not as inducers of the cytochrome P-450 system but as inhibitors of that system. Such drugs will slow the rate at which vitamin K antagonists are destroyed in the liver. The result is that a lower dose of anticoagulant is required to achieve a therapeutic effect. Patients on vitamin K antagonists who begin to take such drugs will require downward adjustment in their anticoagulant dose to avoid becoming overanticoagulated.

Displacement of the Anticoagulant from Plasma Albumin. In the circulation, anticoagulants are present in two freely exchangeable pools: a pool of unbound drug, and a pool of drug bound to plasma albumin. Although by far most of the drug is in the albumin-bound pool, it is the size of the tiny unbound pool that determines the degree of anticoagulation, because it is from this pool that the drug is taken up by the liver to exert its effect. When a patient on anticoagulants is given another drug that binds to albumin, the pool of unbound anticoagulant increases as the new drug displaces some of the albumin-bound anticoagulant from the protein into free solution. Such a drug has the effect of increasing the potency of the anticoagulant and will throw the patient into an overanticoagulated state unless the dose of anticoagulant is cut.

Alterations of Intestinal Bacteria by Oral Antibiotics. A small amount of vitamin K is manufactured by the bacteria in the gastrointestinal tract. This makes no difference in patients on a normal diet, but in malnourished patients the intestinal bacteria can represent a significant source of the vitamin. Vitamin K deficiency can develop in these patients if their intestinal flora are suppressed by oral antibiot-

Table 16-2. Interactions Between Vitamin K Antagonists and Other Drugs

Promotion of Anticoagulant Effect		Opposition of Anticoagulant Effect	
Inhibition of cytochrome P-450	Displacement of anticoagulant from albumin	Alteration of intestinal bacteria	Induction of cytochrome P-450
Chloramphenicol Allopurinol	Long-acting sulfonamides Phenylbutazone Phenytoin Aspirin (3g/day)	Neomycin	Barbiturates Glutethimide

ics. If these patients are placed on vitamin K antagonists, they will become overanticoagulated as the developing deficiency shifts the balance between the vitamin and the anticoagulant drug.

In Table 16-2, some of the more commonly used drugs that take part in these interactions are classified according to mechanism.

Liver Disease

Patients receiving anticoagulants are extraordinarily sensitive to the effects of liver disease on clotting factor production. Accordingly, the development of liver disease (e.g., drug-induced or viral hepatitis) is an occasional cause of sudden overanticoagulation in patients on vitamin K antagonists.

Change in Diet

In a patient on vitamin K antagonists, the level of anticoagulation depends on the balance between the dose of anticoagulant and the amount of vitamin K in the diet. A change in the diet may therefore throw an anticoagulated patient out of control and should be considered as a possibility whenever a patient on vitamin K antagonists lapses from control in either direction.

Noncompliance

The most common cause of poor control in an anticoagulated patient is noncompliance: The patient fails to take the drug. The best way to diagnose noncompliance is to measure the level of anticoagulant in the blood. It takes several days for most of the commonly used vitamin K antagonists to be eliminated from the body, so a very low blood level suggests that the patient has not taken the anticoagulant for a number of days.

Complications

Bleeding

Bleeding is a common complication in patients receiving oral anticoagulants. It is particularly common in the overanticoagulated patient, but it may take place when the level of anticoagulation is in the therapeutic range. In the latter case, bleeding generally occurs from a preexisting lesion such as a healed duodenal ucler or an intestinal polyp. Bleeding in overanticoagulated patients, however, can occur even in the absence of an underlying lesion.

Management of Bleeding Caused by Vitamin K Antagonists

Stop the anticoagulant

Replace depleted clotting factors with fresh frozen plasma or, less desirably, with factor IX concentrate

Give Vitamin K if necessary

Give transfusions as indicated

Minor bleeding can sometimes be managed by withholding the anticoagulant for a while and restoring the depleted clotting factors with fresh frozen plasma (or, if fluid overload is a problem, with factor IX concentrate, which in fact contains all the vitamin-K-dependent clotting factors; the concentrate is a poor second choice, however, because it carries the risk of hepatitis as well as that of thrombosis due to contaminating activated clotting factors). It is often necessary, however, to neutralize the anticoagulant by giving vitamin K. A single dose of vitamin K is all that is needed to correct the clotting defect. Because correction requires the synthesis of new clotting factor, it takes 24 to 48 hours to reach completion. During this interval it may be necessary to give fresh frozen plasma (or factor IX concentrate) as a stopgap measure. Blood transfusions should be given as needed.

Decisions as to how to treat bleeding in chronically anticoagulated patients can be very difficult. Whereas stopping the bleeding is obviously essential, anticoagulation may be indispensable to prevent intravascular clotting in a high-risk patient (e.g., one with an artificial heart valve). The words of Hippocrates apply: "Art is long and life is short; the occasion instant, decision difficult and experiment perilous." Choosing among the therapeutic alternatives, with their uncertain benefits and imponderable risks, can tax the skills of the most able and experienced physicians.

Anticoagulation during Pregnancy

There are unusual hazards to the use of vitamin K antagonists during pregnancy. Vitamin K antagonists cross the placenta and enter the fetal bloodstream, leading to congenital anomalies if they are used during the first trimester. Maternal bleeding during delivery is also a problem. For these reasons, vitamin K antagonists should not be used during pregnancy, especially in the first and last trimesters. Long-term anticoagulation in pregnant women is generally carried out with heparin, which does not cross the placenta.

Other Anticoagulants

Two other agents are occasionally used as anticoagulants, one obtained from snake venom and the other from bacteria.

Ancrod

Ancrod is a highly specific protease isolated from the venom of the Malayan pit viper, *Agkistrodon rhodostoma*. It acts like reptilase, splitting fibrinopeptide A from the fibrinogen molecule. Fibrinogen altered in this way can no longer be acted on by thrombin. The blood is thus effectively stripped of fibrinogen (this process is called *defibrination*) and in this way is rendered unclottable.

The fibrinlike molecule produced by the action on fibrinogen is able to form a sort of clot, but the clot is weak and cannot be cross-linked by factor XIII. Its formation can be detected in clotting assays, but it is too weak to survive the powerful shearing forces in the circulation, so it breaks up in the blood vessels.

Dextran

Dextrans are mixtures of high-molecular-weight glucose polymers secreted by certain bacteria. Dextran for clinical use is isolated from the medium in which these bacteria are grown. It exerts its anticoagulant effect mainly by coating the red cells, thereby reducing blood viscosity and decreasing stasis in the circulation. It also has an antiplatelet action. It is occasionally used to prevent venous thrombosis, especially postoperatively.

FIBRINOLYTIC AGENTS

Like heparin, the fibrinolytic agents are used to treat acute thrombosis and embolism. They work by activating plasmin, the fibrin-dissolving enzyme of plasma. The plasmin opens

Table 16-3. Fibrinolytic Agents

Agent	Source	Antigenicity	Cost
Streptokinase	Streptococci	High	Moderate
Urokinase	Human	None	High
Tissue plasminogen activator	Cloned human	None	Very high

clogged vessels by digesting any clot that has already formed, in addition to slowing further clotting by digesting factors V and VIII and by releasing fibrin-split products.

Three fibrinolytic agents are currently in use: streptokinase, urokinase, and tissue plasminogen activator. Each has advantages and disadvantages (Table 16-3).

Streptokinase

This protein is made by group C streptococii, from which it is purified for clinical use. In the bloodstream, it combines with plasminogen (the precursor of plasmin), to form a complex with new and cannibalistic properties: The plasminogen in the complex is converted by the streptokinase into a highly specific protease that is able to convert free (i.e., not complexed to streptokinase) plasminogen into plasmin (Fig. 16-6). In practical terms, streptokinase has the disadvantage of being a foreign protein against which patients may have developed antibodies during a previous streptococcal infection. On the other hand, it is much less expensive than urokinase or tissue plasminogen activator.

Fig. 16-6. How streptokinase and urokinase activate plasmin.

Urokinase

This protein is made by the kidney and is isolated from human urine. It is a protease that acts directly on plasminogen, converting it to plasmin (Fig. 16-6). As a human protein, urokinase is not antigenic, so patients do not make antibodies against it. However, it is about 10 times as expensive as streptokinase. In fact, it is so expensive that streptokinase is preferred over urokinase unless the patient to be treated has an allergy that prevents its use.

Tissue Plasminogen Activator

Tissue plasminogen activator (t-PA), a major initiator of fibrinolysis in the normal circulation (see Ch. 13), has recently become available in large quantities through gene cloning. It has attracted a great deal of attention as a fibrinolytic drug because, unlike streptokinase and urokinase, t-PA binds specifically to the fibrin in a blood clot, a process that both restricts its mobility and results in a sharp increase in its activity. As a result, t-PA will generate plasmin mainly at the site of a clot undergoing dissolution, whereas in contrast, streptokinase and urokinase will generate plasmin throughout the general circulation. Because the action of t-PA is localized whereas that of streptokinase and urokinase is generalized, the latter two have to activate much more plasmin than the former in order to dissolve the same amount of clot. This means that t-PA should theoretically generate the same clot-lysing power as streptokinase or urokinase with much less risk of bleeding. Recent clinical trials have shown, however, that the risk of bleeding is just as high in patients treated with t-PA as in those treated with other fibrinolytic agents. These findings, together with its very high cost, suggest that t-PA is probably not the fibrinolytic agent of choice, at least at the present time.

Clinical Use

Acute myocardial infarction is on its way to becoming the major indication for fibrinolytic therapy. Patients with fresh myocardial infarctions clearly benefit from a single intravenous dose of a fibrinolytic agent given within 3 to 6 hours of the onset of the illness: Clots in the coronary arteries dissolve, myocardial damage is decreased, and survival improves. Although treatment is often complicated by bleeding, sometimes severe, the overall results are promising, and the use of a fibrinolytic agent in myocardial infarction—investigational at the moment—is likely to become standard treatment in the near future.

Fibrinolytic agents are also used in the treatment of severe thrombophlebitis. For this condition, the agent is usually given intravenously in fixed doses for 24 to 48 hours, after which the patient is switched over to heparin. In contrast to practice with other anticoagulants,

treatment is generally not followed in the laboratory, because the dose is fixed. The existence of a fibrinolytic state, however, should be established once early in treatment by some laboratory measure of fibrinolysis: a shortened euglobulin lysis time, a prolonged thrombin time, elevated levels of fibrin-split products, or any other convenient test.

For treating thrombophlebitis, fibrinolytic agents appear to be the most effective of all the anticoagulants, but they are also the most dangerous with respect to bleeding. Even arterial lines can begin to leak blood in patients being given fibrinolytic agents. Consequently, these agents are rarely used for thrombophlebitis, and then only in its most serious forms, as in massive pulmonary embolism or very extensive thrombophlebitis in young patients, for example. Fibrinolytic agents should be avoided in any patient with an increased risk of bleeding (e.g., postoperative patients, who can be anticoagulated with heparin or vitamin K antagonists under some circumstances but who should not as a general rule receive fibrinolytic agents).

Bleeding from Fibrinolytic Agents

When a patient on fibrinolytic therapy begins to bleed, the chances are overwhelming that the fibrinolytic agent is primarily responsible and treatment should be directed accordingly. If bleeding is minor (e.g., a leak around an arterial line), it can sometimes be handled by local compression. If it is severe, or if it does not respond to local measures, fibrinolytic therapy should be stopped. This will restore fibrinolysis to normal levels within an hour or two, but a bleeding problem may still exist because of the secondary effects of fibrinolysis (i.e., low plasma fibrinogen, factors V and VIII, and circulating fibrin-split products). Fresh frozen plasma or cryoprecipitate can be used if necessary to treat these secondary problems. Blood transfusions should be given as required.

Clinical Use of Fibrinolytic Agents

Acute myocardial infarction
Give a single intravenous dose if infarction is less than 3 to 6 hours old

Thrombophlebitis
Use at fixed doses for 24 to 48 hours, then switch to heparin

Document the existence of a fibrinolytic state early in therapy

Use only for the most serious forms of thrombophlebitis, because there is a high risk of bleeding with fibrinolytic agents

Management of Bleeding Caused by Fibrinolytic Agents

Stop fibrinolytic therapy

Give blood transfusions

Administer fresh frozen plasma or cryoprecipitate if necessary to correct plasmin-induced deficiencies of fibrinogen and factors V and VIII

Give ε-aminocaproic acid for life-threatening bleeding

Occasionally bleeding caused by fibrinolytic therapy is massive or occurs in a critical location (e.g., inside the skull). This sort of bleeding problem constitutes a major emergency and requires the most rapid possible reversal of fibrinolysis. This is accomplished by giving ε-aminocaproic acid, an inhibitor of plasminogen activation. This treatment carries with it the hazard of thrombosis and should only be used for the most serious forms of fibrinolysis-associated bleeding.

ANTIPLATELET DRUGS

In addition to the anticoagulants, which interfere with the formation and maintenance of the fibrin clot, a number of agents in clinical use work by interfering with platelet function. These antiplatelet agents are used mainly to prevent thrombosis on the arterial side of the circulation, where clots are generally thought to originate as intravascular platelet aggregates. They are less useful against thrombosis on the venous side, because venous thrombosis appears to result mainly from inappropriate activation of the clotting cascade, with platelets playing only a secondary role.

The antiplatelet agents in current use include aspirin, sulfinpyrazone, and dipyridamole (Table 16-4). They are all much less potent than the anticoagulants, but they are also much less hazardous. Bleeding caused by impaired platelets is only a minor problem with aspirin (although its ability to cause serious GI bleeding through local irritation is well known) and is never seen with the other two drugs.

Aspirin

Aspirin blocks thromboxane production by irreversibly inactivating platelet cyclooxygenase. Through its effect on thromboxane production, aspirin prevents the secondary wave of aggregation undergone by platelets responding to direct stimuli. Its use as an antiplatelet agent is based on this effect.

In very high doses, aspirin blocks the production of prostacyclin, a natural inhibitor of platelet aggregation, by inactivating the cyclooxygenase of the vascular endothelium. In the absence of prostacyclin, platelet aggregation is extremely efficient—enough to more than offset the direct effect of aspirin on the platelets. Theoretically, then, high doses of aspirin would have an effect diametrically opposed to that desired—that is, the drug would act to promote platelet aggregation, not inhibit it. However, doses of aspirin sufficient to achieve this reversed effect are not used in practice.

Sulfinpyrazone

Sulfinpyrazone, like aspirin, is an inhibitor of platelet cyclooxygenase, although its action, unlike aspirin's, is reversible. Its anti-platelet effect is the result of its ability to block thromboxane formation.

Table 16-4. Antiplatelet Agents

Agent	Effect	Mechanism of Action
Aspirin	Decreased thromboxane production	Inactivation of cyclooxygenase (*ir*reversible)
Sulfinpyrazone	Decreased thromboxane production	Inhibition of cyclooxygenase (reversible)
Dipyridamole	Increased cAMP	Inhibition of phosphodiesterase

Fig. 16-7. Cyclic AMP metabolism. For the sake of clarity, some phosphate-bound oxygen atoms have been omitted.

Dipyridamole

As with many tissues, the function of platelets is controlled in part by the internal concentration of a special regulatory nucleotide known as *cyclic adenosine monophosphate* (cAMP) (Fig. 16-7). This nucleotide is made from adenosine triphosphate (ATP) by adenyl cyclase, an enzyme whose activity is influenced by external stimuli such as hormones. It is broken down by phosphodiesterase, which opens its ring to convert it to AMP. Its concentration inside the platelet depends on the relative activities of the cyclase and the phosphodiesterase: A high cyclase/phosphodiesterase ratio favors its accumulation; a low ratio favors its depletion.

In the platelet, cAMP acts as a general suppressant, inhibiting aggregation and release. It follows that any drug that can promote the accumulation of this nucleotide is likely to interfere with platelet function. Dipyridamole is such a drug, causing cAMP to accumulate in platelets by inhibiting phosphodiesterase. It is in this way that dipyridamole exerts its anti-platelet effect.

Because aspirin and dipyridamole work through different mechanisms, they act synergistically to inhibit platelet function. These two drugs used in combination offer a particularly effective form of anti-platelet therapy.

INDICATIONS FOR TREATMENT

Venous throbosis and pulmonary embolism are the most frequent indications for anticoagulant treatment (Table 16-5). Because they are so subtle, so often difficult to diagnose, and especially because they are so common, they will be discussed more fully than the other indications for anticoagulation.

Venous Thrombosis

Venous thrombosis usually involves the veins of the legs and pelvis. It occurs most often when there is stasis of blood in the veins —notably, in pregnant women and in patients placed at bed rest. The likelihood of this event is increased if the patient has had a recent

---

Uncommon Causes of a Hypercoagulable State

Coagulation disorders
    Antithrombin III deficiency
    Protein C deficiency
    Protein S deficiency
    Abnormal plasminogen
    Defective release of plasminogen activator
    Dysfibrinogenemia
    Increased factor V or VIII (?)

Stem cell diseases
    Polycythemia vera
    Essential thrombocythemia
    Thrombocythemia secondary to myelofibrosis or chronic myelogenous leukemia
    Paroxysmal nocturnal hemoglobinuria

Vessel wall disease
    Homocystinuria

Table 16-5. Indications for Anticoagulants and Antiplatelet Drugs

	Full-dose Anticoagulation	Antiplatelet agents	Low-dose heparin	Fibrinolytic agents
Prophylactic				
Against arterial thrombosis				
Postmyocardial infarction		+		
Postcerebrovascular thrombosis		+		
Saphenous vein bypass grafts		+		
Against arterial embolism		+		
Valves and grafts	+	+ (mechanical)		
Other				
Against venous thrombosis				
Patients put to bed			+	
Before chest or abdominal surgery			+	
Broken hip or before hip surgery	+			
Therapeutic				
Venous thrombosis and pulmonary embolism	+			
Arterial embolism	+ (old)			+ (fresh)
Atherosclerosis				
Myocardial infarction			+	+ (new)
Unstable angina		+		
Stroke-in-evolution	+			
Transient ischemic attacks		+ (aspirin)		
Thrombocytosis		+		

operation or suffers from congestive heart failure or any of the conditions associated with chronic DIC. In addition, there are certain uncommon diseases, almost all hematologic, in which venous thrombosis may be a major problem. All these conditions that predispose to venous thrombosis are said to induce a "hypercoagulable state."

The diagnosis of venous thrombosis is difficult to make on clinical grounds. The leg on the affected side may ache and swell, and there may be tenderness over the course of the vein, but these symptoms are seen in other conditions as well. Moreover, venous thrombosis often occurs without any clinical manifestations whatsoever. It is therefore important to be able to make the diagnosis by more accurate techniques. A number of methods are available to establish the diagnosis of venous thrombosis (Fig. 16-8). These include the following.

Venography

In venography, radiography is used to visualize obstructed vessels after the injection of a radiopaque dye into the veins of the legs. This procedure is the surest way to diagnose venous thrombosis, but it is an invasive technique and may sometimes be complicated by thrombosis of a previously normal vein.

^{125}I-Fibrinogen Scanning

When given intravenously to a patient with ongoing venous thrombosis, ^{125}I-fibrinogen will be incorporated into the clot, where it can be detected by external radiation monitoring. This is a less invasive procedure than venography and is commonly used in some areas of the world to diagnose venous thrombosis. Its disadvantages are that (1) it takes about 3 days for enough radioactivity to be incorporated so the clot can be seen by external monitoring, and (2) it is unreliable in picking up clots in the deep veins of the pelvis and thigh, although it is quite accurate for calf vein thrombosis.

Impedance Plethysmography

In this procedure, the leg is made to fill with excess blood by occluding the veins of the upper thigh through the use of an inflatable cuff. The cuff is then abruptly deflated, and the rate at which the excess blood drains from the leg

Venography

^{125}I-fibrinogen
scanning

A

B

Impedance
plethysmography

Doppler
ultrasound

C

D

Fig. 16-8. Methods of diagnosing venous thrombosis. (**A**) Venography. Veins are visualized by radiography after the intravenous injection of a radiopaque dye. (**B**) ^{125}I-fibrinogen scanning. ^{125}I-figrinogen taken up into a clot is detected by external radiation monitoring. (**C**) Impedence plethysmography. When the cuff is inflated, venous drainage from the leg is blocked, causing the leg to swell as it fills with excess blood. Deflation of the cuff permits excess blood to drain off, restoring the leg to its original size. The rate at which the leg returns to its original size is measured electrically. (**D**) Doppler ultrasound. A beam of ultrasound is directed at the vein in the leg. The pitch of the echo from the beam indicates whether blood is flowing through the vein.

is determined by measuring the rate of fall in the volume of the engorged leg is it returns to its original size, using the electrical resistance across the leg (i.e., the impedance) as the volume indicator. This method is best for detecting obstructing thrombi in the large veins of the thigh and pelvis; it is not reliable for calf vein thrombosis.

Doppler Ultrasound

This test uses high-frequency sound (ultrasound) to determine whether blood is flowing in a vein. A beam of ultrasound is aimed at the vein, causing some of the sound to be reflected from the red cells in the vein as an echo. If the red cells are moving, the pitch of the echo will be different from that of the original beam be-

cause of the Doppler effect (the same effect that causes the pitch of a locomotive whistle to drop as the train passes). If, however, the red cells are at rest because of a clot in the vein, the beam and the echo will have the same pitch. Like impedance plethysmography, the ultrasound test is sensitive to thrombi in the large veins of the thigh and pelvis, but it cannot pick up calf vein thrombi.

Pulmonary Embolism

The real danger posed by a clot in the veins of the leg or pelvis is that a piece of the clot can break away from its original mooring, travel to the lungs, and lodge there as a plug in the pulmonary circulation. A piece of clot that breaks loose in this way is known as an *embo-*

lus, and the occlusion of a pulmonary vessel by such a piece of clot is called *pulmonary embolism*.

The symptoms of pulmonary embolism usually begin abruptly and include various combinations of cough, chest pain, and breathlessness. A large embolus blocking both main branches of the pulmonary artery (a so-called saddle embolus) will cause acute, crushing chest pain like that of a heart attack and can prove fatal within minutes unless treated immediately. A smaller embolus can present with cough, shortness of breath, or both; if small enough, it may cause no symptoms at all. If an embolus affects a region of lung with an already impaired blood supply, it can cause the death of a segment of lung tissue (pulmonary infarction). Symptoms in this case are hemoptysis and "pleuritic" chest pain (i.e., pain aggravated by respiration, attributable to inflammation of the pleura overlying the dead lung). Chronic recurrent pulmonary emboli can lead to pulmonary hypertension and ultimately right heart failure.

Like the diagnosis of venous thrombosis, the diagnosis of pulmonary embolism must be established by special techniques, either lung scan or pulmonary angiography.

Lung Scan

The lung scan shows the distribution of blood and air in the lungs. Both are determined by giving the patient a suitable radioactive tracer and then measuring the distribution of the radioactivity in the lungs with a scanning device. To look at the distribution of blood, ^{125}I-labeled aggregated albumin given by vein is often used as a tracer; the distribution of air is determined with ^{133}Xe given by inhalation. Certain abnormalities in the distribution patterns will indicate a high likelihood of pulmonary embolism.

Pulmonary Angiography

In pulmonary angiography, the pulmonary blood supply is directly visualized by radiography after the injection of a radiopaque dye into the pulmonary artery through a right heart

Fig. 16-9. Pulmonary angiogram showing cut-off left pulmonary artery (*arrow*). A column of dye that should normally fill that artery and its branches is abruptly blocked by an embolic plug located at the point of the cut-off. This x-ray finding is virtually diagnostic of pulmonary embolism. (From Shuck, J.W., Walder, J.S., Kam, T.H. & Thomas, H.M. (1980) Chronic persistent pulmonary embolism: Report of three cases. Am J. Med. *69*:790–794, with permission.)

catheter. The presence of cut-off vessels (Fig. 16-9) is virtually diagnostic of pulmonary embolism. Pulmonary angiography is much less dangerous than it sounds and is used frequently to establish the diagnosis of pulmonary embolism with certainty before committing a patient to a hazardous course of anticoagulant therapy.

Treatment

Once the diagnosis of venous thrombosis or pulmonary embolism is made, anticoagulant therapy is started. As a general rule, patients are begun on heparin (or, less frequently, fibrinolytic drugs followed by heparin), then switched to a vitamin K antagonist after 7 to 10 days. Treatment with a vitamin K antagonist is continued for 3 months or so, then stopped.

Other Indications

Arterial Embolism

Arterial embolism (i.e., obstruction of an artery by a clot that has traveled there from somewhere else) is always an indication for anticoagulation. If the embolus is fresh, fibrinolytic agents should be used. Otherwise, treatment is similar to that used for pulmonary embolism. If the patient has an underlying condition that is regularly associated with arterial embolism—for example, an artificial heart valve, or a prolapsed mitral valve with chronic atrial fibrillation—prophylactic anticoagulation should be started with a vitamin K antagonist for an indefinite period to prevent the first episode of embolism from occurring.

Fractured Hip and Hip Surgery

Venous thrombosis and pulmonary embolism are especially common in patients who have fractured their hips or who require hip surgery. These patients should be anticoagulated with full doses of vitamin K during their convalescence.

Low-Dose Heparin

Low-dose heparin is an unusually benign method for preventing venous thrombosis that should be considered in all patients at risk of developing this condition. Examples are patients about to undergo chest or abdominal surgery and patients on bed rest because of chronic heart failure or malignancy.

Atherosclerotic Heart Disease or Cerebrovascular Disease

Whether to anticoagulate patients for angina, heart attacks, or strokes has been a vexing question since anticoagulants were first introduced into medical practice. Opinion has cycled over the years, depending on the results of the most current studies. Very large scale clinical trials, however, are just now beginning to provide some reasonably firm answers to these difficult questions. Currently there appears to be no indication for heparin or vitamin K antagonists in any form of atherosclerotic disease affecting the brain, except perhaps in stroke-in-evolution. In myocardial infarction,

treatment with low-dose heparin is now recommended unless the risk of embolism is high (e.g., in a patient with atrial fibrillation); in these patients, low-level warfarin anticoagulation (PT $1.2-1.5 \times$ normal) is used. Further recommendations will depend on the results of future clinical trials.

Antiplatelet Drugs

Thrombocytosis

Intravascular clotting is a problem when there are too many platelets in circulation, particularly if the platelets are functionally abnormal. Antiplatelet agents are often given to control clotting in thrombocytosis. Evidence as to their effectiveness is scanty, but their use under these conditions constitutes a valid approach to therapy.

Artificial Valves and Blood Vessel Grafts

Clots will always form on artificial valves and blood vessel grafts, with arterial embolism as the inevitable sequel, unless patients with such valves and grafts are anticoagulated prophylactically. The need for vitamin K antagonists in these patients has been demonstrated. For mechanical valves, antiplatelet agents should probably be used as well, because they have been shown to provide an extra measure of protection beyond that afforded by vitamin K antagonists. The best regimen for such patients probably consists of full doses of a vitamin K antagonist, plus dipyridamole to cripple the platelets. Saphenous vein bypass grafts are kept open with aspirin plus dipyridamole, and atrioventricular (A-V) shunts with aspirin alone.

Atherosclerotic Heart Disease or Cerebrovascular Disease

Antiplatelet agents have been studied as intensively as anticoagulants in an effort to find a role for them in the treatment of heart attacks and strokes. These studies show that aspirin is useful in cerebrovascular disease (1) to reduce the frequency of attacks and prevent full-blown strokes in patients who suffer from so-called transient ischemic attacks (i.e., brief episodes of neurologic symptoms caused by atherosclerosis of the blood vessels that supply the brain) and (2) to reduce the likelihood of second strokes in patients with prior cerebral thrombosis. In coronary artery disease, antiplatelet agents (1) are useful in unstable angina and (2) will reduce the mortality rate after a heart attack. Beyond these limited indications, no other use has yet been found for antiplatelet agents in managing the complications of atherosclerosis.

Prevention of Atherosclerosis

The role postulated for platelets in the development of atherosclerosis has raised considerable interest in the possibility that antiplatelet drugs might be useful in preventing this disease. Despite the claims of certain widely publicized studies, however, the answer to this question is not clear. Although aspirin may well turn out to be an effective prophylaxis against heart attacks, it remains to be seen whether this benefit will result in an increased life expectancy, or offset the dangers of acute GI bleeding in patients receiving long-term aspirin therapy.

SUGGESTED READINGS

ACCP-NHLBI National Conference on Antithrombotic Therapy (1986) Chest *89*:25.

Bauer, K.A. & Rosenberg, R.D. (1987) The pathophysiology of the prethrombotic state in humans: Insights gained from studies using markers of hemostatic system activation. Blood *70*:343.

Brozovic, M. (1976) Oral anticoagulants, vitamin K and prothrombin complex factors. Br. J. Haematol. *32*:9.

Graham, D.Y. & Smith, J.L. (1986) Aspirin and the stomach. Annu. Rev. Med. *104*:390.

Hirsh, J. (1981) Blood tests for the diagnosis of venous and arterial thrombosis. Blood *57*:1.

Kelton, J.G. & Hirsh, J. (1980) Bleeding associated with antithrombotic therapy. Semin. Hematol. *17*:259.

Lewis, S.M. (1987) Thromboplastin and oral anticoagulant control. Br. J. Haematol. *66*:1.

Oates, J.A., Wood, A.J.J. & FitzGerald, G.A. (1987) Drug therapy. Dipyridamole. N. Engl. J. Med. *316*:1247.

Preston, F.E. (1985) Platelet suppressive therapy in clinical medicine. Br. J. Haematol. *60*:589.

Schaefer, A.I. & Handin, R.I. (1980) The role of platelets in thrombotic and vascular disease. Progr. Cardiovasc. Dis. *22*:31.

Schafer, A.I. (1985) The hypercoagulable states. Ann. Intern. Med. *102*:814.

Sharma, G.V.R.K., Cella, G., Parisi, A., et al. (1982) Drug therapy: Thrombolytic therapy. N. Engl. J. Med. *306*:1268.

Verstraete, M. & Collen, D. (1986) Thrombolytic therapy in the eighties. Blood *67*:1529.

SECTION III

White Blood Cells
and Their Diseases

Although white blood cells are no whiter than any other unpigmented tissue cells, the term *white cell* was concocted by nineteenth century microscopists to distinguish these actually colorless cells from the red-tinted erythrocytes. The blood contains three principal types of white blood cells: the polymorphonuclear leukocytes, the monocytes, and the lymphocytes. These white cells or leukocytes arise from pluripotent stem cells in the bone marrow (Ch. 1) and differentiate into those forms that are easily distinguished and different numbers of which circulate in the blood (Table III-1). Each type has a very different life history, function and fate. The enumeration of leukocytes, usually called the *white blood cell count* is one of the most frequently obtained laboratory values in medicine, because it is extremely informative as to the state of health of the host. The total white blood cell count is determined automatically by means of an electronic counter in most laboratories in the United States. The differential count, which identifies the different blood cell types, is usually done by an examination of Wright's stained smears, although automated counters for this purpose are being developed. The physician obtaining a white blood cell count and differential count receives a report of (1) the white blood cell count in cells per microliter (μl) or, as sometimes stated, per cubic millimeter (mm^3) and (2) percentage differential of the total of each white blood cell type. A convention being promoted for expressing laboratory values in medicine, known as the *SI system* (International System of Units; le Systeme International d'Unites), recommends that the number of white blood cells be expressed as cells per liter and that the *fraction* rather than the *percentage* of blood cells be enumerated. In other words, 5000 white blood cells per microliter becomes 5×10^9 cells per L, 50% neutrophils becomes 0.5 neutrophils, or 3% eosinophils becomes 0.03 eosinophils.

Table III-1. Numbers of White Blood Cells in Normal Blood

Total white blood cells	4,500–11,000/μl
Band-form (immature) Neutrophilic Polymorphonuclear Leukocytes	3%
Segmented (mature) Neutrophilic Polymorphonuclear Leukocytes	40–70%
Lymphocytes	25–45%
Eosinophilic Polymorphonuclear Leukocytes	3%
Basophilic Polymorphonuclear Leukocytes	0.5%
Monocytes	4%

The principal known function of white blood cells is in defending the organism against microbes. In this activity, the white blood cells are deployed in two major categories: the phagocytes and the lymphocytes. To defend against infection, there is considerable cooperation between these classes of white blood cells.

SUGGESTED READING

Young, D.S. (1987) Implementation of SI units for laboratory data. Ann Intern Med *106*:114.

Immunoproteins and Immunoprotein Disorders

IMMUNOPROTEINS: PLASMA PROTEINS IMPORTANT TO THE PHAGOCYTIC AND LYMPHOID SYSTEMS

A discussion of the plasma immunoproteins is introduced at this point for two reasons. First, the major class of circulating immunoproteins, the immunoglobulins, is produced by a set of lymphoid cells, the plasma cells. Other lymphocytes produce but do not secrete immunoglobulins, and the production and disposition of immunoglobulins by lymphocytes is intimately linked to their state of differentiation. Therefore, a comprehension of the stucture and function of immunoglobulins aids considerably in understanding lymphoid cell development. Second, the cells of the phagocytic and lymphoid systems depend to a large extent on recognition mechanisms that help them identify and respond to foreign invasion. In large measure, this surveillance is mediated by circulating immunoproteins. These proteins are remarkably versatile in that they can be involved simultaneously with white blood cells and pathogens.

Normal Structure and Function of the Immunoproteins

Immunoglobulins

Immunoglobulins, or antibodies, are a class of proteins of very similar structure that are secreted by plasma cells. The composition of all normal immunoglobulins is an assembly of two pairs of polypeptides; two larger ones are called *heavy chains* and two smaller ones are designated *light chains* (Fig. 17-1). Disulfide bonds connect the heavy chains to each other, and each heavy chain to one light chain. Despite the general similarity in the structure of immunoglobulins (Igs), small differences in the amino acid sequences of the heavy chains create important variations in the function of the immunoglobulins in their specific interactions with the immune system. These variations determine five classes of heavy chains, designated μ, γ, α, δ, and ε, which comprise immunoglobulins classified as IgM, IgG, IgA, IgD, and IgE, respectively (Fig. 17-2). Similar small differences in the amino acid sequences

Fig. 17-1. The structure of immunoglobulin.

of the light chains define two classes called $\varkappa$ and λ. The importance of $\varkappa$ and λ light chains in immune functions is unknown, but as amplifed in Chapter 20, they are very relevant for defining an origin of immunoglobulins from a single clone of lymphoid cells and for diagnosing certain neoplasms of lymphoid cells.

Alterations in the primary structure of the heavy chains and light chains near the region of the immunoglobulin where the heavy chains and light chains overlap confer the most remarkable feature on the immunoglobulin— their incredibly specific binding to all sorts and conditions of substances—which become defined as antigens. The domains in which the binding to antigen takes place is known as the *Fab region*. Bound to antigens by their Fab sites, the class of heavy chain and the opposite end of the immunoglobulins called the *Fc region* determine what will happend to the antigen–antibody complex (Fig. 17-1). The very similar amino acid sequences of about one-half the light chains and heavy chains in the Fab region and all the Fc region define what is called the *constant domains* of immunoglobulin molecules (shaded area, Fig. 17-1). The specificity for antigens arises from very different amino acid sequences in the other half of the Fab regions of the light chains and heavy chains, de-

noted as the variable domains. Most of the differences are clustered into four sequences of the variable regions, called the *hypervariable domains*. These combinations and permutations of amino acid sequences modify the final folding of the Fab region of the immunoglobulin molecule sufficiently to confer the exquisite specificity for antigen-binding characteristic of antibody molecules. A current theory describing how immunoglobulins are synthesized and how their antigen binding specificity is achieved is outlined in Chapter 20.

Immunoglobulins are found in all protein-containing internal body fluids. External secretions, such as tears, saliva, and gut fluids, contain principally immunoglobulin A (IgA) because of a unique carbohydrate-containing sequence called *secretory piece* that enables the immunoglobulin to be secreted. The function of secretory IgA is not known with certainty. IgG and IgA, but not IgM, cross the placenta. Therefore, newborns have maternal IgG and IgA in their plasma, but not IgM. On the other hand, IgM is made by newborns before they have the capacity to produce IgA or IgG.

The catabolism of immunoglobulins is proportional to their concentration in the plasma. Therefore, persons with high concentrations of

Class	Heavy Chain Class	Serum Concentration mg/ml	Structure		Major Functions
IgG	γ	12		Monomer	Antitoxin Virus neutralization Opsonization } Divided into subclasses IgG$_1$ - IgG$_4$ with different participation in these functions
IgA	α	3		Dimer, joined by "J-chain"	Immune functions in Secretions ? Prevent attachment of pathogens to mucosal surface
IgM	μ	1		Pentamer	Complement activation Agglutination reactions
IgD	δ	0.03	 B-cell membrane	Monomer	Unknown
IgE	ε	0.0001	 Mast cell & Basophil membrane	Cell bound "Cytophilic"	Mediator release

Fig. 17-2. Classes of immunoglobulin.

immunoglobulins in their plasma degrade these molecules more rapidly than do those with low concentrations of the proteins.

Complement

At least 20 proteins make up the *complement system* (Fig. 17-3); most of the proteins are designated by a number preceded by the capital letter C. Complement resembles the coagulation system (Ch. 13) in that it operates as a cascade, wherein proteins become sequentially activated. The consequences of activation of parts of the cascade are directed, like antibody, toward conferring recognition on foreign objects so they can be dealt with by white blood cells or, in some cases, even to cause the lysis of the foreign cells. In certain circumstances, immunoglobulin antibodies

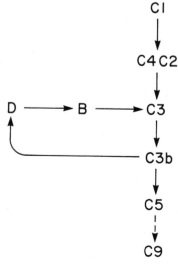

Fig. 17-3. (**A**) Classic complement sequence. Components within boxes remain entirely or partly attached to the target cell surface. (**B**) Alternative complement pathway and its relationship to the classic sequence.

cause the initial activation of the complement system (Fig. 17-3A). In such instances, antibody provides recognition, whereas complement generates or amplifies the effector response initiated by the recognition with antibody.

The Fc region of certain immunoglobulins bound to an antigen that usually is on a cell surface binds C1, which is actually a complex of protein subunits. The assembly of the C1 complex on the cell surface activates an enzymatic activity in the C1 complex called *esterase* of the C1 protein. This enzyme catalyzes the splitting of the C2 and C4 complement components into fragments. Pieces of C2 and C4 called C2b and C4b bind to the cell surface. C3 is the complement protein found in highest concentration in the blood. The C4b–C2b complex, known as the *classic pathway C3 convertase*, binds and splits C3 into fragments called C3a and C3b. C3a leaves the site at which it was cleaved, but it has the capacity to cause contraction of smooth muscle and to increase permeability, rendering it a mediator of inflammation. C3b bound to the cell surface is recognized by phagocytes and can cause phagocytosis or destruction of the cell to which it is bound by phagocytic cells. Of chemical interest in the binding of C3 to target objects is the fact that C3 cleavage results in the exposure of a previously buried cysteinyl sulfydryl group esterified to a nearby glutamate residue and the scission of this internal thioester linkage. The exposed glutamate then becomes covalently linked by a transacylation reaction to a hydroxyl or amino group on the target surface.

C3b is also an initiator of a more primitive limb of the complement pathway, the *alternative pathway* (also known as the properdin system (Fig. 17-3B). In this system, proteins called *factor B* and *factor D*, which are similar to C2 and C4, enter the complement sequence without a requirement for antibodies. These and other alternative pathway proteins complete a loop by eventually binding and cleaving C3. The surfaces of microorganisms such as the lipopolysaccharide that is the endotoxin of gram-negative bacteria, yeast cell walls, and membranes of certain mammalian cells, espe-

cially after damage or alteration in various diseases, bind the components of the alternative pathway that cause the fixation of C3, the alternative pathway C3 convertase. C3b binds and cleaves C5 to C5a and C5b. The former is a potent chemotactic factor for attracting phagocytic cells. The latter reacts with the rest of the complement components, C6–C9. The C6–C9 aggregate can punch holes in membranes of susceptible cells; it is called the *lytic* or *membrane attack complex*. The actual lytic agent is a a circular polymer of C9 molecules the assembly of which forms a pore, 10 nm in diameter, in the target cell plasma membrane.

Complement components are found in most protein-containing body fluids. The major source of plasma C3 is synthesis by hepatocytes. The origin of other circulating complement proteins is not entirely certain, but macrophages are capable of synthesizing many of them.

To counteract the possibility of uncontrolled complement activation, the plasma contains inhibitor proteins that block the complement sequence at various control points. Acting as dampers, these inhibitors prevent low levels of complement activation when the inciting stimulus is small, but do not stop activation by strong stimuli.

An inhibitor of C1 esterase prevents the cleavage of C1. Persons who are genetically deficient in C1 esterase suffer from recurrent attacks of edema (hereditary angioneurotic edema). Two other proteins, factors H and I, respectively, act to dissociate activated factor B from C3b, thereby inhibiting the autocatalytic feedback loop that initiates the alternative pathway of complement activation. The decay of the alternative pathway C3-converting complex is also enhanced by a molecule on the surface of target cells called *decay-accelerating factor* or *DAF*. DAF is interesting because it is one of a class of surface membrane proteins anchored to the lipid bilayer through a sugar–inositol linkage and because its deficiency contributes to the pathogenesis of a blood disease called paroxysmal nocturnal hemoglobinuria (Ch. 28). In addition to dissociating the C3 convertase, H and I promote the sequential degradation of C3b to a number of fragments called iC3b, C3c, and C3d. Phagocytes and lymphocytes, respectively, have surface receptors that bind objects to which iC3b and C3d are affixed. Deficient expression of a receptor for iC3b is the cause of a genetic disorder (see Ch. 18). C3c is released from the surface of the target cell and has no known functional significance. The plasma antiproteases and a plasma carboxypeptidase inhibit the action of the complement chemotactic factor, C5a. Another inhibitor, known as *protein S* (a different protein S than the vitamin-K-dependent protein S that is a component of the coagulation system!), binds to C6, preventing binding of C7, and therefore the completion of the formation of a lytic complex. In addition there is a C8-binding protein that inhibits the contribution of this C component to lytic activity.

Measurement of Plasma Immunoproteins

Complement

In the clinical setting, blood complement components are commonly assayed by two techniques. The first is a functional test for the entire sequence of components C1–C9 that measures the capacity of the system to lyse susceptible cells. Sheep red cells are coated with IgM antibody and reacted with a test serum; the quantity of hemoglobin released from the red cells after a suitable incubation period is then determined. This release of hemoglobin depends on the entire complement sequence being activated and producing lysis of the cell; this assay can be standardized in various ways. Usually the quantity of serum required to lyse 50 percent of the erythrocytes is measured, and the result is reported as CH_{50} units. This test serves as a screening assay for reductions in the levels of one or more components of the complement sequence. It is also possible to measure levels of certain complement components immunochemically as described for immunoglobulins.

Immunoglobulins

The concentration of immunoglobulins can be measured immunochemically by using specific antibodies directed against them. The immunochemical measurement of the immunoglobulin concentration is determined by the density of precipitate formed in mixtures of test serum and specific antibody.

The concentration of plasma immunoglobulin, and of certain other plasma proteins, can also be assayed by the electrophoretic technique, *protein electrophoresis*. For convenience, blood is permitted to clot and the serum rather than plasma is analyzed. Serum is placed in a narrow strip on a porous matrix, such as paper or an agar gel, and then subjected to an electrical field. The proteins migrate in the electrical field according to their net charge. After an appropriate time, the matrix is fixed and stained, enabling the position of the separated proteins to be visualized (Fig. 17-4A). Albumin is well separated from the more cationic serum proteins collectively called *globulins*. The globulin fraction of plasma is further classified into α, β, and γ regions on the basis of distance migrated (Fig. 17-4A). Immunoglobulins migrate in the γ range and are referred to as γ-globulins, although not all γ-globulins are immunoglobulins.

From the information gained by electrophoresis of purified proteins, the position of normal serum protein components is known. The relative concentrations of the components can be quantified by shining a light through the matrix as it moves across a photometer. The stained regions absorb light in proportion to the amount of protein present, and the changes in absorbance of light by the stain are charted on a strip recorder (Fig. 17-4A). The total protein in the serum can be measured chemically, allowing its absolute quantity to be determined. For example, if the total protein is 6 g/dl and the albumin is 60 percent of the density of the scan, the albumin concentration in the sample is 3.6 g/dl.

Immunoglobulins in an electrophoretic field

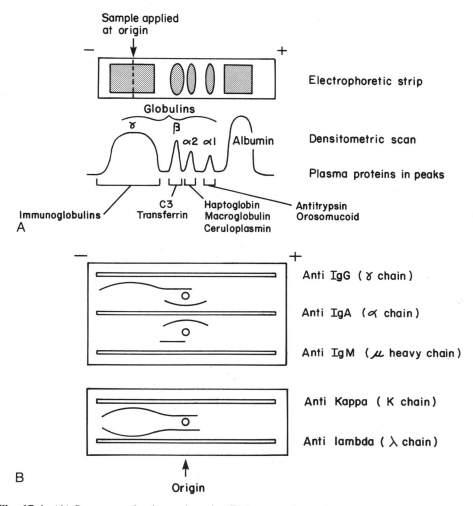

Fig. 17-4. (**A**) Serum protein electrophoresis. (**B**) Immunoelectrophoresis. Serum samples are put in wells at the origin, subjected to electrophoresis, and then allowed to diffuse toward specific antibodies added to the troughs. The arcs indicate the position of precipitin reactions.

remain as a diffuse band near the negative electrode and even move in the opposite direction, as demonstrated in Figure 17-4A. This finding indicates that immunnoglobulins tend to have a relative net positive charge. Figure 17-4A also shows that the immunoglobulins form a broad band in comparison with other components of the serum. This indicates that normal plasma contains a wide range of antibodies with various specificities. The reason for this lack of homogeneity is the wide repertoire of primary structures of serum im-

munoglobulins programmed in the variable sequences of the normal immunoglobulin molecules.

This electrophoretic technique is only sensitive enough to detect the major serum protein classes; it does not discriminate among the different classes, subclasses, or subunits of immunoglobulins. To detect these entities, an immunological method, *immunoelectrophoresis*, is used. This technique combines the separate powers of electrophoresis with the specificity of antigen–antibody reactions. A serum sample is subjected to electrophoresis in an agar matrix and then reacted in a different direction against antibodies specific for components being sought, for example, an antibody class or a light chain type. The presence of a precipitin arc demonstrates the existence and electrophoretic mobility of the serum protein in question (Fig. 17-4B). Immunoelectrophoresis is sufficiently sensitive to distinguish the different antibody classes when whole serum is reacted against antibodies acting with whole serum. To achieve a better resolution, monospecific antibodies, raised in animals injected with purified proteins, are used. The resulting immunoelectrophoretic pattern is much simpler and easier to interpret quantitatively (Fig. 17-4B).

DISORDERS OF PLASMA PROTEINS

Reactive Changes in Plasma Proteins and Immunoproteins

In response to infection or inflammation, changes occur in the concentration of certain serum proteins. The magnitude of the variation is a function of the nature, intensity, and duration of the provocation. Proteins that alter their concentrations in this way have been named *acute-phase reactants*. Of the proteins mentioned in Chapter 1, haptoglobin, macroglobulin, ceruloplasmin, complement proteins, and immunoglobulins increase during inflammatory diseases. The concentration of the coagulation protein, fibrinogen, also rises. This protein is elongated in structure and has a tendency to coat red blood cells, causing them to clump. The clumped red cells settle rapidly when anticoagulated blood is left standing. This phenomenon is the basis of the long-known fact that the red cell sedimentation rate rises in inflammatory diseases.

The increased immunoglobulin levels may reach extremely high values, as much as four to five times the baseline normal concen-

---

Diseases Associated with Serum M Components

Plasma cell neoplasms: Multiple myeloma, plasmacytoma

Non-Hodgkin's lymphoma: Macroglobulinemia of Waldenström, heavy chain disease

Chronic lymphocytic leukemia

Other neoplasms

Cirrhosis of the liver

Chronic infections

Autoimmune disorders

Immunodeficiency disorders

---

trations. Examples of chronic infections or inflammatory diseases associated with hypergammaglobulinemia are listed below. Occasionlly the stress of these processes on the immunological system can lead to the expression of abnormal immunoproteins called *paraproteins*, as will be seen later in this chapter.

The changes in complement proteins are variable, depending on the disease process. Chronic infections usually promote a moderate rise in the complement components. However, in disorders characterized by immune complex formation, for example, systemic lupus erythematosus (SLE), complement components can be consumed and their levels may actually fall if production does not keep up. In contrast to other acute-phase proteins, the concentration of transferrin falls during infection and inflammation (see also Ch. 4).

Paraproteins

A given immunoglobulin molecule is the product of a single clone of lymphocytes (Ch. 20). The many immunoglobulins in normal plasma and other body fluids reflect the production of numerous lymphoid clones. Therefore, normal serum immunoglobulins and hypergammaglobulinemia are said to be *polyclonal*. Under certain conditions, a single clone of immunoglobulin-producing cells can proliferate sufficiently to result in the accumulation of significant amounts of immunoglobulins with the identical primary sequence, constituting a paraprotein.

Types of Paraproteins

The monoclonal immunoglobulin detected by electrophoresis of the serum is a single band of protein in the diffuse γ-globulin region (Fig. 17-5), the paraprotein is called an *M component*, and when the M component is associated with disease, its presence defines a monoclonal gammopathy.

Further analysis of the M component by immunoelectrophoresis characterizes it as to its class of heavy chains and light chains (Fig. 17-5). The heavy chains may be of any class (i.e., μ, α, γ, δ, ε), but the light chains of a given M component will be only either γ or ϰ. In some cases, the abnormal clone will produce only heavy chains, heavy chain fragments, or only light chains. The light chains, being of relatively low molecular weight, are filtered readily by the glomerulus, and enter the urine. The presence of immunoglobulin light chains in the urine has historically been called *Bence Jones proteinuria*. It is worth noting that Bence Jones protein in the urine is not detectable by commercial "dip-stix" used to screen the urine for albumin, but can be detected by heat coagulation or sulfosalicylic acid tests for urine protein. Sometimes the paraprotein will be present in small amounts, and it is necessary to concentrate the serum or urine in order to detect it.

M components made up of isolated heavy chains of the γ, α, or μ class or fragments thereof may migrate in an electrophoretic field to a region other than that characteristic of immunoglobulins. By the process of immunoelectrophoresis, the M component can be identified as being immunoglobulin by its immunologic reaction in forming a precipitin line with anti-immunoglobulin of the appropriate class. However, the protein will not form a precipitin arc against anti-λ or anti-ϰ antibodies, indicating that only heavy-chain determinants and not light-chain sequences are present.

Fig. 17-5. Protein electrophoresis and immunoelectrophoresis of a paraprotein-containing serum. Protein electrophoresis shows M component in the γ region. Immunoelectrophoresis defines M component as having γ heavy chains and ϰ light chains. Paraprotein is therefore an IgG–K.

Causes of Paraproteins

An M component is often the product of a malignant neoplasm of the antibody-secreting cells. The lymphoid cell neoplasm most often associated with paraproteins is *multiple myeloma*, which is described in Chapter 27. Under these circumstances, the M component is present in fairly high concentrations, greater than 2 g/dl (or greater than 6 g/dl of Bence Jones protein in the urine). Its concentration increases with time, and there is other evidence of the underlying malignancy. In the setting of lymphoid neoplasms producing M components, the "normal polyclonal" immunoglobulin levels are often reduced.

M components can also appear in various inflammatory and degenerative immunologic disorders. In these situations, the balance of regulatory factors that ordinarily prevent any one clone of immune cells from expressing itself above the background of its fellows becomes deranged, and for some reason, a clone of antibody-forming cells becomes unusually active. M components are also found in a few apparently healthy persons. In this setting, the concentration of the M component is usually less than 1 g/dl (or less than 6 g/dl of Bence Jones protein in the urine), and the level remains constant with time. The incidence of this benign monoclonal gammopathy rises with age, reaching nearly 6 percent of the population of octogenarians and their older brethren. Most persons with such incidentally detected M components do not proceed to develop lymphoid neoplasms, but in slightly more than 10 percent of cases a malignant lymphoid disease does appear with time.

Effects of M Components

Kidney Damage

Bence Jones proteins can accumulate in renal tubular cells. This accumulation may result in obstruction of the tubular lumen and can lead to necrosis of the tubular cells. In some cases, there is a selective preference for damage to proximal convoluted tubules giving rise to amino aciduria, glucosuria, uricosuria, and phosphaturia. Light-chain deposition can also damage distal convoluted tubules, leading to acidosis and inability to concentrate the urine. Progressive necrosis of renal tissue can eventuate in chronic renal failure.

It is not clear why the toxicity of immunoglobulin light chains for the kidney is so variable in its incidence and distribution of effect within the organ. Presumably, the differences in the primary structure of the various light chains account for this variability.

In addition to the direct toxicity of light chains for the kidneys, amyloidosis, a complication of paraprotein production, described in detail below, can produce renal damage.

Hyperviscosity Syndrome

The viscosity of the blood is determined by the concentrations of formed elements and of the plasma proteins. The molecular dimensions of normal immunoglobulin molecules are sufficiently small that they do not appreciably affect the flow properties of the blood. However, if the immunoglobulins aggregate, they can significantly impede blood flow. IgM, because it exists as a pentamer and therefore has the highest molecular weight, is the paraprotein most frequently associated with hyperviscosity syndrome (see Fig. 17-2). IgA molecules also have some tendency to aggregate, and therefore IgA paraproteins are sometimes also associated with hyperviscosity syndrome. IgM aggregates increase the viscosity of the blood to a marked degree over five times that of normal plasma, when their concentration rises to levels of 5–8 g/dl. Once these levels are achieved, symptoms begin to appear.

The clinical effects of hyperviscosity are usually manifested by impaired blood flow to the brain. A patient with the hyperviscosity syndrome will complain of dizziness, loss of consciousness, and visual disturbances. Ophthalmoscopic examination of the microcirculation in the retina can detect engorged vessels, dilated to form what are termed "sausages." A patient with a hyperviscosity syndrome may also have impaired circulation to the fingers and toes and complain of numbness and coldness at the periphery of the extremities. The association of serum hyperviscosity with high serum IgM concentrations in the setting of a lymphoid neoplasm was first described by the Swedish hematologist Jan Waldenström; this entity continues to bear the designation macroglobulinemia of Waldenström. In nonneoplastic inflammatory or immunological disorders such as SLE, the increased concentration of polyclonal immunoglobulins can occasionally aggregate to produce a hyperviscosity syndrome.

Impaired Hemostasis

Paraproteins, especially IgM, can have deleterious effects on platelet function and on the actions of coagulation proteins, leading to hemorrhages of the skin and mucous membranes. The clinician may be able to see these hemorrhages as well as the dilated vessels on ophthalmoscopic examination of the retina.

Impaired Phagocyte Function

Paraproteins, especially IgA aggregates, interfere with the movement of wandering phagocytes. Immunoglobulin paraproteins have also been shown to bind to complement components, thereby impeding the activation of complement required for optimal phagocytic function.

Inflammation. The normal function of immunoglobulins and complement proteins is to confer the ability to recognize foreign substances as nonself, when appropriate, and to attact cells of the immune system to the foreign matter so these cells can kill, degrade, and eliminate pathogens. It is extremely unusual for paraproteins associated with lymphoid neoplasms to have true specificity for any particular substance. Insofar as paraproteins are products of disordered cellular machinery, that is, of malignant lymphoid cells, sometimes these immunoglobulins begin to react with normal proteins, as well as with each other. The abnormal immunoglobulins of the IgM class occasionally form complexes with IgG, a phenomenon seen in rheumatoid arthritis, in which case the IgM is designated a rheumatoid factor.

Paraproteins or aggregates of paraproteins and other proteins can react with complement components to initiate inappropriate inflammatory responses in the skin, kidney, blood vessels, or for that matter, anywhere. Occasionally, lowering of the temperature of the blood below the core body temperature of 37°C causes these reactions to occur. If the cooling produces a frank precipitate of plasma protein, a cryoprecipitate is said to be present.

The structure of a paraprotein will determine its reactions with other components of the immune system. Because the possible permutations of structure of these proteins are so vast, the manifestations of cryoprotein states, such as immune complex disease, can be truly protean, ranging from none to a fulminant vasculitis. The paraproteins are not directed against known specific antigens, so these cryoprotein complexes are not usually, strictly speaking, immune complexes. The M component can be detected by immunoelectrophoresis in such complexes, provided the various components in the complex can be appropriately dissolved. These autoaggressive inflammatory expressions of paraproteins arise most often in non-Hodgkins lymphomas.

In one unusual and interesting case, a patient with a lymphoid neoplasm developed yellow coloring of the skin and mucous membranes, because the IgG M component present in high concentrations bound the yellow vitamin riboflavin with high affinity. The riboflavin–protein complex deposited in the skin was responsible for the peculiar pigmentation of the patient. In another case, an IgG paraprotein was believed to have had some specificity for peripheral nerve myelin and was thought responsible for a peripheral neuropathy in that patient.

The reactive biological effects of paraprotein complexes cited here are encountered in non-neoplastic conditions associated with abnormal concentrations or structures of immunoglobulins, as well as in diseases primarily affecting antibody-forming cells. For example, cryoprecipitates can be demonstrated in patients with circulating hepatitis B virus antigen; the antigen appears in the cryoprecipitates along with IgG. This finding suggests that the chronic presence of certain infectious antigens can modify the behavior of immunoglobulins so as to promote these abnormal reactions.

Some Manifestations of Systemic Amyloidosis

Peripheral neuropathy

Cardiomyopathy

Nephrotic syndrome

Purpura

Macroglossia

Polyarthropathy

Coagulation factor $\times$ deficiency

Amyloidosis. Amyloidosis is a rather non-specific pathological entity in which tissues become infiltrated with a waxy substance having a fibrillar ultrastructure and that stains green after reacting with Congo red dye. This infiltration can impair the function of organs and, depending on the extent of the process and the organs involved, amyloidosis can be a serious and fatal condition. This disorder can arise in a number of unrelated settings. This fact and the finding that the infiltrative material has a variable chemical composition suggest that amyloidosis is really more than one disease. In one instance in which the amyloidosis is a genetic disorder, for example, and in which the patients suffer a progressive neuropathy, the amyloid is a polymer of a mutant plasma protein called *transthyretin* (or *prealbumin*), a thyroid hormone-binding protein.

Nevertheless, it is clear that (1) most amyloid deposits of importance in hematology contain pieces of immunnoglobulin molecules, and (2) amyloid appears in patients with high circulating levels of immunoglobulins, including patients with paraprotein M components. The pattern of tissue deposition in such patients is variable. Any tissue or organ can be affected, but certain characteristic syndromes are relatively common. In patients with Bence Jones protein in the urine, amyloid deposits are found in the kidney parenchyma and can impair renal function. The damage primarily affects the renal glomerulus such that proteinuria sufficient to cause the nephrotic syndrome is common. Amyloid deposition in the peripheral nerves causes a neuropathy with a stocking-glove distribution. Cardiac involvement may lead to congestive cardiac arrhythmias. Infiltration of the skin can cause it to lose its elasticity and render it susceptible to hemorrhage, especially in intertriginous regions. In some cases the joints are affected and are even seen to become enlarged and limited in range of motion. A classic finding is enlargement of the tongue, known as macroglossia, a complication that can impair the ability to swallow. A complication of special interest to the hematologist is the development of coagulation factor X deficiency. For some reason, amyloid deposits absorb this coagulation factor.

Our understanding of the mechanism of immunoglobulin-derived amyloid formation is far from complete. It appears that the final common pathway of amyloid formation is the assembly of protein fragments into a linear array called a β-pleated sheet structure. Something about the primary and secondary characteristics of amyloidogenic proteins causes them to aggregate in this fashion. In patients with circulating Bence Jones protein, these immunoglobulin fragments form the bulk of the amyloid structure. The amyloid in such cases is

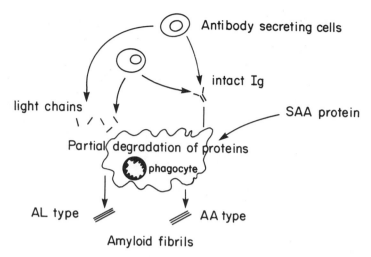

Fig. 17-6. Pathogenesis of amyloidosis.

designated AL type. In other patients, the source of the precursor subunits, called SAA protein, is a mixture of serum proteins of undetermined origin and intact immunoglobulin molecules. The amyloid in these patients is said to be of the AA type. It is now believed that abnormalities in the degradation of immunoglobulins and other proteins by mononuclear phagocytes plays an intermediate role in the pathogenesis of secondary amyloidosis (Fig. 17-6). These cells normally are responsible for the degradation of serum proteins (Ch. 18). The presence of abnormal immunoglobulin fragments secreted by neoplastic plasma cells presents the macrophages with proteins that they cannot degrade appropriately. This situation leads to the accumulation of protein breakdown products that have the chemical propensity to form the amyloid deposits.

Treatment of Paraproteins

When the presence of a paraprotein is the result of an underlying infectious, inflammatory, or neoplastic disorder, the ideal treatment is to eradicate the underlying disease. In such cases, treatment may reverse amyloid deposition in tissues, when it is present. However, such definitive treatment is not always possible and, in the case of lymphoid neoplasms, may only be of temporary benefit. In these circumstances, it may be possible literally to wash the paraprotein out of the patient by means of a procedure called *plasmapheresis*. With this technique, whole blood is removed from the patient in amounts that are tolerable, the formed elements and plasma are separated, and the formed elements are returned to the patient. The fluid volume removed with the paraprotein-containing plasma is repleted by infusion of normal plasma, albumin, or electrolyte solutions. Depending on the cardiovascular status of the patient, the distribution of the paraprotein, and the intensity of symptoms, this type of treatment can be repeated for long periods of time. With plasmapheresis, it is possible to alleviate the symptoms of the hyperviscosity syndrome or to reduce the manifestations of cryoproteinemia. IgG antibodies are distributed throughout the extracellular fluid, whereas IgM is localized to the vascular system. Therefore, it is clearly easier to remove IgM by plasmapheresis than it is to remove IgG or IgA.

SUGGESTED READINGS

Alper, C.A. (1974) Plasma protein measurements as a diagnostic aid. N. Engl. J. Med. *291*:287.

Bloch, K.J. (1979) Antibodies and their functions. pp. 31–40. In Textbook of Immunology. Benacerraf, B., & Unanue, E.R., Eds. Williams & Wilkins, Baltimore.

Fuks, A., & Zucker-Franklin, D. (1985) Impaired Kupffer cell function precedes development of secondary amyloidosis. J. Exp. Med. *161*:1013.

Glenner, G.G. (1980) Amyloid deposits and amyloidosis. The β-fibrilloses. N. Engl. J. Med. *302*:1283, 1333.

Greipp, P.R. (1984) Amyloidosis (AL). An approach to early diagnosis. Arch. Intern. Med. *144*:2145.

Kyle, R.A. (1978) Monoclonal gammopathy of undetermined significance, natural history of 241 cases. Am. J. Med. *64*:814.

Müller-Eberhard, H.J. (1988) Molecular organization and function of the complement system. Ann. Rev. Biochem. *57*:321.

Phagocytes and Nonneoplastic Phagocyte Diseases

Phagocytosis, the capacity to engulf particulate matter, is a property possessed by many types of cells. Certain cells are uniquely adept at this function—the polymorphonuclear leukocytes and the mononuclear phagocytes— and therefore have been called "professional" phagocytes. Phagocytes develop from a common committed stem cell called the *granulocyte-macrophage stem cell*. This stem cell differentiates into branches that lead to the formation of three classes of polymorphonuclear leukocytes and to mononuclear phagocytes (Fig. 18-1).

POLYMORPHONUCLEAR LEUKOCYTES

The class of phagocytes called *polymorphonuclear leukocytes* are called such because the nuclei of the cells in the circulation are segmented to form two or more lobes. The polymorphonuclear leukocytes are also called granulocytes for the numerous granules in their cytoplasm. The coloration of these granules after reaction with Wright's stain determines the further subdivision of polymorphonuclear leukocytes into three classes: *neutrophilic* polymorphonuclear leukocytes, in which the gran- ules are essentially colorless; *eosinophilic* polymorphonuclear leukocytes, in which the granules stain red, and *basophilic* polymorphonuclear leukocytes in which the granules are blue-black after staining. These cells may also be called neutrophils, eosinophils, and basophils, respectively. The hematological importance of these three classes of polymorphonuclear leukocytes is quite different, as are their numbers in the peripheral blood.

Neutrophils

The neutrophilic polymorphonuclear leukocytes, often called "polys" by physicians, are the most numerous polymorphonuclear leukocytes, normally making up 50 to 80 percent of the leukocytes. Their function is to enter the tissues and to kill invading microorganisms. The mature polymorphonuclear leukocyte in the circulation is a cell capable of sticking to the capillary wall adjacent to such sites of invasion, passing through the capillary into the tissues by active ameboid motion, and finding and killing pathogens in these tissues. The life cycle of the neutrophilic polymorphonuclear leukocyte is geared toward the development and execution of these functions.

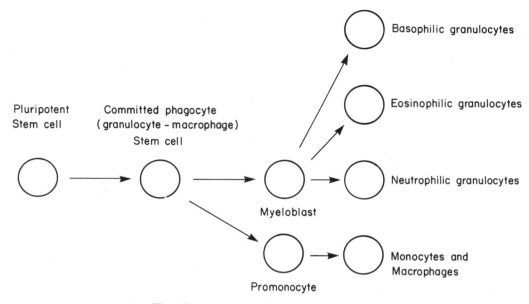

Fig. 18-1. Pathways of phagocyte maturation.

Development of Neutrophilic Polymorphonuclear Leukocytes

The neutrophilic polymorphonuclear leukocyte matures from the bone marrow committed phagocyte stem cell. During this time, ordinarily requiring 10 days, the cells undergo characteristic changes in appearance that have arbitrarily led to the classification of stages of maturation (Fig. 18-2). The major characteristics permitting the identification of the developmental stages are nuclear shape and the presence or absence of granules.

The first stage of maturation recognizable by the appearance of the cells in stained bone marrow smears is the *myeloblast*. The myeloblast is a large cell having a large nucleus and multiple distinct nucleoli. The normal marrow contains few myeloblasts, and the myeloblast is not highly distinctive in appearance in comparison with other very immature cells. Therefore, it is not always easy to identify myeloblasts with certainty. After a time, the myeloblast begins to synthesize granules. This granulated myeloblast is designated the *promyelocyte*. The granules in the promy-

elocyte arise from the Golgi apparatus by the same mechanism described for various secretory cells, such as the pancreas or the salivary gland, in which secretory products are packaged in granules. Being the first granules to appear, they are called *primary granules*. Because the promyelocyte granules stain with an azure hue, they are also called azurophilic, as well as primary granules. These granules contain enzymes that can degrade protein (proteases), fats (lipases), and carbohydrates (glucosidases and mannosidases), as well as a heme-containing peroxidase, often called *myeloperoxidase*, important in killing microorganisms. This enzyme has a green color, which is responsible for the greenish hue of pus.

In the next developmental stage, the nucleus becomes rounder and the nucleoli less distinct. Azurophilic granule synthesis ceases. The cells of this stage, *myelocytes*, continue to divide as they synthesize another set of granules that will have the distinct staining characteristics of mature neutrophilic eosinophilic or basophilic polymorphonuclear leukocytes. Therefore, these granules are called *specific* or *secondary granules*. The myelocytes continue to undergo

Stage of Maturation		Percent of Total Nucleated Bone Marrow Cells
Myeloblast		0.2 – 1.5
Promyelocyte		2 – 4
Myelocyte		8 – 16
Metamyelocyte		10 – 25
Band form		10 – 15
Polymorphonuclear leukocyte		6 – 12

Fig. 18-2. Maturation of neutrophils.

cell division after ceasing to make azurophilic granules. This process dilutes the concentration of azurophilic granules relative to that of specific granules. Therefore, azurophilic granules are not visible in stained smears of mature polymorphonuclear leukocytes. As can be expected from their variable staining properties, the content of the specific granules differs among the different classes of polymorphonuclear leukocytes. Depending on the appearance of the specific granules, myelocytes can be designated neutrophil, eosinophilic, or basophilic. In the neutrophilic polymorphonuclear leukocyte, the secondary granules are smaller than the azurophilic granules. They contain lysozyme, an enzyme that degrades cell wall mucopeptides of certain gram-positive bacteria, a vitamin B_{12}-binding protein, and an iron-binding protein called *lactoferrin*.

Myeloblasts, promyelocytes, and myelocytes can divide. They make up the mitotic compartment of granulocyte development. Beyond the myelocyte stage, the granulocytes are incapable of cell division and therefore constitute the postmitotic compartment. The major changes from this point on in the development of neutrophilic polymorphonuclear leukocytes involve progressive segmentation and condensation of the nucleus. An indentation of the round nucleus of the myelocyte defines the neutrophilic *metamyelocyte*. Further nuclear condensation and development of the indentation make the nucleus bilobed, indicating the *band form* or *stab form*. The final polymorphous form of the nucleus heralds the complete development of the neutrophilic, polymorphonuclear leukocyte. It is possible that the segmented nucleus permits the neutrophil

External membrane receptors
for IgG, complement fragments,
chemotactic factors

Submembrane meshwork of
actin filaments involved in
movement and pseudopod
formation

Membrane oxidase enzyme –
when stimulated converts
oxygen to superoxide anion (O_2^-)
and hydrogen peroxide (H_2O_2)

Segmented nucleus

Specific and primary granules

Fig. 18-3. Functional anatomy of the mature neutrophil.

to fit through small spaces as they crawl in the tissues.

In addition to the changes in appearance during maturation, polymorphonuclear leuko-cytes develop biochemical and functional characteristics important for their actions against microorganisms (Fig. 18-3). During maturation, the cells acquire the ability to move accurately and ingest particulate matter. They also develop the capacity to kill microorganisms.

The ability of the cells to move is probably a major factor that enables them to exit from the bone marrow sinuses. A system of fibers beneath the plasma membrane, composed of the protein actin, interact with myosin and other proteins to drive active ameboid motion of the cells. Glycolysis is the source of metabolic energy that powers these movements. Receptors on the outer surface of the membrane develop that are capable of reacting with a number of substances that activate adhesion of the cells with surfaces and neutrophil movement, phagocytosis, and metabolic reactions important in killing microorganisms. The metabolic reaction arises from an enzyme system that takes electrons from the reduced pyridine nucleotide (NADPH) and adds them to oxygen sequentially to form reactive metabolites. The

first product of oxygen metabolism is the superoxide anion (O^2-), a one-electron reduction product of oxygen; the second product is hydrogen peroxide (H_2O_2).

Rapid motility, the capacity to phagocytize, and the ability to produce bactericidal oxygen metabolites become manifest at the myelocyte phase of development. These functions are fully ripe by the stage of band and segmented forms.

Occasionally, the majority of peripheral blood neutrophils are found to have a peculiarity of nuclear shape. Instead of being organized into several lobes, the segmentation is limited to two lobes that appear quite round (Fig. 18-4A). These two lobes may overlap to give the appearance of a single round nucleus with the dense staining of the usual mature neutrophil nuclei (Fig. 18-4B). This nuclear configuration, called the Pelger-Huet anomaly, appears in two circumstances. One is inherited. It is passed as an autosomal recessive trait and is not associated with any significant abnormalities in the functioning of the mature neutrophils. The second setting in which these so-called Pelger-Huet cells appear is in the blood of some patients who have acute non-lymphocytic leukemias or who have preleu-

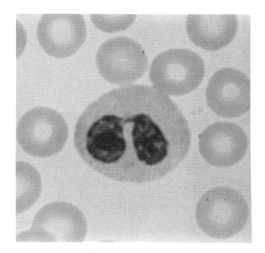

Fig. 18-4. Pelger-Huet cell.

kemia. In this context, the anomaly appears to be the result of an acquired derangement in the genetic material of the phagocytic stem cell.

Fate and Function of Neutrophilic Polymorphonuclear Leukocytes

The maturation of the neutrophil from myeloblast to a segmented form in the bone marrow takes about 1 week (Fig. 18-5). After

release from the bone marrow into the circulation, some polymorphonuclear leukocytes traverse the axial stream, the main column of formed elements coursing in the middle of blood vessels. These cells are readily removed during venipuncture and measured as the peripheral blood neutrophil count. Such cells are said to constitute part of the *circulating neutrophil pool*. In a person of average size, this pool contains 25 billion cells (Fig. 18-6). Other neutrophils roll along the sides of the vessels, peripheral to the main column of streaming cells in the center of the lumen. At any given time, about one-half the given neutrophils in the vascular compartment are not found in samples of peripheral blood. This hidden population of neutrophils has been called the *marginal pool*, with the idea that it is the cells that roll along the vessel walls. Probably most of the marginated neutrophils are actually sequestered in the lungs, spleen, and elsewhere. These cells mix freely with the circulating cells. Rolling along the endothelium, the neutrophilic polymorphonuclear leukocytes are in a position to respond to substances diffusing into the vessels from the tissues. Molecules emanating from microorganisms or from the interaction between microorganisms or injury to the host alter the endothelial surface of the

Fig. 18-5. Neutrophil life cycle.

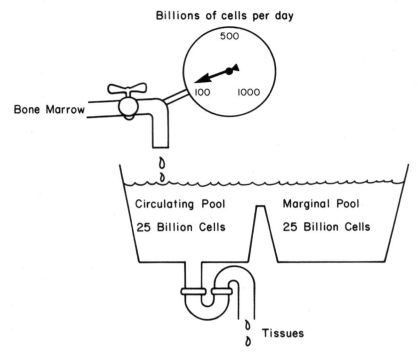

Fig. 18-6. Neutrophil turnover. From the standpoint of the neutrophil, a standard 70-kg person can be viewed as a laundry tub having two compartments—a circulating pool and a marginal pool. Mature neutrophils enter these two peripheral pools from the bone marrow and leave them for tissues within 12 hours. Note the large number of neutrophils turned over in a day indicated on the meter. This amount can increase tenfold on demand.

vessels, rendering it sticky, so that the polymorphonuclear leukocytes stop rolling and become stationary. The neutrophils then act on the endothelial cells, causing them to separate, permitting the neutrophilic polymorphonuclear leukocytes to crawl into the surrounding connective tissues. The molecules that enhance the ability of the polymorphonuclear leukocytes to stick to the endothelium also have the capacity to attract the polymorphonuclear leukocytes toward the source of inflammation. This sensing and response by polymorphonuclear leukocytes to the gradient of factors elaborated by microbial invasion or injury is called *chemotaxis*, and the molecules in the gradient are termed *chemotactic factors* (Fig. 18-7).

The chemotactic factors that have the ability to attract polymorphonuclear leukocytes are many and varied. This abundance is reasonable in light of the importance of polymorphonuclear leukocyte chemotaxis for survival against infection. Figure 18-7 lists some important chemotactic agents. These include organic molecules released by microorganisms. In addition, the systems of inflammatory mediators elaborate compounds that attract polymorphonuclear leukocytes. These systems include the complement system, the coagulation system, and a series of arachidonic acid oxidation reactions that occur in the membranes of many cells, including phagocytes and platelets.

Chemotactic factors act by binding to receptors on the outer surfaces of the membranes of the polymorphonuclear leukocytes. The poly-

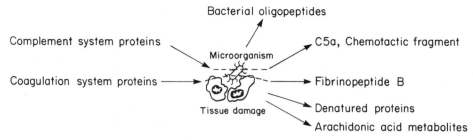

Fig. 18-7. Generation of chemotactic factors.

morphonuclear leukocytes attach themselves to fibers of the interstitial spaces and move toward the source of the chemotactic factor gradient. They crawl rather than swim and use a tank-tread mechanism to move the sites on their membranes that are adherent to collagen fibers and tissue mucopolysaccharide fibers to the rear of the cell, whereupon the adhesive sites become detached. The system of actin fibers beneath the cell membrane provides the motor forces for this translational movement.

The total number of polymorphonuclear leukocytes going through this emigration process out of the circulation into the tissues, called *diapedesis*, is on the order of 100 billion cells per day in a 70-kg person (Fig. 18-6). It follows that to maintain the normal level of circulating polymorphonuclear leukocytes, an equivalent number of cells must leave the bone marrow. The life cycle of the polymorphonuclear leukocyte therefore depends on a high turnover. The average polymorphonuclear leukocyte circulates in the blood for less than 12 hours. Compare this short circulation time of the neutrophil with those of red blood cells (120 days) and of platelets (7 days).

Should the cells leaving the circulation encounter microorganisms, they will ingest them if they recognize the microbes appropriately as foreign. An important mechanism for rendering microbes recognizable is a process whereby serum components coat the microbes. The molecules that coat organisms are called *opsonins* (from the Greek, meaning "to prepare for dining.") These molecules are normal con-stituents of plasma. The major plasma opsonins are IgG and the C3 fragments C3b and iC3b, which become deposited in the microorganisms by the action of the classic or alternative pathways of complement activation, as described in Chapter 17. The opsonins bound to microorganisms engage membrane receptors on the surfaces of the polymorphonuclear leukocytes. These interactions cause the membrane to extend pseudopodia that envelop the opsonized objects. As in locomotion, these movements are driven by the actin system of fibers beneath the cell membrane. Concomitantly, the granules are secreted into the forming phagolysosome. The membrane of this structure generates superoxide anion and hydrogen peroxide. The microorganism is exposed to these products while it is still outside the cell and ultimately in an enclosed vacuole that is in a sense outside the phagocyte (Fig. 18-8). The environment is therefore also exposed to granule enzymes and to reactive oxygen metabolites. These neutrophil products are believed to damage normal tissues and therefore may be important mediators of inflammation. In this region, the toxic properties of the lytic granule enzymes, the oxygen metabolites, and a potent microbicidal system composed of the azurophil granule enzyme myeloperoxidase and hydrogen peroxide work to kill the microorganism (Fig. 18-9).

The segregation of degradative enzymes and oxygen metabolites away from the cytoplasm of the polymorphonuclear leukocyte helps prevent damage to the phagocyte as it attacks

Fig. 18-8. Phagocytosis.

$$H_2O_2 \qquad\qquad 2H_2O$$

Peroxidase

Cl^-

Genetic material
of microbe oxidized
and destroyed

Fig. 18-9. Hydrogen peroxide–halide–peroxidase microbicidal system.

microbes. However, superoxide anions and hydrogen peroxide diffuse easily across membranes. The cytoplasm of the neutrophil contains the enzymes superoxide dismutase and catalase and the metabolite reduced glutathione (GSH), which detoxify these compounds should they enter the cell. Superoxide dismutase converts superoxide to hydrogen peroxide; catalase and reduced glutathione destroy hydrogen peroxide. Recall that these are the same protective systems that operate in erythrocytes for destroying oxidants. Reduced glutathione is regenerated, as in the erythrocyte, by reactions coupled to the hexosemonophosphate shunt of the glycolytic pathway (Fig. 18-8).

Another important effector system activated by phagocytic recognition is the elaboration of bioactive arachidonic acid metabolites known as *icosanoids*. The initial steps in this process are identical to those described for platelet icosanoid metabolism in Chapter 14 (Fig. 14-6) and involve the release of arachidonic acid from membrane phospholipids. Instead of the dominance of cyclooxygenation that converts arachidonate to prostaglandins and thromboxanes in platelets, a different set of enzymes converts arachidonic acid to compounds known as *leukotrienes*, although phagocytes can also produce the prostaglandins (Fig. 18-10). A large number of leukotriene inter-

mediates have been identified. A few of these are of particular interest; leukotrienes B_4, C_4, and D_4 (LTB$_4$, LTC$_4$, and LTD$_4$). LTB$_4$ is a potent chemotactic factor for neutrophils and monocytes. LTC$_4$ and LTD$_4$, historically known as "slow-reacting substances of anaphylaxis," have strong smooth muscle constricting effects. Therefore, these agents contribute importantly to the inflammatory effects of phagocytic infiltration of tissues during infection and injury.

How does the reaction of chemotactic factors and opsonins with phagocytes result in so many effects: locomotion, secretion of lytic enzymes, elaboration of toxic oxygen metabolites, and release of leukotrienes and prostaglandins? The step between the binding of chemotactic factors and opsonins with cell surface receptors and this panoply of effector mechanisms is called *signaling* or *stimulus-response coupling*. This signaling process has been extensively analyzed in phagocytes because of the many rapid and easily measurable responses elicited by agonists, and the findings are in large part also applicable to the way in which agonists stimulate platelets to undergo shape changes and secretion and in which a large variety of cells are induced to undertake mitosis in response to growth factors.

Two major and interrelated classes of signals are generated when agonists such as chemotactic factors or opsonins engage receptors (Fig. 18-11). One of these signal systems is the breakdown and resynthesis of a class of membrane phospholipids, the *phosphoinositides*. Another is a change in the cytosolic concentration of *ions*, especially *calcium*. The initial event in phosphoinositide metabolism following receptor perturbation involves the hydrolysis of *phosphatidylinositol-bis-phosphate* (*PIP$_2$*) by an enzyme called *phospholipase C*. Phospholipase C attacks the phosphodiester bond between the phosphorylated inositol ring in PIP$_2$ and its diacylglycerol backbone, generating *diacylglycerol* (*DAG*) and *inositol triphosphate* (*IP$_3$*). Phospholipase C ordinarily requires higher concentrations of

Fig. 18-10. Pathways for the production of prostaglandins and leukotrienes in phagocytes. An enzyme called *phospholipase A₂*, releases arachidonic acid from the second carbon in the glycerol backbone of membrane phospholipids. Corticosteroids are believed to inhibit this reaction. A cyclooxygenase enzyme sensitive to inhibition by nonsteroidal anti-inflammatory chemicals such as ibuprofin converts arachidonate to prostaglandin H_2 (PGH_2) via an intermediate, 11-hydroxy pentaeonic acid (11-HPETE). PGH_2 is then further metabolized to other prostaglandins. A different pathway involves an enzyme called 5Clipoxygenase, which oxidizes arachidonate into 5C hydroxypentaeonic acid, the precursor of the leukotrienes. LTC_4 and LTD_4 are sulfur-containing lipids, and the source of the sulfur is glutathione.

calcium than are found in the unstimulated (resting) phagocyte for significant activity, but following stimulation of the receptor, a cytosolic gaunosine triphosphate (GTP)-binding protein, known as a *G-protein*, associates with the receptor and the phospholipase C, permitting the latter to be very active at low calcium concentrations. The IP_3 released by the breakdown of PIP_2 diffuses to cytoplasmic vesicles that contain abundant calcium (*calciosomes*) and cause these structures to release the stored calcium into the cytoplasm. This rise in cytosolic calcium, in addition to potentiating the activity of phospholipase C, activates a number of intracellular reactions involved in phagocyte responses, such as the contractile activity

of myosin. The other product of PIP_2 hydrolysis, DAG, activates an enzyme called *protein kinase C*, and this enzyme presumably stimulates other reactions by phosphorylating key intracellular proteins. DAG is also the substrate for the enzyme phospholipase A_2, which generates arachidonic acid for disposal into the leukotriene and prostaglandin pathways.

A different set of reactions terminates or reverses the processes set in motion by the breakdown of PIP_2. A series of kinases catalyze the phosphorylation of phosphatidylinositol (PI) and phosphatidylinositol monophosphate (PIP), resulting in the resynthesis of PIP_2. ATP-dependent pumps in the plasma membrane and possibly in the intracellular calcium storage vesicles efficiently restore the increased cytosolic calcium levels to baseline values.

Eosinophilic Polymorphonuclear Leukocytes

The eosinophilic polymorphonuclear leukocytes develop in the bone marrow through the same maturation steps as the neutrophilic polymorphonuclear leukocyte. The specific granules of the eosinophilic polymorphonuclear leukocyte are very large. The red staining of the eosinophil granule arises from its abundant quantities of a basic protein, that is, one having many positively charged amino acids. The segmentation of the nucleus of the mature eosinophil tends to be less marked than that of the other granulocytes, so that the mature eosinophil has a bilobed nucleus with a thinner stalk between the lobes than that observed for the band form of the neutrophil.

The eosinophilic polymorphonuclear leukocyte has capabilities similar to those of the neutrophilic polymorphonuclear leukocyte for chemotaxis, phagocytosis, and microbicidal activity. Nevertheless, representing ordinarily a small proportion of the total polymorphonuclear leukocyte population, its role in defense against bacterial infection is uncertain. Because the eosinophil count rises in certain parasitic infestations and allergic states, it has been theorized, although not proved, that the eosinophil has a special role in combating parasites or in controlling allergic insults.

Basophilic Polymorphonuclear Leukocytes

The specific granules of the basophil are also very large. The blue staining of the basophilic specific granules derives from large amounts of acidic (negatively charged) poly-

saccharides with many sulfate and carboxyl groups, such as heparin.

The basophil contains the bulk of the histamine found in the blood. When appropriately stimulated, the basophil releases histamine. The circulating basophil has receptors for IgE on its surface. Antigens reacting with IgE on the basophil surface are potent inducers of histamine release. It may be that the tissue mast cell, which also releases histamine and other vasoactive substances after exposure to IgE and antigens reactive with it, is related to the circulating basophil. The consequences of release of these mediators are manifestations of allergy, such as rhinitis, bronchospasm, urticaria, angioedema, and anaphylaxis. The function of basophils in humans has not yet been determined.

MONONUCLEAR PHAGOCYTES

In many ways the mononuclear phagocytes behave like the polymorphonuclear leukocytes. Both arise from the bone marrow, circulate, enter the tissues in response to chemotactic factors, are actively phagocytic, and kill microbes by means of an oxygen-dependent mechanism. The major difference between these phagocytes is the longevity of the mononuclear phagocytes, in contrast with the brief, hectic life span of the polymorphonuclear leukocytes.

Development of the Mononuclear Phagocyte

The mononuclear phagocyte does not develop through a series of morphologically discrete stages as does the polymorphonuclear leukocyte, but rather appears to mature continuously. The marrow phase of mononuclear phagocyte development is ordinarily much less distinctive than that of polymorphonuclear leukocytes. The promonocyte, the monocyte precursor, is very difficult to find or identify in the bone marrow. It is believed that this cell

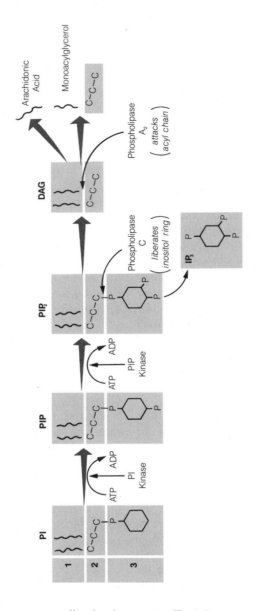

Fig. 18-11. Stimulus-response coupling in phagocytes. **(Top)** Structures and reactions of phospholipids involved in transmembrane signaling. Phosphatidylinositol (PI), the source of signal phospholipids has two fatty acids (1) linked to a glycerol backbone (2) and an inositol ring (3) bound to the third carbon by a phosphodiester bond. Sucessive phosphorylation of the inositol ring in the 4 and 5 positions by ATP-requiring kinases generates phosphatidylinositol phosphate (PIP) and phosphatidylinositol *bis*-phosphate (PIP$_2$) respectively. PIP$_2$ is the target of a phosphodiesterase enzyme, phospholipase C, which liberates the inositol ring containing three phosphates, inositol triphosphate (IP$_3$) into the cytoplasm, leaving diacylglycerol (DAG) at the plasma membrane. The phospholipids are all potential substrates of phospholipase A$_2$ enzymes, which attack the second acyl chain, usually an arachidonic acid, producing free arachidonic acid and, depending on the species hydrolyzed, monoacylglycerol or else a phospholipid missing one fatty acid (called a lysophospholipid). For simplicity, only the hydrolysis of DAG is shown in the dia-

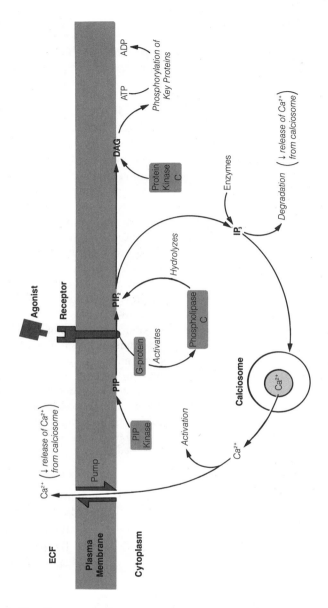

gram. **(Bottom)** Signaling reaction cycles. Agonist binding to the external portion of a receptor causes a conformational change in the transmembrane portion of the receptor such that the cytoplasmic region interacts with a G-protein which in turn activates phospholipase C. Phospholipase C hydrolyzes PIP_2 to produce IP_3 and DAG. IP_3 interacts with calciosomes to release ionized calcium into the cytoplasm where it activates a variety of enzymes and structural proteins involved in phagocyte responses. A cytoplasmic enzyme, protein kinase C, binds DAG at the plasma membrane and phosphorylates other enzymes or structural proteins important in phagocyte responses. Dissipation of the activation signals is brought about by membrane pumps that extrude calcium, by enzymes that degrade IP_3, thereby stopping the release of calcium from calciosomes, and by the enzymatic breakdown of DAG. Activation of PI kinases regenerate PIP_2 for further signaling. PIP_2 also interacts with cytoplasmic actin-regulating proteins.

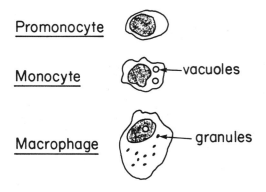

Promonocyte

Monocyte ——vacuoles

Macrophage —— granules

Fig. 18-12. Development of the mononuclear phagocyte.

remains in the marrow only a few days and then enters the circulation as a monocyte.

The blood monocyte is recognizable in Wright's stain smears on the basis of certain characteristic features. The nucleus seems to wrap around itself. The cytoplasm is gray and occasionally contains vacuoles and granules. The cell shape is oval or irregular. In the transition to the tissue macrophage, the mononuclear phagocyte becomes progressively larger than the monocyte. The nucleus becomes round, and distinct nucleoli appear. The cyto-plasm becomes blue and may contain azurophilic granules (Fig. 18-12).

Function and Fate of Mononuclear Phagocytes

The mononuclear phagocytes have much in common with neutrophilic polymorphonuclear leukocytes. They have the same receptors for, and response to, chemotactic factors and opsonins as polymorphonuclear leukocytes. They kill microorganisms by immolating them with degradative enzymes, derived from cytoplasmic granules, superoxide, and hydrogen peroxide. Monocytes, like polymorphonuclear leukocytes, crawl to sites of infection and injury (Fig. 18-13).

After 24 to 36 hours, the monocyte leaves the capillary system, entering either the tissues, as does the polymorphonuclear leukocyte, or certain organs important for filtering and immunologic function, such as the liver, spleen, lymph nodes, and lungs. The macrophages in the liver, spleen, and lymph nodes are organized so as to be in intimate contact with matter percolating through the blood and

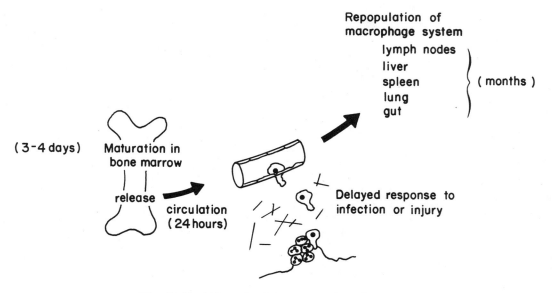

Repopulation of
macrophage system
  lymph nodes
  liver
  spleen   } (months)
  lung
  gut

(3-4 days)   Maturation in
               bone marrow

               release
               circulation   Delayed response to
               (24 hours)   infection or injury

Fig. 18-13. Life cycle of the mononuclear phagocyte.

Fig. 18-14. Fluid phase pinocytosis (**A**); adsorptive pinocytosis (**B**).

lymphatic circulation of these organs. Constituting a sentry network to engulf microbes that gain access to the gates and alleyways of the body, they also trap and destroy aged or prematurely damaged blood cells. This filtering function of mononuclear phagocytes was called the reticuloendothelial system for many years, although this term is now relatively meaningless, as it is now known that macrophages, not endothelial cells, are responsible for this filtering function.

The large mass of macrophages in contact with the circulation is also strategically located to interact with normal and abnormal plasma proteins. In the former case, the macrophages have the capacity to internalize large quantities of soluble proteins by the process of pinocytosis (Fig. 18-13). The cells pinch off tiny vesicles of membrane containing the plasma and carry it to the cell interior, from which granules containing proteolytic enzymes fuse with the vesicles. The ingested proteins are then rapidly degraded. In this way, the mononuclear phagocyte system is responsible for catabolizing plasma proteins. The internalization of soluble material is called *fluid-phase pinocytosis*. Macrophages also take up other proteins that bind to their membranes. This process is called *adsorptive pinocytosis*. The difference between fluid phase and adsorptive pinocytosis is illustrated in Figure 18-14. Aggregated proteins, immune complexes, and complexes of activated clotting factors are cleared from the circulation in this way. Macrophages also cooperate with lymphoid cells to assist them in performing complex immunological functions, such as the generation of specific antibodies and the mounting of cell-mediated immune reactions. In many in-

stances, the macrophages have a role in containing and inactivating certain parasites, such as mycobacteria, viruses, and trypanosomes. In such cases, the lymphoid system arms the macrophages by enabling them to secrete large quantities of hydrogen peroxide after phagocytosing these parasites.

REGULATION OF THE PHAGOCYTE LIFE CYCLE

The principal purpose of phagocytosis is to defend against microorganisms and to clean cellular debris after injury. It is therefore reasonable that a major stimulus for phagocytic maturation, release, and disposition to the tissues is the presence of chemotactic factors or substances released from microorganisms, such as cell-wall endotoxins. In addition, infection induces the synthesis and release of phagocyte growth factors, G-CSF, GM-CSF, and others (Chap. 1). These substances can be found in both serum and urine. The presence of infection, tissue damage, or other inflammatory states markedly increases—as much as tenfold—the maturation rate, the size of the marrow precursor pool, and the daily turnover rate of phagocytic cells.

REACTIVE CHANGES IN PHAGOCYTES

The number of peripheral blood phagocytes, principally the neutrophils, change rapidly in response to stress. Depending on the magnitude and type of stress, the counts rise or fall variably within a matter of hours. An increase in the neutrophil count above 10,000/μl defines a neutrophilic leukocytosis or *neutrophilia*; a drop below 1500/μl is designated *neutropenia*, although this definition is somewhat arbitrary. *Monocytosis* describes an elevation of the monocyte count above normal, *monocytopenia* is a decrease below normal. The set at which the peripheral blood neutrophil count is maintained in the "normal" state depends on the population studied. The normal values given in Table III-1 are based on samples of blood taken from white persons of European origin. Although the range of normal thus established is applicable to many populations, many blacks and certain Mideastern populations have average neutrophil counts considerably lower than the normal levels listed here. This fact must be kept in mind when evaluating neutrophil counts. A healthy black person displaying no evidence of blood disease but having a neutrophil count below the normal range is actually normal. Some of the usual stresses that affect phagocytes encountered in medical practice are described below.

Adrenergic Stimulation

Adrenergic agents such as epinephrine raise the peripheral white blood cell count as much as twofold within minutes. Both neutrophilic polymorphonuclear leukocyte and lymphocyte counts increase. The rise in neutrophils is the result of a mobilization of the cells from the marginal pool. This shift in distribution occurs because the stimulation of adrenergic receptors on the leukocytes reduces their intrinsic stickiness. The elevation in neutrophil and lymphocyte counts may persist for hours. On the other hand, the eosinophil count falls, rather than rises, in response to adrenergic stimulation.

Infection, Inflammation, and Necrosis

The presence of microbes or damaged tissues releases certain chemotactic factors, eliciting polymorphonuclear leukocytes from the bone marrow as well as the marginal pool. If the stimulus is persistent, bone marrow production of phagocytes increases and contributes to the elevated circulating level of neurophilic polymorphonuclear leukocytes and monocytes, that is, neutrophilia and monocytosis. If the stimulus is strong, the level of circulating neutrophils may rise as much as tenfold, and immature forms may appear in the blood. Such extreme elevations in the blood neutrophil count, especially if associated with the appearance of immature forms, are sometimes called a *leukemoid reaction*. When nucleated red cell precursors are present together with the immature neutrophils, the picture is defined as a *leukoerythroblastic reaction*. Leukoerythroblastic reactions occur in states of acute hypoxia and in some disorders involving invasion of the bone marrow. Processes of this kind that characteristically cause leukoerythroblastic reaction are cancers that invade the bone marrow and fibrosis of the bone marrow.

The emergence of immature neutrophils usually occurs in reverse order of maturation, bands being most frequently encountered, but metamyelocytes, myelocytes, and even promyelocytes and myeloblasts can appear in extreme states of stress. This peripheral blood neutrophilic polymorphonuclear leukocyte immaturity is commonly called a "shift to the left." Presumably this terminology arose from a convention wherein developing forms were diagrammed in textbooks from left to right in order of increasing maturity. This parlance, which is not only unfair to left-handers and to writers of oriental languages but is also uninformative, ought to be abandoned.

Sometimes infections and related stresses cause a drop rather than a rise in the neutrophil count. This falls occurs most often in cases of viral infections. The decrease in counts is presumably the result of a direct toxic effect of the virus infection on the production of phagocytes in the bone marrow. A drop in the neutrophil count may occasionally take place in bacterial infections, especially of an overwhelming nature. A bacterial infection characteristically displaying this effect is septicemia caused by gram-negative organisms, especially typhoid fever. The mechanism of the fall in the neutrophil count is an increase in the fraction of cells that become too sticky for proper function and that enter the marginal pool. Toxins produced by the infection may also inhibit the production of neutrophils in the bone marrow.

The eosinophil counts may or may not parallel changes of neutrophil counts during bacterial infection. In parasitic infections caused by worms, such as trichinosis (but not protozoa), the eosinophils may increase and may become the major blood white cells. This state is called *eosinophilia*. The eosinophil count can also rise in allergic states such as asthma.

The monocyte count usually rises somewhat in parallel with the neutrophil counts in acute infection and inflammation. However, a marked monocytosis, elevation of the monocyte concentration, does not ordinarily occur. Persistent increases in the monocyte count are encountered in chronic inflammatory diseases, such as tuberculosis, sarcoidosis, and subacute bacterial endocarditis.

In addition to changes in neutrophil numbers and in the appearance of immature forms in the blood during infection, inflammation, and necrosis, some alterations in the appearance of neutrophilic polymorphonuclear leukocytes can also take place. Greenish blotches can be seen in the cytoplasm of some neutrophilic polymorphonuclear leukocytes. These are aggregates of rough endoplasmic reticulum called *Döhle bodies* in deference to their first observer. Ordinary granules are barely visible in neutrophilic polymorphonuclear leukocytes because of their neutral staining characteristics. However, in these states of stress, blue-black granules become visible in the neutrophil cytoplasm. These so-called *toxic granules* are much smaller than the specific granules of basophils and are therefore not easily confused with the latter. The toxic granules may be remnants of circulating matter that were ingested and partially degraded by the neutrophil.

Alkaline phosphatase is an enzyme of unknown physiological function that splits phosphate off from a variety of synthetic esters at a very alkaline pH. The hydrolysis of phosphate esters can be measured chemically in extracts of polymorphonuclear leukocyte or, more conveniently, can be semiquantitatively estimated on fixed blood smears by means of a histochemical staining reaction. The phosphate liberated is colored by suitable reagents, and the number of cells so stained and the intensity of the staining are noted to establish an alkaline phosphatase score. This alkaline phosphatase activity of neutrophilic polymorphonuclear leukocytes in reactive states, polycythemia vera, and idiopathic myelofibrosis is usually elevated above normal, but is low or absent in chronic granulocytic leukemia (Ch. 28).

MEDICATIONS AND PHAGOCYTE DISEASES

The first or major side effect of many medications is often a change in the leukocyte count. Often, the toxic effect of medications is to lower the leukocyte count either by a direct toxic effect on the production of neutrophils in the bone marrow or by generating antibodies that can react with phagocytic white blood cells.

A few drugs raise the phagocyte count. Corticosteroids increase the neutrophil count by releasing neutrophils from the bone marrow and stimulating the bone marrow production of neutrophils. The mechanism for this effect is in part the action of corticosteroids to inhibit neutrophils from sticking to endothelium and crawling into the tissues. The reduction in tissue neutrophils secondarily causes an increase in the release of tissue chemotactic factors.

The effect of corticosteroids on eosinophils is the opposite of the effect on neutrophils. Corticosteroids lower the eosinophil count, whereas corticosteroid deficiency, as observed in Addison's disease (adrenal insufficiency), causes a rise in the eosinophil count.

Lithium carbonate, a drug used by psychiatrists to treat manic-depressive disease, raises the blood neutrophil count without impairing neutrophil delivery to the tissues.

ALTERATIONS IN PHAGOCYTE ACTIVITY

The concept of phagocyte activity refers to the process whereby microorganisms and phagocytes come into contact with one another, killing or containing the microbes. Normal phagocyte activity requires both adequate numbers and proper functioning of phagocytic cells. The activities of phagocytes in the defense against microorganisms can be summarized by two generalizations.

The first rule is that the defense against high-grade encapsulated pathogens, such as the Streptococcus, Pneumococcus, Meningococcus, and Haemophilus, primarily involves macrophages of the filter organs, the spleen, liver, and lung, and the opsonins of serum, IgG, and opsonic fragments of C3 (Fig. 18-15).

The second generalization about phagocytes in host defense against infection is that the protection against low-grade resident microorganisms, microbes that infest the skin and mucosal surfaces, for example, *Staphylococcus aureus* and gram-negative enteric flora, requires a constant flow of wandering phagocytes, the monocytes and especially the polymorphonuclear leukocytes into the tissues (Fig. 18-16).

Patients with congenital or acquired abnormalities of opsonins of macrophages acquire unusually frequent and severe infections, specifically septicemias, pneumonias, and meningitis, caused by the encapsulated organisms.

Disorders of Opsonins

Immunoglobulin deficiency is encountered as a physiological concomitant of infancy. Maternal IgG crosses the placenta but is depleted before the infant is able to mount an antibody response with IgG. The low point of infant

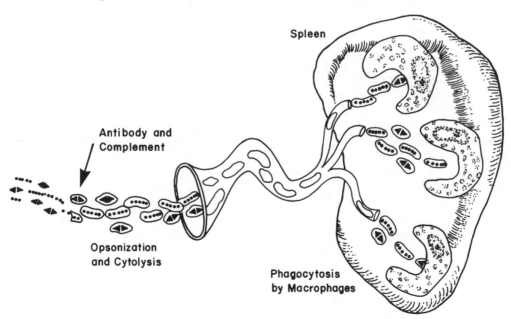

Fig. 18-15. Normal defenses against infection by encapsulated high-grade pathogens. These defenses include serum immunoproteins, antibodies, and complement components that react with microorganisms and either lyse them or coat (opsonize) them to make them attractive to macrophages for phagocytosis in filter organs of the reticuloendothelial system (spleen, liver, lymph nodes).

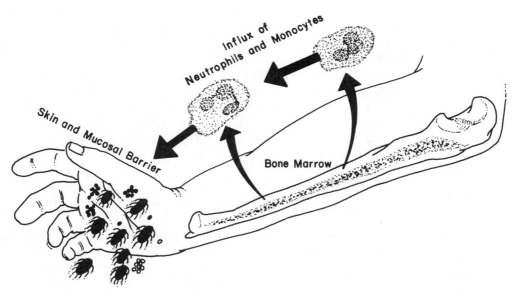

Fig. 18-16. We are continually infested with potentially pathogenic resident organisms. These organisms are normally kept at bay by mucosal and cutaneous barriers and by constant influx of wandering phagocytes—neutrophils and monocytes generated by bone marrow.

IgG occurs at about 6 weeks of age. Therefore, the 6-week-old infant is at high risk of infection with the encapsulated pathogens cited. Furthermore, even older infants and children lack a well-developed repertoire of anticapsular antibodies, as compared with adults, and are therefore more susceptible to such infections than are adults. A pathological diminution or absence of immunoglobulins occurs in the congenital antibody deficiency syndromes and acquired disorders of antibody formation associated with diseases of the lymphoid system. Some diseases of complement predispose to recurrent infections with encapsulated pathogens. For example, patients having the rare genetic diseases in which the major opsonin of complement C3 is not synthesized or is destroyed with abnormal rapidity suffer from recurrent infections caused by high-grade microorganisms. Infection is occasionally the presenting problem in an immune complex disorder such as systemic lupus erythematosus, in which the C3 protein gets consumed abnormally.

Disorders of Clearance by Macrophages

Splenectomy

Because of its abundant blood flow and its unique circulation, which puts blood in contact with many macrophages, the spleen is an efficient organ of clearance. Other clearance organs such as the liver can match the efficiency of the spleen only if the material to be cleared is very recognizable to the hepatic macrophages. Such recognition is possible only with heavily opsonized cells or microorganisms, that is, those that have been massively coated with IgG, C3b, or both. Removal of the spleen creates a small but definite risk of serious bloodstream infection by encapsulated pathogens. These infections may be fulminant and rapidly fatal. The danger of such infections is greater in splenectomized infants and young children than in adults, because the former have lower quantities of specific anticapsular

Disorders Often Leading to Serious Recurrent or Severe Infections with Virulent Encapsulated Pathogens

Antibody deficiency syndromes
    Transient infantile antibody deficiency
    Congenital antibody deficiency
    Acquired antibody deficiency
        Associated with lymphoid neoplasms
        Protein-losing syndromes

Complement disorders
    Congenital deficiency of C3 or other components
    Acquired deficiency of C3 or other components caused by immune complex diseases (systemic lupus erythematosus, acute glomerulonephritis)

Mononuclear phagocyte disorders
    Macrophage ablation: Splenectomy
    Macrophage bypass: Hepatic cirrhosis
    Macrophage diversion: Sickle cell anemia; other hemoglobinopathies with unstable erythrocytes

Combined disorders
    Hepatic cirrhosis: Macrophage bypass and impairment of C3 synthesis

antibodies, which permit the liver and other macrophage-rich organs to compensate for the absence of the more efficient spleen. Splenectomy is an example of macrophage ablation.

Cirrhosis of the Liver

Although a less efficient clearance organ than the spleen, the liver contains a large number of macrophages that can clear microorganisms from the portal blood. In severe liver cirrhosis, a sizeable fraction of the portal circulation circumvents the liver parenchyma and its macrophages, reducing the total clearance function of this macrophage system. Hepatic cirrhosis is therefore an example of macrophage bypass. Patients with certain forms of severe liver disease may have low levels of C3 in their serum as well, because the hepatocyte is the source of C3 and many other proteins that circulate in the blood. It is not surprising, therefore, that patients with advanced cirrhosis of the liver are highly susceptible to bacterial infections.

Hemolytic Disorders

In diseases characterized by large numbers of chronically damaged red blood cells, such as sickle cell anemia or the thalassemia syndromes, the macrophage system is diverted from its task of clearing microorganisms. The macrophages have to ingest the abnormal red blood cells, eventually depleting membrane from their surfaces and saturating their capacity to ingest anything else. The association between infection and hemolysis is most frequently seen in sickle cell anemia, in which the hemolytic state is constant and lifelong. Furthermore, the diversion of the macrophage system is further exacerbated by infarction of the spleen, which follows frequent occlusions in the splenic circulation. As in the case of splenectomy alone, the susceptibility to infection in severe hemolytic anemia is most marked in infancy and early childhood.

Disorders of Neutrophil and Monocyte Activity

The flow of neutrophils and monocytes into the tissues on which normal neutrophil and monocyte phagocytic activity depends is equivalent to the large turnover of polymorphonuclear leukocytes and monocytes. A sufficient diminution in the number of available wandering phagocytes or in the ability of these cells to function properly, predisposes the patient to unusually recurrent or severe infections with low-grade pathogens.

Decreased neutrophil turnover can be caused by impaired neutrophil production, destruction of mature neutrophils, or a combination of these mechanisms. Destruction of mature neutrophils sufficient to predispose to recurrent infections occurs infrequently, because of the immense productivity of the bone marrow for neutrophils. However, a reduction of neutrophil formation frequently results from many causes of bone marrow failure. In these disorders of neutrophil synthesis, the neutrophil blood count can reflect the turnover directly, and the risk of infection begins to mount when the neutrophil count falls below 500 cells/µl. The infections occur most frequently in those areas where microorganisms are in contact with the tissues: the skin, the anus, the mouth, and the respiratory passages.

In the presence of a normal neutrophil production rate, the flow of neutrophils into the tissues can be reduced if the neutrophils are defective in their ability to leave the circulation and enter the tissues. Theoretically, failure to elaborate chemotactic factors could cause such an impairment in neutrophil turnover, but in fact the great number of chemotactic factors produced during infection prevent this possibility from being a real problem. On the other hand, congenital and acquired abnormalities of neutrophils can prevent these cells from responding properly to chemotactic factors. In that case, the blood neutrophil count increases, tissue neutrophils decrease, and skin and mucosal infections occur. Corticosteroids have this effect on neutrophils. In addition, a rare genetic disorder exists in which this situation arises because structural components of neutrophils are defective.

White blood cells have a family of membrane glycoproteins called *Leu-CAMs* ("leukocyte-cell adhesion molecules"). Phagocytes and lymphocyte Leu-CAMs consist of two polypeptide chains designated alpha and beta. The beta chains are identical in structure whereas the alpha chains are cell-type specific. In the phagocyte, the principal Leu-CAM mediates the binding of the cell to the complement fragment iC3b and also to various molecules found in the extracellular tissue matrix.

Disorders Often Leading to Recurrent or Severe Infections with Resident Pathogens

Deficiency of neutrophils and monocytes
    Congenital neutropenia
    Autoimmune neutropenia
    Medication-induced neutropenia
    Generalized bone marrow failure secondary to aplastic anemia, metastatic cancer, acute leukemia, marrow fibrosis, effects of toxins, and ionizing radiation

Disorders of phagocyte structure and function
    Various genetic diseases in which neutrophil adhesion, locomotion, and phagocytosis are impaired
    Chronic granulomatous disease
    Chediak-Higashi syndrome

Reductions in Neutrophil Turnover

It cannot be overemphasized that the neutrophil count of the peripheral blood may not be a reliable indication of the neutrophil turnover from blood to tissues. For example, a low neutrophil count in the blood could result from a redistribution into the marginal pool, in which case the delivery of neutrophils into the tissues might be normal. One way to test for tissue penetration of neutrophils into peripheral tissues is to make an abrasion on the forearm that scrapes off the superficial epidermis without causing bleeding and to place a glass coverslip over the abrasion. The tissue damage produced by this technique releases chemotactic factors that attract neutrophils. The neutrophils stick to the glass coverslip. By 5 hours, the coverslip should be covered with neutrophils. If this coverslip is replaced with another, monocytes as well as neutrophils will be on it by 12 to 24 hours. This dermal abrasion technique is called the *Rebuck skin window*.

For this reason, phagocyte Leu-CAM (also known as the Mo1 antigen) is important for the adhesion necessary for leukocyte locomotion and for phagocytosis of iC3b-opsonized particles. A number of families have been described in which members suffer from recurrent infections caused by low-grade pathogens. The phagocytes of these patients are defective in adhesion to surfaces and in phagocytosis of iC3b-coated particles, because the cells express variably diminished amounts of Leu-CAMs. The degree of expression of Leu-CAM correlates inversely with the susceptibility to recurrent infections. The heterogeneity of this disorder and analysis of affected leukocytes at the molecular level indicate that Leu-CAM deficiency (or "anchor disease") is actually a variety of specific genetic defects in which either the beta chain of phagocyte Leu-CAM is not synthesized or an abnormal chain is generated.

If the neutrophils that reach the tissues have a reduced capacity to kill microorganisms, susceptibility to infection is also increased. Such a reduction in killing capacity is found in the genetic disorder *chronic granulomatous disease*, usually inherited as an X-linked recessive trait. In this condition, the polymorphonuclear leukocytes and monocytes do not produce superoxide and hydrogen peroxide, the toxic products of oxygen required for efficient killing of bacteria and fungi. This failure is the result of a variety of possible molecular defects. In different families with the disease, the enzyme system that couples NADPH oxidation to oxygen reduction to superoxide is either missing, incapable of activation, or qualitatively defective in the affected cells. Alternatively, in rarer instances in which the leukocytes have nearly a complete deficiency of the enzyme glucose 6-phosphate dehydrogenase, the capacity of the cells to regenerate NADPH from NADP, thereby providing reducing equivalents for the superoxide-forming enzyme, may be sufficiently impaired to render the neutrophil unable to synthesize superoxide and hydrogen peroxide. Patients with all these variants of chronic granulomatous disease may suffer from recurrent episodes of lymphadenitis,

pneumonia, osteomyelitis, and abscesses affecting the skin, liver, and other organs. Histologically, the affected tissues frequently contain granulomas, hence the name of this disease. The microorganisms causing the infections in these patients are gram-positive and gram-negative bacteria and fungi, predominantly of low grade, that is, organisms that do not ordinarily cause infections in normal persons. Interestingly, phagocytes in these patients have the capacity to kill streptococci, pneumococci, and a variety of other organisms. This ability is explained by the role of oxygen metabolites in the pathogenesis of this disease (Fig. 18-17).

Aerobic organisms such as *Streptococcus* and *Pneumococcus* elaborate hydrogen peroxide as part of their normal metabolism. In the free-living state this production of potentially toxic compounds does not appear to harm the microorganisms. However, in the narrow confines of phagocytic vacuoles of phagocytes from patients with chronic granulomatous disease, the hydrogen peroxide synthesized by the bacteria is sufficient to cause their own suicide. The granule enzyme myeloperoxidase enters the phagocytic vacuole by fusion in the normal fashion in phagocytes of patients with chronic granulomatous disease and works with hydrogen peroxide to kill the bacteria. However, many aerobic microbes, including *Staphylococcus aureus* and most gram-negative enteric organisms, produce the enzyme catalase. This enzyme destroys the hydrogen peroxide generated by the bacteria. Unlike catalase-negative microbes, these microbes therefore do not destroy themselves. Therefore, chronic granulomatous disease neutrophils and monocytes cannot kill catalase-producing organisms, and the patients afflicted with this disorder suffer from recurrent infections with such microorganisms.

The diagnosis of chronic granulomatous disease can easily be made by means of biochemical and histochemical techniques that detect the ability of blood neutrophils to metabolize oxygen. One such test, called the NBT test, mixes blood neutrophils with a dye called ni-

Fig. 18-17. Pathogenesis of chronic granulomatous disease. *Streptococcus* and other aerobic catalase-negative organisms accumulate hydrogen peroxide in phagocytic vacuole of chronic granulomatous disease (CGD) phagocyte and are killed by it. The catalase-positive organisms have no net accumulation of hydrogen peroxide and are not killed. A normal phagocyte makes enough hydrogen peroxide to overcome the protective effect of catalase produced by the micro-organism.

troblue tetrazolium (NBT) in the presence of microorganisms. If the phagocytes are normal, they reduce the yellow dye to a blue product called *formazan*, and precipitates of this material can be seen in the light microscope. Neutrophils of patients with chronic granulomatous disease fail to reduce the dye. Female carriers of the disease will show that approximately one-half their cells possess the chronic granulomatous disease gene, because only one-half their cells reduce the dye in this test.

Two other genetic diseases affecting phagocyte function are interesting and worthy of brief description. In hereditary myeloperoxidase deficiency, an autosomal recessive condition, the azurophilic granules lack the enzyme myeloperoxidase. The microbicidal power of myeloperoxidase in the presence of hydrogen peroxide is missing in the affected neutrophils, and they are somewhat impaired

in their capacity to kill microbes. Unlike chronic granulomatous disease, however, this deficiency is not associated with serious susceptibility to bacterial infection, but may predispose to infection by the fungus *Candida albicans*. It may be inferred that the main role of the peroxidase system is in the killing of this ubiquitous fungal organism.

The Chediak-Higashi syndrome is an autosomal recessive disorder of unknown cause. The most distinctive feature of the Chediak-Higashi syndrome is the fact that white blood cells and many other cells possess large abnormal granules that represent fusions of certain normal cytoplasmic granules. This granule aggregation in dermal melanocytes causes a partial albinism and a silvery gray hair color. The giant granules in mature neutrophils fuse abnormally slowly with phagocytic vacuoles after ingestion of microorganisms, causing a small delay in microbicidal activity by the cells.

The major clinical consequences of the Chediak-Higashi syndrome relate to cellular dysfunctions that cannot as yet be explained either anatomically or enzymatically. Patients with this disease have variable degrees of neutropenia and impairment of neutrophil locomotion, leading to decreased neutrophil activity in the tissues. The result is recurrent infections with low-grade pathogens. There are also minor abnormalities of platelet function, renal tubular function, and variable changes in neuronal function, which can sometimes lead to neurological deficits. Many patients with the Chediak-Higashi syndrome develop what has been called an accelerated phase of the syndrome, characterized by fever, pancytopenia, and organ enlargements caused by proliferations of macrophagelike cells. The accelerated phase leads inexorably to death by infection and wasting. Genetic diseases closely resembling the Chediak-Higashi syndrome exist throughout the animal kingdom. Species known to carry the genes include mice, cattle, mink, and even killer whales.

STORAGE DISEASES

Storage diseases encompass a large family of genetic disorders caused by the absent or significantly reduced activity of enzymes that reside in cellular lysosomes. The consequence of this hypoactivity is the accumulation within cells of substances ordinarily degraded by these enzymes, usually complex lipids, glycolipids, or mucopolysaccharides. This accumulation is often toxic, and the susceptibility of a given cell type to this toxicity determines the clinical manifestation of the storage disorder. Nearly all lysosomal storage diseases are inherited in an autosomal recessive manner.

Many storage diseases cause neurological and skeletal dysfunction. Only one, a variant of Gaucher's disease, is frequently encountered by the hematologist, because this form of Gaucher's disease is characterized by splenomegaly and hypersplenism or bone marrow failure, or both. The blood, however, is often

relevant in other types of storage diseases, because blood leukocytes may also lack the enzyme in question, permitting biochemical measurements of peripheral blood leukocytes to establish the diagnosis. In addition, products accumulating abnormally in leukocyte lysosomes can cause visibly distinct inclusions or cytoplasmic vacuoles to appear in blood cells. The inclusions appearing in leukocytes of patients with storage diseases carry the name Alder-Reilly bodies. In mucopolysaccharide storage disorders the inclusions are metachromatic, that is, they appear bluish-purple after the cells are stained with toluidine blue dye.

The bone marrow contains foam cells in many storage diseases. Foam cells are macrophages laden with vacuoles containing undigested matter (Fig. 18-18). Although not entirely specific for storage disorders, the appearance of foam cells in a bone marrow aspirate or biopsy specimen may help establish the diagnosis in the appropriate clinical setting.

Gaucher's Disease

The first storage disease was recognized by Philip C.E. Gaucher in 1882 as an epithelioma of the spleen. The variant of Gaucher's disease encountered by the hematologist is type I; its clinical manifestations are caused by deficiency of glucocerebrosidase activity in cells of the phagocyte system. The recessive gene for Gaucher's disease is most prevalent in Ashkenazi Jewish populations.

Sphingolipids are components of normal plasma membranes. They consist of the alcoholic compound sphingosine linked to fatty

Fig. 18-18. Foam cell (**A**); Gaucher cell (**B**).

acids. They may be linked to sugars, phosphate, or sulfate. This general compound is also designed a ceramide. The enzyme glucocerebroside B-glucosidase (glucocerebrosidase) creates a glucose residue from the one-carbon of sphingosine. This degradation is part of the general digestive process that occurs after senescent blood cells are internalized by macrophages of the spleen and other clearance organs and during the normal turnover of blood cells in the bone marrow comprising the effective hematopoiesis. The inability to degrade a variety of blood cell glycolipids by the enzyme-deficient macrophages results in an accumulation of the undigested glycolipid in the cytoplasm of the macrophages. The undigested matter takes on the appearance of a series of wrinkled tubules, 6 nm in diameter, which contain cholesterol, phospholipid, and protein as well as glucocerebroside. The wrinkled inclusions are distinctive, and macrophages laden with them are called *Gaucher cells* (Fig. 18-18).

Gaucher cells may also be seen in bone marrow specimens of patients with diseases associated with very high blood cell turnover, such as in the homozygous β-thalassemias or in chronic granulocytic leukemia. In this setting, it may be that the mass of blood cell membranes to be processed outstrips the digestive capacity of normal macrophages and that glucocerebroside or other membrane constituents accumulate in these macrophages.

The clinical manifestations of type I Gaucher's disease vary in severity and are the result of an accumulation of Gaucher cells in the spleen, liver, and bone marrow. Splenic enlargement may cause either discomfort in the left upper quadrant or gastric compression, or both. Anemia, leukopenia, and/or thrombocytopenia can occur as a consequence of hypersplenism. The accumulation of Gaucher cells in the bone marrow may superimpose an element of bone marrow failure on the shortened survival of blood cells due to hypersplenism.

The nonhematological consequences of Gaucher's disease occur in the liver and the skeleton. Enlargement of the liver and impairment of liver excretory function are secondary to encroachment on the liver parenchyma by Gaucher cells. Erosion of long bones by Gaucher cells originating in the marrow can lead to pathological fractures and to deformities. A characteristic bone abnormality visible on x-ray films of the limbs is a widening on the epiphyses, called the *Erlenmeyer flask deformity*.

The clinical manifestations of Gaucher's disease are extremely variable. This disorder usually presents in mid- to late childhood and early adulthood. It is often not progressive and may be compatible with a normal life span. The hematological complications of anemia or thrombocytopenia with attendant bleeding frequently respond to splenectomy. However, if bone lesions are a prominent feature of the disease, considerable morbidity can occur.

Gaucher's disease types II and III are uncommon and involve the nervous as well as the mononuclear phagocyte systems. Except for splenectomy and supportive management of skeletal damage, there is no known treatment of this storage disorder.

SUGGESTED READINGS

Brady, R.O., & Barranger, J.A. (1983) Glucosylceramide lipidosis: Gaucher's disease. pp. 842–856. In The Metabolic Basis of Inherited Disorders. Stanbury, J.L., Wyngaarder, J., Frederickson, D.S., et al., Eds. McGraw-Hill, New York.

Gallin, J.I., Goldstein, I., & Snyderman, R., Eds (1988) Inflammation. Basic Mechanisms and Clinical Correlates. Raven Press, New York.

Gleich, G.J., & Adolphson, C.R. (1986) The eosinophil leukocyte: Structure and function. Adv. Immunol. *39*:177.

Rotrosen, D., & Gallin, J.I. (1987) Disorders of phagocyte function. Adv. Immunol. *5*:127–130.

Stossel, T.P. (1987) The molecular biology of phagocytes and the molecular basis of nonneoplastic phagocyte disorders. pp. 499–533. In The Molecular Basis of Blood Diseases. Stamatoyannopoulos, G., Nienhuis, A.W., P. Leder, & Majerus, P.W., Eds. WB Saunders, Philadelphia.

Neoplastic Disorders of the Phagocytic Leukocytes

A change in the genetic makeup of dividing cells normally committed to develop into phagocytes is a neoplastic transformation of phagocytes if it leads to (1) uncontrolled growth; (2) failure of, or disorderly, differentiation; (3) uncontrolled or inappropriate invasion of normal tissues; and (4) inhibitory influences on the growth or development of normal cells in the bone marrow. The neoplastic transformation of phagocytic cells causes a class of diseases operationally defined as the nonlymphocytic leukemias. The specific names of the disorders depend on the predominant neoplastic cell type, usually determined by its appearance (Fig. 19-1). Most of the phagocytic neoplasms are first diagnosed when extensive infiltration of the bone marrow with leukemic cells has occurred, and they tend to be rapidly fatal when untreated. Therefore, these disorders are called *acute leukemias*. A more indolent neoplasm, *chronic granulocytic leukemia*, usually presents as a proliferation of relatively mature as well as immature phagocytic cells. It is actually a neoplasm of the uncommitted stem cell and is described in Chapter 28. It is interesting to reflect that the normal phagocyte life cycle involves large-scale proliferation and invasive behavior resembling the leukemic cell. However, nature has built into the mature invasive form of the normal phagocyte a total lack of the capacity to divide, so that it dies (the neutrophil) or remains dormant (macrophage) in the tissues.

CAUSES OF AND PREDISPOSITION TO PHAGOCYTE NEOPLASIA

Various forms of injury to immature, dividing bone marrow phagocyte precursors predispose to the development of acute nonlymphocytic leukemia by causing mutations in the genetic makeup of the dividing cells. The kinds of injury include those known to produce alterations in nucleic acids, such as ionizing radiation, exposure to organic solvents, and alkylating chemicals used in cancer chemotherapy. The normal cell has a variable capacity to resist and repair such genetic damage; this accounts for why this kind of injury does not invariably lead to neoplasia. However, in some genetic conditions, the resistance to such injury may be reduced, predisposing to a higher-than-normal incidence of acute leukemia.

In two rare autosomal recessive diseases—Bloom's syndrome and Fanconi's anemia—bone marrow failure occurs early in life and the affected patients have a high probability of developing acute nonlymphocytic leukemia. The incidence of acute leukemia is also ele-

Fig. 19-1. **(A)** Developmental origin of acute (nonlymphocytic) leukemias of the phagocyte lineage. **(B)** Leukemic myeloblasts, two of which contain Auer rods.

vated in trisomy 21, also known as Down's syndrome, a common congenital disorder caused by abnormalities in the separation of chromosomes after fertilization of the ovum. All cells of affected persons have an extra chromosome number 21, which is somehow associated with mental retardation. The connection between the genetic disorder and the predisposition to the development of acute leukemia (which can be lymphocytic as well as nonlymphocytic) is not understood, but presents another association between a known genetic abnormality and the leukemic process. Finally, in acute nonlymphocytic leukemias, the neoplastic cells have aberrations in their chromosomal architecture, another finding indicative of genetic damage. Although viruses can cause leukemias in animals and are now strongly implicated in the causation of at least one lymphoid neoplasm in humans, there is no evidence that viruses produce acute nonlymphocytic leukemia in humans.

CLASSIFICATION OF THE ACUTE NONLYMPHOCYTIC LEUKEMIAS

As fine a classification as is possible is important with diseases in general and in neoplastic diseases in particular. The better the classification of the disease, the more accurately can physicians evaluate the prognosis and response to therapy. An indolent disorder, for example, might appear to be more responsive to treatment than an aggressive one, whereas the differential responses reside in the intrinsic nature of the two diseases rather than the effectiveness of the therapy.

The hallmark of acute nonlymphocytic leukemia is a relatively monotonous infiltration of the bone marrow and sometimes the blood with a population comprising at least 20% immature phagocytes. The appearance of the predominant cell type on Wright-stained smears was for many years the basis of the classification of the acute leukemia. A predominance of myeloblasts defined acute myeloblastic leukemia; promyelocytes, acute promyelocytic leu-

kemia; and monocytes, acute monocytic leukemia, respectively. Although in comparison with the heterogeneity of normal bone marrow, the morphology of leukemic cells is relatively uniform, often the appearance of the leukemic cells is bizarre and variable, reflecting abnormal differentiation. The cells may have features of both myeloblasts and monocytes, defining the entity *myelomonocytic leukemia*. Even in what was called acute myelogenous leukemia, myeloblasts may vary in size and shape, may demonstrate partial differentiation to form strange promyelocytes, or may look like monocytes or macrophages. The peculiarities in the morphology of differentiation are defined as myelodysplastic changes and consist of oddities in nuclear morphology, including large size and marked variation in the aggregation state of the chromatin and alterations in the size and shape of cytoplasmic granules. One may occasionally see large basophilic and eosinophilic granules in the same cell, a highly unusual occurrence in normal granulocytopoiesis. In one particular configuration, granules form elongated needles called Auer rods (see Fig. 19-1). Because these granules are all azurophilic, they contain the enzyme peroxidase. Therefore, the peroxidase stain will sometimes help detect granules in leukemic cells where they are sparse, identifying such cells as being of the granulocytic lineage. Occasionally, no granules can be discerned at all, and the cells do not resemble either lymphoid or phagocyte origin by morphological criteria. The disease in this case was called acute undifferentiated leukemia and may be a neoplasm derived from stem cells.

The variability in morphology of leukemic cell populations meant that earlier efforts at classification were fairly crude. One important event in the classification of acute nonlymphocytic leukemias was the coming together of experts in the 1970s to achieve a consensus relating the morphology and clinical behavior of the leukemias with the markers available at the time, for the most part histochemical enzyme reactions. This classification was called the *French-American-British* or *FAB* classifi-

Table 19-1. Classification of Acute Nonlymphocytic Leukemias

FAB Designation	Characteristics
M1	Myeloblastic (immature neutrophilic) lineage detected by > 3% blasts with azurophilic granules, Auer rods, or staining with peroxidase histochemical reaction. No further maturation noted. Surface antigens reactive with neutrophil-specific lineage markers may be present
M2	> 50% of bone marrow cells are myeloblasts or promyelocytes. Neutrophil-lineage-specific surface antigens present
M3	Most cells are promyelocytes with many azurophilic granules and/or aggregated Auer rods. Neutrophil-lineage-specific surface antigens present
M4	> 20% of marrow cells are myeloblasts or promyelocytes in addition to which > 20% are promonocytes and monocytes. Both monocyte- and neutrophil-lineage-specific markers present
M5	> 90% of the phagocyte lineage cells are monocytes of variable maturity. Monocyte-lineage-specific surface markers present
M6	Hallmarks of acute nonlymphocytic leukemia (myeloblasts and promyelocytes with or without Auer rods) plus easily detectable numbers of bizarre erythroid precursors
M7	Pleomorphic blasts with markers for platelet peroxidase, platelet glycoproteins and factor-8-related antigen; frequent fibrosis of the bone marrow

cation and divided the acute nonlymphocytic leukemias into six classes, M1 through M6 (Table 19-1). Classes M1 through M3 represent leukemias in which cells of the neutrophilic lineage with different degrees of maturation prevail and in which the enzyme myeloperoxidase can be detected. M4 and M5 have monocytic cells of differing maturity that express a nonspecific esterase. M6 is a leukemia with immature cells with erythroid features. The discrimination of nonlymphocytic leukemias from lymphocytic leukemias and of the different subtypes of nonlymphocytic leukemia was markedly improved by the introduction of monoclonal antibodies (see Ch. 20) reactive against surface antigens of neutrophil-lineage precursors (M1 through M3) or monocyte-lineage precursors (M4 and M5). An M7 has recently been added to the FAB list. This leukemia expresses markers associated with megakaryocytes and platelets and is therefore called *acute megakaryoblastic leukemia*.

Further evidence in support of the importance of genetic alterations in leukemia has come from leukemic cell chromosomal analysis (or karyotypes). Clonal chromosomal defects are detected by cultivating cells in the presence of a DNA synthesis inhibitor that synchronizes the cells so as to permit analysis

of a large number of metaphases. The fine structure of the chromosomes is then visualized by means of fluorescent dyes that bring out a band pattern in the chromosomal arms. These high resolution techniques have shown that a majority of phagocytic cell lineage leukemias demonstrate chromosomal abnormalities. This information has provided further evidence for the clonality of acute nonlymphocytic leukemia and has also defined additional syndromes of acute nonlymphocytic leukemia that are characterized by distinct chromosomal abnormalities.

A variant of M4 leukemia, for example, is the finding of an admixture of myelomonocytic blasts and eosinophils. Distinctive for this variant is a cytogenetic abnormality consisting of inversion, translocation, or sometimes deletion of the long arm of chromosome number 16. The most common aberration is an inversion between the short and long arms, designated [inv(16)(p13;q22)] where p and q indicate the short and long arms, respectively, and the numbers the specific bands involved. This disorder accounts for about 5 percent of acute nonlymphocytic leukemias and may be somewhat more responsive to therapy than the other types. Another syndrome with a characteristic chromosomal aberration is an M2 variant with frequent Auer rods in which mature neutrophils may express the Pelger-Huet anomaly. The cytogenetic finding is a translocation from the long arm of chromosome 21 to the long arm of chromosome 8 [t(8;21) (q22;q22)]. A monoblastic leukemic syndrome is associated with the translocation of a segment of chromosome 11 to the chromosome 9 [t(9;11) (p22;q23)]. Promyelocytic (M3) leukemia is nearly always accompanied by a translocation between chromosome 15 and 17 [t(15; 17)(q22;q21)]. About 70 percent of acute nonlymphocytic leukemias arising in persons previously exposed to chemotherapy or radiation (see Ch. 31) demonstrate deletions of the long arm of chromosomes 5 or 7 (5q⁻) or (7q⁻). Finally, a rare variant in which elevated platelet counts are encountered expresses inversions or translocations on chromosome 3 [t(3;3)(q21;q26.2)] or [inv(3;3)(q21;q26.2)].

PATHOGENESIS OF ACUTE NONLYMPHOCYTIC LEUKEMIA

Contrary to the commonly held idea, leukemia cells do not necessarily engage in wildly rapid multiplication. In fact, the multiplication rate of leukemic cells is often slower than that of normal hematopoietic stem cells. The ill effects of leukemia stem more from the failure of the neoplastic cells to differentiate, to crowd out and suppress normal bone marrow cells, and from their tendency to invade normal tissue than from rapid growth.

Clonal Growth

The continued reproduction of the transformed cell leads to what is termed a *clonal expansion*. The clonal and genetic nature of the neoplastic process was first documented by studying the electrophoretic mobility of the enzyme glucose 6-phosphate-dehydrogenase of the leukemic cells in persons heterozygous for the A and B isozymes. Recall that these enzymes have different mobilities in an electric field. The body cells of persons inheriting genes for both isoenzymes will be either A or B because of random inactivation of the X chromosome. This means that the dividing bone marrow phagocyte precursors will have an equal chance of making either A or B glucose 6-phosphate dehydrogenase isozymes, and their progeny will yield on average an equal mix of these enzymes. On the other hand, a clonal proliferation of a single cell will contain only one or the other enzyme, and the leukemic cells of such patients with acute nonlymphocytic leukemia are either of the A or B type (Fig. 19-2).

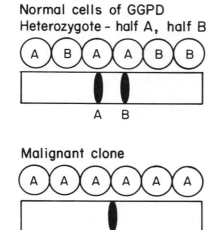

Fig. 19-2. Glucose 6-phosphate dehydrogenase activity in cells as a marker of clonal expansion.

ONCOGENES: THE MOLECULAR BASIS OF PHAGOCYTE LEUKEMIA

General Features

A major dividend of molecular cloning techniques has been the discovery that changes in the structure or expression of one or more of a limited number of normal cellular genes can cause cells to exhibit the characteristics of malignancy defined above. These genes have therefore been named *oncogenes*. Oncogenes were actually first identified as the parts of the genetic material of certain viruses responsible for malignant transformation of infected cells in animals. Most of these viruses are so-called *retroviruses*, which have RNA as their genetic material and use a reverse transcriptase enzyme to make complementary DNA in infected cells that then integrates into the host DNA. The integrated DNA either has no effect, programs the synthesis of more virus using the cell's synthetic machinery, or causes the cell to undergo malignant transformation. An important aspect of the discovery of cellular oncogenes was the ability to transfer DNA from tumors into nonmalignant cells in tissue cultures, a process called *transfection*, and to observe a change in the target cell from normal to transformed phenotype. Definition of this phenotype included piling up of the transformed cells on the surface of the tissue culture dish, increased motility, and the ability to form tumors in immunodeficient (nude) mice. Subsequent study of the transforming DNA revealed the identity between the regions important for transformation, the structure of viral oncogenes, and the presence of similar genes in normal cells.

The nomenclature of oncogenes has arisen from the historical identification of such genes and depends on the source of the genetic material. Cellular genes homologous to viral oncogenes usually bear the name related to the viral system such as *src* (the "sarc" or sarcoma-producing gene of Rous sarcoma virus of fowl) *abl* (the Abelson virus first discovered as a cause of lymphoid tumors in rodents) or *fes*

(feline sarcoma virus). The prefix *v-* or *c-* (e.g., *v-abl* or *c-abl*) denotes whether the gene is viral or cellular. In some cases, more than one related viral oncogene is known, in which instance a prefix denotes the specific viral gene: examples are *ras* genes related to Kirsten murine sarcoma virus (*Ki-ras*), Harvey murine sarcoma virus (*Ha-ras*), or Rasheed rat sarcoma virus (*Ra-ras*). The presence of oncogenes in viruses and cells raises the question of where these genes first arose. It is generally believed that the cellular genes came first and that it is somehow adaptive for the viruses to influence the growth characteristics of their target cells, a feat accomplished by stealing cellular growth-control coding sequences.

Although oncogenes are increasingly implicated as the basis of neoplasia, the mechanism of oncogene action is less clear. Oncogenes are believed to transform by working through aspects of the normal cellular equipment regulating cell growth and movement and hence can be no better understood than those mechanisms. In general, cell division can be triggered by growth factors that bind to receptors on the external surface of the plasma membrane. This binding elicits signals in the cytoplasm that interact with cellular factors (transducers) that further react with components in the nucleus that regulate genes controlling cellular proliferation. Therefore, oncogene products can theoretically function at any of these control points inside or outside the cell to induce' the malignant phenotype (Fig. 19-3). Cells ordinarily express the products of their own oncogenes under carefully regulated circumstances, but the constitutive expression of these genes following transformation or the expression of altered gene products can result in neoplastic cell behavior. It is important to emphasize, however, that it is not yet established that the action of any one oncogene is the sole basis of most human tumors. Most information concerning the development of human tumors is consistent with the involvement of more than one genetic event, and it may require the concerted action of many genes in order to evolve a frank cancer.

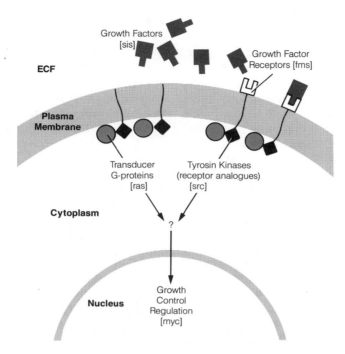

Fig. 19-3. Action of oncogenes.

One class of oncogenes, for example, programs the synthesis of secreted substances nearly identical to normal factors that elicit cell growth and division. These growth factors chronically stimulate the cell to divide. An example of such an oncogene that acts in this so-called "autocrine" fashion is *c-sis*, which produces a product resembling platelet-derived growth factor. Another set of oncogenes encodes molecules that act as receptors for growth factors. However, unlike normal receptors, which are active only when ligated by their specific agonist, these oncogene-derived receptors behave as if activated constitutively. An example of this class is the product of *c-fms*, which resembles the receptor for the phagocyte growth factor GM-CSF. The activation of a growth factor receptor transmits (transduces) a signal to the nucleus that induces cell division. One phase of this signaling involves plasma-membrane-associated enzyme activity that attaches phosphorus atoms to tyrosine residues of certain proteins, and *src* oncogenes encode such tyrosine-kinases. Another

"transducer" oncogene product is a set of guanosine-triphosphate-binding proteins that interact with plasma membrane (and possibly other) enzymes, the so-called G proteins described in the previous chapter. A different class of oncogenes, the *ras* genes, are postulated to be aberrant G proteins that behave as if stimulated by activated receptors. The ultimate target of signaling is in the nucleus, and some oncogenes act at that site. Examples of such oncogene products are *myc, fos, myb*, and the large T antigen of polyoma virus.

Because oncogenes are indigenous to all cells, some change in their composition or expression is required for neoplastic behavior. *Ras* oncogenes isolated from tumor cells, for example, have been shown to have single base substitutions, the consequence of point mutations, that result in the encoding of altered gene products. In this instance it is the abnormal product that presumably affects the cellular phenotype. A more frequent finding is that an oncogene has a normal primary sequence, but its expression is greatly increased. This situation arises from another event common to neoplastic cells, especially in leukemias, the rearrangement of chromosomes. This rearrangement can put DNA sequences that promote or enhance the expression of cellular genes inappropriately in the proximity of oncogenes, causing the oncogenes to be excessively expressed. Presumably, the causes and predispositions to genetic damage increase the frequency of point mutations and/or chromosomal rearrangements, leading to the recombinations that express abnormal oncogenes or normal oncogenes inappropriately.

Oncogenes and Acute Nonlymphocytic Leukemia

The most frequently detected oncogene abnormality in this disease is the presence of *N-ras* mutations, which have been detected in about a third of the cases examined thus far. A type of cell called HL-60, which resembles the promyelocyte, was originally isolated from a patient with acute nonlymphocytic leukemia. HL-60 cells grow in tissue culture and have, in addition to a *N-ras* mutation, marked hyperexpression of *c-myc*, a transforming oncogene (especially when combined with *N-ras* mutations) encoding a nuclear protein. The HL-60 cells can be induced to differentiate into mature neutrophils by a variety of agents. One of the first events accompanying differentiation and loss of the capacity to divide is a marked decrease in expression of the *c-myc* gene product.

Oncogenes or possible oncogenes reside at or near points of chromosomal abnormalities in certain acute nonlymphocytic leukemias. The oncogene *c-ets* 1, a homologue of an avian viral leukemia oncogene resides on chromosome 22, which translocates to chromosome 9 in the M5 variant described above. The genes for hematopoietic growth factors GM-CSF and M-CSF and also the receptors for M-CSF (which is also an oncogene *c-fms*) and for platelet-derived growth factor (PDGF) all reside on the long arm of chromosome 5 (5q),

which is deleted or otherwise abnormal in a number of acute nonlymphocytic leukemias. A loss of differentiating factors or their receptors that drive phagocyte progenitors to mature and lose proliferative potential might predispose such cells to malignant transformation. Finally, the myeloperoxidase gene is located on chromosome 17; this gene is transcriptionally activated early in neutrophil development. It is possible that this makes this region of the chromosome susceptible to mutation or else that myeloperoxidase promoter elements contribute to the expression of other factors contributing to the leukemic state. Furthermore, the myeloperoxidase gene is rearranged in the t(15;17) translocation. The accumulating data about chromosomal aberrations and the detection of oncogenes in acute nonlymphocytic leukemia is very exciting and suggestive, but it is not at all certain how these facts fit together at the present time.

CONSEQUENCES OF THE ACUTE NEOPLASMS OF PHAGOCYTES

The major clinical problem engendered by acute leukemia is bone marrow failure. Indeed, the pathological definition of acute leukemia requires that more than 20 percent of the bone marrow nucleated cells be malignant "blasts." With further clonal expansion of the neoplastic cells, the normal marrow elements diminish in number, possibly because some leukemic cells release inhibitors of normal hematopoiesis. The consequences of bone marrow failure are anemia, hemorrhage, and infection because of diminution in the numbers of normal erythrocytes, platelets, and phagocytes, respectively.

Although "leukemia" means "white blood," implying the presence of large numbers of malignant leukocytes in the blood, this "leukemia" only occurs in a few cases of acute leukemias of phagocytes at the time of diagnosis. In most patients the total white blood cell count is initially decreased and the bone marrow is packed with leukemic cells. A "leukemia" with high peripheral blood white cell concentrations is prevalent in leukemias with monocytic and myelomonocytic morphology (M4 and M5), but these are a few of the total cases encountered. The presence of large numbers of immature phagocytes in the blood does not invariably indicate a diagnosis of acute nonlymphocytic leukemia, as reactions to stress or other processes irritating the bone marrow can cause a reactive phagocytic leukocytosis in the blood. In contrast to a *leukemoid reaction*, however, in which all stages of neutrophil maturation populate the blood, the leukemic disorders exhibit mature polymorphonuclear leukocytes and very immature cells with an absence of maturational stages in between. This phenomenon is called *the leukemic hiatus*. When the leukemic cell count in the blood becomes very high (greater than 100,000 cells/ml), a leukemic sludge can actually impair blood circulation, causing pulmonary insufficiency and neurological symptoms because of defective tissue oxygenation.

The neoplastic cells have a propensity to invade normal tissues. The most frequently ravaged organs are those that come into intimate contact with the circulation, such as the spleen, liver, bone, and lymph nodes; these organs are often enlarged and painful in the acute leukemias. Actually, no organ is immune to infiltration. The central nervous system and other sites can serve as sanctuaries where leukemic cells lie dormant, possibly protected from antileukemic therapy. Leukemic cells can cause organ dysfunction by diffuse infiltration of a given organ or can establish a solid tumor mass called a *chloroma*. The term chloroma arises from the greenish color these lesions sometimes have. The green hue is caused by the presence of the enzyme peroxidase in the malignant cells.

The metabolic effect of leukemic proliferation takes its toll on the organism in terms of inanition, presumably because the leukemic cell burden robs the host of nutrients and elaborates substances that derange metabolic regulatory mechanisms.

In addition to the general effects of leukemic proliferation, specific subtypes of acute nonlymphocytic leukemias are associated with special clinical features. In acute promyelocytic leukemia (M3), the patient is invaded by a large burden of malignant cells bearing azurophilic granules. Apparently the contents of these granules leak into the circulation and nonspecifically activate the coagulation system, causing disseminated intravascular coagulation, which results in generalized bleeding (Ch. 15). The malignant cells in acute monocytic leukemia (M5) are uniquely invasive of body tissues. Patients with this disorder have considerable organ enlargement, including painful enlargement of the gums. Presumably the cells are capable of responding to chemotactic factors in the bacteria-rich milieu of the oral cavity. Another feature of acute monocytic leukemia is that the malignant cells release large quantities of the enzyme lysozyme.

Mature macrophages have a limited capacity to proliferate. It is therefore not surprising that neoplasms of this cell line are relatively rare. *Histiocytic medullary reticulosis* is a disorder in which macrophages appear to undergo a malignant transformation. Unlike most other forms of malignant transformation of phagocytes, the cells in histiocytic medullary reticulosis are quite capable of phagocytosis. In some cases, this phagocytosis is uncontrolled and the malignant macrophages engulf normal blood cells. Therefore, some of the anemia, thrombocytopenia, and neutropenia associated with this disease may be attributable to abnormal clearance of these cells by the malignant macrophages.

TREATMENT OF NEOPLASMS OF PHAGOCYTES

Currently, the only treatment for these disorders is to destroy or suppress the malignant clone. Chemotherapeutic agents are used for this purpose, with the strategy of achieving some selective toxicity against the leukemic cells without destroying all the normal stem cells. That such selectivity is possible is evidenced by the fact that various combinations of drugs temporarily restore the bone marrow and blood of patients with acute leukemia to a normal state. Some of the drugs used and their mechanisms of action are described in Chapter 31. This normalization by means of chemotherapy is called *induction of a complete remission*. This treatment is successful in about two-thirds of patients with acute nonlymphocytic leukemia. In the remaining one-third, either the leukemic cells do not disappear at all in response to the drugs or do not completely disappear. The latter situation is called a *partial remission*. Unfortunately, the induction of a complete remission in these diseases is preceded by a period in which the production of normal blood cells is totally abolished. This temporary aplasia of the marrow results from the effect of the preexisting leukemia and of the chemotherapy on the bone marrow stem cells. For 2 to 3 weeks after completion of chemotherapy, the patient suffers from progressive anemia and profound thrombocytopenia and granulocytopenia and is subject to hemorrhage and infection. Therefore, during the period of bone marrow aplasia, the patient requires supportive care in the form of erythrocyte, platelet, and occasionally white blood cell transfusions and treatment of infections with appropriate antibiotics. Unfortunately, some patients otherwise destined to achieve a complete remission may die in this interval because of infection or hemorrhage. Researchers are trying to shorten this dangerous period of pancytopenia by administering hemotopoietic hormones such as GM-CSF to stimulate recovery of the normal bone marrow.

After the period of bone marrow suppression, the surviving normal stem cells regenerate populations of erythrocytes, polymorphonuclear leukocytes, monocytes, and platelets. The state of remission lasts for a variable length of time, usually months to a couple of years, but goes on for many years in a minority of cases. The reappearance of leukemic cells in bone marrow or blood heralds the onset of relapse. Possible reasons for relapse are that (1) not all leukemic cells were killed but are present in numbers too small to be visible in the bone marrow sample viewed during the complete remission; (2) dormant leukemic cells are resistant to the chemotherapy and become active; (3) leukemic cells are protected from the drugs because they hide in tissues such as the brain and testis, which are poorly penetrated by the chemotherapeutic drugs; and (4) whatever damaged the bone marrow stem cells causing the development of leukemia in the first place also transforms the remaining normal cells, and they eventually become malignant. In other words, even after the first leukemic clone is eradicated, a new one emerges. To combat the first possibility, researchers are trying different combinations of drugs that are more effective in killing leukemic cells. Another approach is to follow induction of a complete remission with one or more courses of combination chemotherapy. This intensification strategy is intended to kill small numbers of residual leukemic cells. Intensification appears to be superior to long-term treatment with lower doses of chemotherapy (maintenance therapy). Against the second possibility, ionizing radiation may be directed at the apparent sanctuaries where leukemic cells are believed to hide. One strategy to prevent relapse is the complete ablation of the marrow and its replacement with completely normal stem cells. This approach, using bone marrow transplantation, is described in Chapter 32.

After relapse, it is possible to induce additional remissions with repetitive chemotherapeutic treatment. However, the probability of complete remission becomes progressively lower with successive attempts at induction, and the duration of the remissions becomes shorter. Eventually resistant to all therapy, patients die of complications of bone marrow failure or of tissue infiltration with leukemic cells.

Eosinophilic Leukemia: Hypereosinophilic Syndrome

The blood eosinophil count very rarely becomes elevated above its normal low level (less than 200/µl) in the absence of infections or allergic disorders. When this elevation occurs, and especially if the eosinophil count becomes very high, the patient is said to have the *hypereosinophilic syndrome*. The blood contains mature eosinophils, and the bone marrow has eosinophils in all stages of maturation. Usually the neutrophil, lymphocyte, and platelet counts are normal, although moderate anemia may be present. Extensive invasion of tissues by eosinophils does not usually occur. This picture clearly differs from acute nonlymphocytic leukemias. Indeed, it is not always certain whether the eosinophil proliferation is a normal response to an unknown stimulus or a primary neoplastic disorder of eosinophil production. This ignorance underlies the use of the noncommittal term hypereosinophilic syndrome in those patients. Changes observed in the chromosomal structure of eosinophils of some patients with this disorder are consistent with a malignant basis of the disease.

The major disability inflicted by the accumulation of eosinophils in some patients is the development of cardiac damage. This damage is expressed as arrhythmias, progressive fibrosis of the endocardium, and eventually heart failure. The basis of this insult to the heart is unknown, but is possibly a toxic effect of substances released from eosinophils.

The rarity and variable severity of this disease has prevented the development of a consensus regarding treatment. In patients with cardiac toxicity, corticosteroids, cytotoxic chemotherapy, and leukopheresis, the removal of eosinophils by attaching the patient to an extracorporeal continuous flow centrifuge has been employed with variable success.

HISTIOCYTOSIS X

The term *histiocytosis X* is given to a collection of uncommon disorders that pathologists classify as a neoplasm of mononuclear phagocytes. The diseases, which mainly affect children and young adults, vary in histology and degree of malignancy. The process is a growth of atypical cells that resemble normal macrophages, although the neoplastic cell has not been well characterized. The proliferation of these cells, called *histiocytes* (as macrophages used to be termed), can occur in any organ, but most frequently takes place in bone. The growth may appear as an isolated lesion affecting one site, or it may involve multiple organs and progress. Often solitary growths contain eosinophils as well as macrophagelike cells; such lesions have been termed eosinophilic granulomas. When the process is more widespread and progressive, bones of the skull are often involved, leading to a constellation of complications including exophthalmos (caused by orbital infiltration), endocrine hormone deficiencies (because of destruction of the pituitary gland after invasion of the sella turcica), and necrotic skin lesions. This progressive form of histiocytosis X also carries the eponym Hand–Schuller–Christian disease. In its most aggressive form, histiocytosis X rapidly evolves to cause extensive organ dysfunction and constitutional deterioration with high fever and prostration and frequently death. Bone marrow infiltration by this process can produce bone marrow failure. This variant has the eponym Letterer–Siwe disease. The progressive variants of histiocytosis X, with their attendant poorer prognoses, are more common in children younger than age 3.

Therapy for histiocytosis X is highly effective for localized disease and involves surgical excision of small lesions or radiotherapy of larger ones. For histiocytosis X of intermediate severity, this treatment together with supportive care, such as endocrine hormone replacement, can prevent death and limit mobidity. Various forms of chemotherapy employed against progressive disease are only marginally successful.

SUGGESTED READINGS

Bennett, J.M., Catovsky, D., Daniel, M.T., et al. (1976) Proposals for the classification of the acute leukemias: French-American-British (FAB) Cooperative Group. Br. J. Haematol. *33*:451.

Bloomfield, C.D., Ed. (1987) Acute myeloid leukemia. Semin. Oncol. *14*:357.

Champlin, R., & Gale R.P. (1987) Acute myelogenous leukemia: Recent advances in therapy. Blood *69*:1551.

Dabich, L. (1980) Acute nonlymphocytic leukemias. Med. Clin. North Am. *64*:683.

Flaum, M., Scholey, R.T., Fauci, A.S., et al. (1981) A clinicopathologic correlation of the idiopathic hypereosinophilic syndrome. I. Hematologic manifestations. Blood *58*:1012.

Greenberger, J.S., Crocker, A.C., Vawter, G., et al. (1981) Results of treatment of 127 patients with systemic histiocytosis (Letterer-Siwe syndrome) Schuller-Christian syndrome and multifocal eosinophilic granuloma. Medicine *60*:311.

Holt, J.T., Morton, C.C., Nienhuis, A.W., & Leder, P. (1987) Molecular mechanisms of hematological neoplasms In The Molecular Basis of Blood Diseases. Stamatoyannopoulos, G., Nienhuis, A.W., Leder, P., Majerus, P.W., Eds. WB Saunders, Philadelphia, pp 347–376.

Koeffler, H.P. (1987) Syndromes of acute nonlymphocytic leukemia. Ann. Intern. Med. *107*:748.

Nimer, S., & Golde, D.W. (1987) The 5q⁻ abnormality. Blood *70*:1705.

Yunis, J.J., Brunning, R.D., Howe, R.B., & Lobell, M. (1984) High resolution chromosomes as an independent prognostic indicator in adult acute nonlymphocytic leukemia. N. Engl. J. Med. *311*:812.

Lymphoid Cells and Reactive Changes of Lymphoid Cells

Lymphoid cells are far more uniform in appearance than are phagocytic leukocytes. However, these cells are exceedingly diverse and complex and are the "brains" of the immune system. They discriminate self from nonself, generate specificity in the attack on offending microorganisms, and are the repositories of memory, permitting a rapid response to invasion. Unlike the phagocytes, that have a life cycle that tends to be a one-way street from bone marrow to blood to tissues, many lymphoid cells circulate and recirculate among bone marrow, blood, lymphatics and lymphoid organs, the lymph nodes, and the spleen.

LYMPHOCYTES IN NORMAL BLOOD AND TISSUES

Most lymphocytes are found in the lymphatic system, or lymphon, a network of channels interspersed by aggregates of lymphocytes together with other cells. These aggregates are lymph nodes of lymph glands and the spleen. The lymphatic system communicates directly with the blood vasculature at the thoracic duct, where the lymph enters the subclavian vein. The blood and lymphatic systems are also in intimate contact in the spleen, where the blood

percolates through rich lymphoid collections, called *white pulp*, of this organ.

Figure 20-1 shows the locations of lymph nodes, the sizes of which can be ascertained by the clinician employing observation and palpation during the physical examination. These nodes include the tonsils and the cervical, axillary, epitrochlear, subclavian, and inguinal glands. Of the internal lymph nodes, the mediastinal nodes may be visualized, especially if enlarged, on x-ray films of the chest. Special procedures including lymphangiography and computed tomography are required to evaluate the size of abdominal lymph nodes.

The architecture of lymph nodes features a capsule surrounding glandular substance divided into outer (*cortical*) and inner (*medullary*) regions (Fig. 20-2A). Lymphatic channels bringing lymph into the gland (afferent vessels) enter the cortex delivering the lymph to a subcortical space. The cortex contains clumps of cells, the *germinal follicles*, the site of antibody-forming lymphoid cells. Lymph percolates into the medulla and leaves by efferent vessels at the hilum of the node. The different types of normal and abnormal lymphocytes prefer to reside in discrete areas of the lymph node (Fig. 20-2B).

In the healthy adult, the blood contains 1500

303

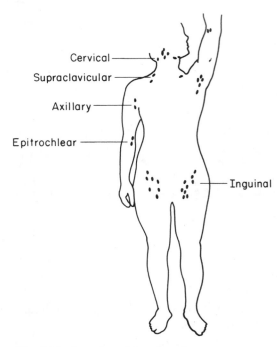

Cervical

Supraclavicular

Axillary

Epitrochlear

Inguinal

Fig. 20-1. Location of lymph nodes.

to 3500 lymphocytes per microliter. Early in life, the number of lymphocytes may be much higher, up to 15,000/µl; the concentration of these cells falls progressively, reaching the adult level by adolescence. Similarly, the lymphoid organs, the lymph nodes and spleen, of young children tend to be relatively large and diminish in size until, by adulthood, they are impalpable or barely so. The typical blood lymphocytes observed on a Wright's-stained smear of the blood is a relatively small leukocyte, essentially characterized as a dense nucleus with clumped chromatin and an indistinct nucleolus with a bit of blue cytoplasm peeking around it (Fig. 20-3). If the nuclear chromatin is less dense, the nucleoli are more obvious and the quantity of cytoplasm is increased, and the lymphocyte is called *atypical* (Fig. 20-3). Up to 5 percent of the lymphocytes of normal persons may be atypical.

What appears simply as typical and atypical lymphocytes to the morphologist in reality represents a complex of many populations of cells having very different life histories and func-

tions. The principal categories of lymphoid cells are thymus-derived lymphocytes (*T cells*) and bone marrow-derived lymphocytes (*B cells*).

Bursa or Bone-Marrow-Derived Lymphoid Cells

In birds, an organ associated with the gastrointestinal tract, the bursa of Fabricius, participates in the education of undifferentiated lymphoid cells into B cells, a function analogous to the activity of the thymus for the development of T cells. Lymphocytes arising from the bone marrow migrate to this organ and acquire the eventual capacity to differentiate into cells that secrete specific antibodies. These cells have been named B cells after the bursa of Fabricius. Birds from which the bursa is removed before hatching have no B cells and no antibodies.

Mammals do not have a bursa of Fabricius; presumably, the bone marrow itself assumes this function of conditioning certain lymphocytes for subsequent antibody formation.

The earliest identifiable cell of B-cell lineage is called a pre-B cell (Fig. 20-4). Mature B lymphocytes circulate in the blood and lymphatics but are found primarily in the germinal centers of the cortex of lymph nodes and in the white pulp of the spleen. Of blood lymphocytes, fewer than one-fifth are B cells. They are typical lymphocytes in their morphological appearance. Responding to antigens, B lymphocytes proliferate and differentiate into clones of plasma cells that secrete specific antibodies directed against the antigens (Fig. 20-5). Plasma cells have a characteristic morphology. They are ovoid to rhomboid in shape. Their nucleus is round, and in an off-center location clumps of nuclear chromatin may be located around the edges of the nucleus in a spoke-wheel pattern. The peripheral cytoplasm stains dark blue in Wright-Giemsa-stained smears because of abundant ribosomes involved in the synthesis of immunoglobulins.

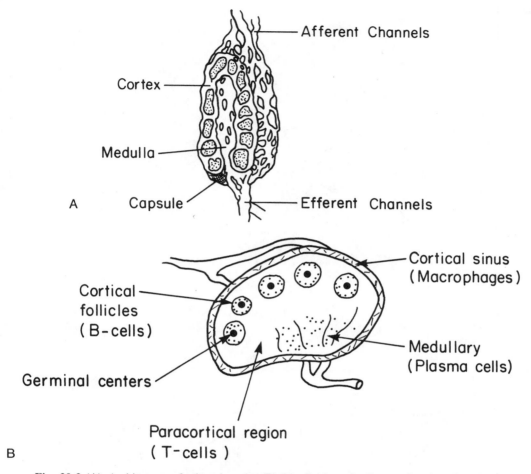

Fig. 20-2 (A) Architecture of a lymph node. **(B)** Distribution of cell types in a lymph node.

A distinct light perinuclear halo is the location of a Golgi complex.

Some antigens are capable of inducing B-cell differentiation into antibody-producing plasma cells without help from other cells. For other antigens, T cells and macrophages interact with the antigens and the B cells to promote differentiation of the B cells in response to antigens. The membranes of the reacting B cells express structures called *Ia antigens*, which are produced under the influence of immune response (Ir) genes. The Ir genes reside within what is called the *histocompatibility complex*, a region of genes on the short arm of chromosome number 6 that program the synthesis of glycoproteins on the surface of cells.

These cell-surface antigens are recognized by the immune system in incompatible situations; this recognition, extremely important in transplantation biology, leads to rejection of the graft (see Ch. 32).

During the course of antibody production against a new antigen, the B-cell system makes IgM first, followed by other classes of immunoglobulin. A mature plasma cell secretes only one class of immunoglobulin, with specificity for only one antigen. This means that the cell makes one class of heavy chains—either μ, γ, α, δ, or ϵ—and one class of light chains ending up as IgM, IgG, IgA, IgD, or IgE antibodies. However, during development, B cells make various classes of immunoglobulin and

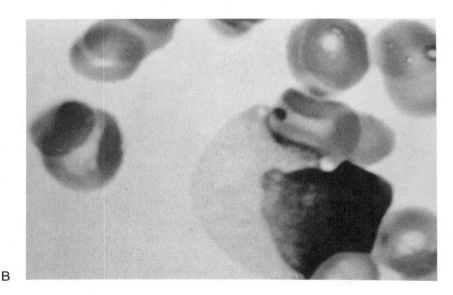

Fig. 20-3. Appearance of typical **(A)** and atypical **(B)** lymphocyte.

express them in different ways. For example, pre-B cells have immunoglobulins in their cytoplasm but not on their membranes, and they do not secrete these immunoglobulins. During maturation, B cells express at varying times IgM and IgD on their surfaces. The surface immunoglobulin of a given B cell will have either x or λ light chains, but the normal B-cell population, like the populations of immuno-globulins in the circulation, will express a mixture of x and λ light chains with a ratio of 2:1. Immunoglobulin is found in the cytoplasm of plasma cells, but not on the external surface. However, the plasma cell secretes large quantities of immunoglobulin. This sequence of changes in the expression of immunoglobulins during B-cell development is diagramed in Figure 20-4.

Fig. 20-4. Functional lymphoid cell differentiation.

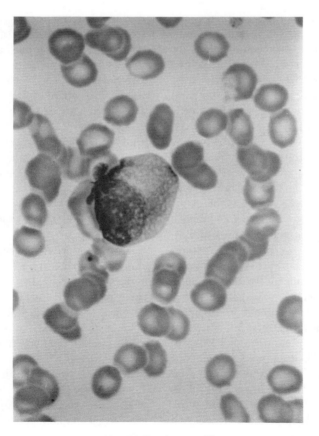

Fig. 20-5. Plasma cell.

How a large but finite number of B cells has the capacity to regenerate clones of plasma cells, producing antibodies to the apparently infinite number of antigents in the environment, and how stimulated T cells acquire the capacity to mount cell-mediated immune responses against specific antigens are among the most fascinating problems in biology. Recent progress in research has made great strides toward solving these problems.

Immature B cells have on their surfaces antigen receptors that serve as crude immunoglobulin molecules. Depending on the conformations of the antigen receptors, certain immature lymphocytes react with varying avidity to antigens. When a threshold in the avidity of binding is achieved, the selected B cell begins to differentiate and proliferate. Usually this process involves the cooperation of macrophages and a subset of T cells (see below). During differentiation and proliferation the specificity of the reaction between the cell and the antigen must increase. In the case of antibody formation (1) gene recombinations or mutations in the genes coding for variable and hypervariable regions of immunoglobulin molecules permit a testing of different immunoglobulins on the surface of the various B cells and (2) the greater avidity of binding between these molecules and the antibody somehow stimulates proliferation of the B-cell clone with the highest specificity.

Advances in genetic technology have generated these insights into how lymphoid cells employ a limited number of genes to produce an enormous quantity of antibody protein molecules, each differing in primary structure. This task is accomplished by the separation of genes coding for regions of immunoglobulin molecules into different parts of cellular DNA and the subsequent recombination of these genes to yield products that code for different immunoglobulins. Not surprisingly, this recombination is restricted to those segments of the gene coding for the variable domain of immunoglobulin molecules. Figure 20-6 shows a scheme for the synthesis of an immunoglobulin light chain. The light chain DNA, located on chromosome 2, contains a small number of base pair sequences that code for the constant region of the molecule, indicated by C, and a larger number of sequences coding for variable region, designated V. In addition, a number of sequences encode the region that joins the constant and variable domains and are shown by the letter J. The recombination of 150 V genes to one of five J genes can yield 750 different genes for the variable region of the light chain. This variability can be increased further by a factor of, say 10, by imprecise splicing at the J–V recombination locus. Following the transcription of the recombined DNA to RNA, intervening sequences, indicated by the broken lines, are spliced out to produce the final RNA product. This RNA can then be translated to synthesize the completed immunoglobulin molecule. The scheme for antibody diversity outlined in the figure for the case of a light chain is even more complex for the heavy chain. The heavy chain gene, located on chromosome 14, also contains sequences involved in recombination, called D for diversity.

Given the information that there may be as many as 80 embryonic heavy chain V genes, 50 D genes, and six J genes, there are 24,000 possible combinations that can be multiplied by another factor of 100 to allow for recombinational variations. These 2.4 million possible different heavy chains combined with 7500 possible light chains lead to the theoretical possibility of 18 million antibodies.

Thymus-Derived Lymphocytes

During fetal development, a population of lymphocytes arises from the bone marrow and migrates to the thymus gland (Fig. 20-4). There, in response to the hormone thymosin, elaborated by the epithelial cells of this organ, the cells acquire the ability to perform their specific immunological functions. The cells leave the thymus and percolate in the blood and lymphatic circulation until they reach specific areas of the spleen and lymph nodes called the *paracortical region* (Fig. 20-2**B**). These T cells recirculate periodically out of the lymphoid organs into the circulation and have

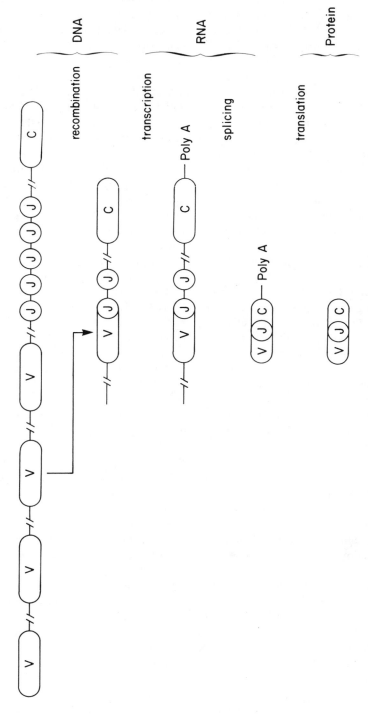

Fig. 20-6. Sequence of changes in the expression of immunoglobulins during B-cell development.

the capacity, like phagocytes, to enter the tissues, although their motility is slower than that of phagocytes. Eventually, the lymphocytes return to the lymph nodes and spleen. Of the blood lymphocytes, about two-thirds are T cells in the normal state. During the course of their meanderings, the cells may encounter an antigen, such as a microorganism, to which they are able to respond. The confrontation causes the lymphocyte to increase in size and undergo division, generating a clone of cells reactive to that antigen. These changes in morphology of the lymphocytes, which correspond to those of the atypical lymphocytes seen in the peripheral blood, are accompanied by DNA synthesis and eventually by cell division. The phenomenon, called *blast transformation*, can be measured in the laboratory by observing the incorporation of radioactively labeled thymidine into cellular DNA.

The way in which T cells acquire specific recognition of targets is analogous to the generation of antibody specificity by B cells. Instead of surface immunoglobulin serving as a crude antigen receptor that undergoes regulated mutation into a specific receptor that eventually becomes secreted to act extracellularly, a family of molecules, known as the *T-cell receptor*, undergoes similar rearrangements but remains affixed to the T-cell membrane. The T-cell receptor resembles immunoglobulin in having two sets of polypeptide chains, each of which has constant and variable regions. The constant regions are anchored in the plasma membrane of the T cell, and the variable domains extend into the extracellular space. As with immunoglobulin genes, a limited number of germ-line T-cell receptor genes rearrange to generate myriad variable sequences in the variable region of the T-cell receptor molecule. The production of antigen specificity involves the selective activation of T-cell clones with T-cell antigen receptors that react progressively more avidly with the antigen.

T cells are particularly important in the destruction of foreign cells and are the principal agents for the rejection of grafts in the setting of purposeful or accidental transplantation of cells and organs.

The particular response of the activated T cell depends on its programming in the thymus. T cells as a whole are functionally very versatile. The many different functions they perform are done by different subsets of T lymphocytes. Certain T-effector cells may directly participate in the killing of facultative intracellular parasites by killing the cells in which the parasites reside, for example, virus-containing cells. Such cells are designated *cytotoxic* or *killer T cells*. Killer T cells may recognize their targets because of the specificity built into them during differentiation. Alternatively, the T cells can recognize and kill target cells that are coated with specific antibodies directed against the target cell. One of the mechanisms by which the killing occurs is the secretion by the cytotoxic or killer T cell of proteins called *perforins*, which punch holes in target cells. The perforins resemble the terminal component of the complement sequence C9 (Ch. 15). A second function of T cells is to elaborate substances, lymphokines that act on other cells. One set of lymphokines activates macrophages, enabling the latter to kill facultative intracellular parasites within them. One of the most important macrophage-activating lymphokines is γ interferon.

Another lymphokine, interleukin 2 (IL 2), acts as a B cell growth factor; in this respect it is important in the setting of a third function of the T cell, where another subclass of these cells, called *helper cells*, cooperate with B cells to stimulate their differentiation into plasma cells producing specific antibodies. Interleukin 2 also induces cytotoxic activity of certain T cells. The attempt to activate such T cells by recombinant IL 2 into "killer (LAK) cells" against tumor cells has been used as a form of experimental cancer therapy. An additional lymphokine, tumor necrosis factor, has multiple toxic metabolic effects. A fourth function of certain T cells is to control or suppress the production of antibodies by B cells, preventing uncontrolled or inappropriate immune reactions. Such cells are designated suppressor cells (Fig. 20-4).

As was mentioned in discussing the cooperative interaction between B cells, helper T cells, and macrophages that occurs during the generation of certain antibody-forming plasma cells, externally disposed histocompatibility molecules are also important in the communication between suppressor T cells and B cells. Suppressor and helper cells use different histocompatibility molecules known as *class I* and *class II*, respectively. The two classes of histocompatibility molecules are desscribed in Chapter 32. In addition to histocompatibility molecules, another set of surface molecules is involved in these complex cellular reactions. In the case of T helper cells, this other molecule is known as *CD4*; for T suppressor cells it is called *CD8*. CD4 is also important as the receptor for the immunodeficiency virus that causes the acquired immune deficiency syndrome (AIDS) (see Ch. 21).

In a system as complex as the immune machinery, obviously a very delicate balance must exist between T-suppressor and T-helper activities in allowing appropriate antibodies, but not autoaggressive antibodies, to form. It follows that imbalances in the number or activity of these T-cell subsets can lead to immunodeficiency and autoimmune phenomena.

If the thymus is removed from or destroyed in an animal or human before or shortly after birth, the subject lacks T cells and lacks the ability to express cell-mediated immunity.

The specificity programmed into B and T lymphocytes persists after an encounter with antigen in the form of immunological memory. Progeny of the specific clones persist for many years in a dormant state. On subsequent encounter with the original antigen, clonal expansion occurs again, but with greater efficiency, and this secondary response in terms of cell-mediated immunity or antibody production is the basis of specific immunity and provides the rationale for vaccination.

Other Cells of the Lymphoid System

A population of lymphocytes that cannot be characterized as either T or B cells as defined by surface Ig expression or cosetting with sheep red cells are designated *null cells*. These cells are very immature lymphocytes, not committed yet to either B- or T-cell lineage. They may even be stem cells. Some of these cells contain terminal deoxyribonucleotide transferase, an enzyme that catalyzes the addition of deoxyribonucleoside triphosphate bases, such as deoxy-ATP, into the 3'-hydroxyl end of single-stranded polynucleotides. This DNA polymerase is unique in mammalian DNA synthesis in not requiring a template for its function. It is a very useful marker for immature cells and for the diagnosis of certain lymphoid neoplasms. Ten to 20 percent of blood lymphocytes are null cells.

A class of cells important in immune reactions are *natural killer cells*. These cells have the ability to kill abnormal cells, such as damaged cells, virus-infected cells, and possibly cancer cells without being primed by previous recognition of the antigen or without requiring a specific antibody for their action. Interferon, the antiviral substance produced by virus-infected cells, stimulates the cytotoxic action of natural killer cells.

Cells with long processes called *dendritic cells* may be important for the complex communication that goes on between B cells, T cells, and macrophages during the generation of specific antibody responses.

IDENTIFICATION OF LYMPHOID CELLS

The different types of lymphocytes can be identified by receptors on their membranes. The receptors may bind particular antibodies or certain types of red blood cells. These surface markers define the various populations of lymphoid cells (Table 20-1).

The most straightforward method for identifying B cells is to detect immunoglobulin molecules in or on them. This can be done by reacting the cells with fluorescein-tagged anti-immunoglobulin antibody, washing off excess reagent, and looking for cell-associated fluorescence in a fluorescence microscope or with a flow cytometer. B cells also bind to erythro-

Table 20-1. Some Functional and Immunochemical Markers of Lymphoid Cells

Cell Type	Functional Marker	Identified by Antibodies
Immature T cell	Terminal deoxynucleotide transferase	Designated T10 or CD3
T cell	IgG(Fc) receptors; form rosettes with sheep red cells; undergo blast transformation following exposure to concanavalin A	Against the sheep erythrocyte receptor. The antibody is designated T3 or CD2
Helper subset	Promote synthesis of antibodies by B cells in tissue culture	Against CD4. The antibody is sometimes designated T4
Suppressor/ cytotoxic subset	Inhibit synthesis of antibodies by B cells in tissue culture	Against CD8. The antibody is sometimes designated T8
Pre-B cell		Against Ig, stains cytoplasm
Immature B cell	Form rosettes with C3b-bearing red cells (i.e., complement receptors present)	Against IgM and IgD, stain the plasma membrane
Plasma cells	Secrete Igs	Designated PCA1, PCA2
Most B cells	Ia antigen	Designated CD19, CD20, Ia
Mature B cells	C3d receptor	Designated CD21

cytes coated with the third component of complement. The erythrocytes surround the lymphocyte. From the floral resemblance, this tableau is called a rosette. Phagocytes also form rosettes with complement-coated erythrocytes, but unlike B lymphocytes, they can phagocytize the complexes under appropriate conditions.

T cells form rosettes with sheep erythrocytes; the formation of these E rosettes has been the principal assay for T lymphocytes. In addition, T cells specifically undergo blast transformation in response to concanavalin A, a lectin, a protein that binds to sugars, specifically to mannose residues. Antibodies can be raised in animals against antigens on the surface of lymphoid cells or unrelated species; these antibodies can be tagged with fluorescein and can be used to identify T cells, B cells, and subsets of T cells, the helper and suppressor cells (Table 20-1). When antibodies against antigens on cells of one species are generated in another species, these antibodies are said to be *heterologous*. The antibodies are generated by the lymphoid system of an organism exposed to the foreign cells. The process that goes into the production of these antibodies involves a selection and the development of multiple clones producing antibodies of varying avidity for the antigen. Furthermore, unless the antigen is perfectly pure, the organism will almost certainly generate antibodies reactive against multiple antigens in the preparation used to immunize the animal. In the case of cells containing multiple surface antigens, this is a serious problem. The development of antibodies for use in detection of certain types of cells by this technique therefore requires that the immunoglobulin preparation be absorbed with various cells until a desired specificity for a particular cell is achieved. With this complex methodology, the specificity of the antibodies is always in question and hard to reproduce from one laboratory to another.

Now it is possible to produce antibodies in tissue culture in large quantities that are specific for a single part of a single antigen. These antibodies are derived from a single clone of B cells. These *monoclonal antibodies* are made by fusing spleen cells from a mouse immunized with the antigen to a mouse lymphoid tumor cell. The tumor cell confers immortality on the fusion product, called a *hybridoma*, which permits it to undergo continuous replication and secrete large quantities of antibody derived from the B-cell genes operative in the hybridoma. In developing a hybridoma antibody, the fusion products must be separated and cultivated separately and analyzed for their antibody specificity. Once the desired antibody is found, its specificity is more definite.

Monoclonal antibodies directed against components of the surface of lymphoid cells are now the principal tools for identification of lymphoid cell subsets. Certain of these antibodies are specific for the various functional subsets of lymphoid cells, for example, for helper T cells, suppressor T cells, and other types of lymphocytes. These antibodies can assist the clinician in determining whether the lymphocyte subpopulations are altered in various disease states and whether an elevation in the blood lymphocyte count or an infiltrate of lymphocytes in the tissues represents the expansion of a particular type of lymphoid cells.

Some of the antibodies are relatively specific for particular stages of lymphoid maturation, whereas others have a broader specificity, for example, for all types of B or T cells. A somewhat confusing situation has arisen from the fact that several commercial sources market monoclonal antibodies and have given them different names. In addition, some of these antibodies may react with different regions of the same surface molecules. Table 20-1 lists some of the different designations as well as a convention called CD (for "cluster of differentiation") adopted by an international workshop.

In normal blood, about one-half the lymphocytes can be identified as T cells and about one-third as B cells. The remainder, bearing neither T- nor B-cell markers, are classified as null cells.

It must be emphasized that the marker systems for identifying lymphoid cells are in constant evolution as new insights develop concerning the complexities of the lymphoid system. The catalog summary of lymphoid cell types and their markers (enumerated in Table 20-1) should therefore be viewed as an initial convenience for learning; the student must be prepared to revise and juggle these concepts. Nevertheless, the use of markers to classify lymphoid cell types is becoming increasingly useful in identifying aberrations in lymphoid cell populations, especially in lymphoid neoplasms.

REACTIVE CHANGES OF LYMPHOID CELLS

Lymphocytes, like phagocytes, respond to infection or inflammation. In many bacterial infections, the lymphocyte count rises, although not usually above 5,000 to 10,000 cells/μl. Responding to the infection, a fraction of the lymphocytes undergoes blast transformation, so that atypical lymphocytes may be common in infection and inflammatory states. Some infections uniquely favor changes in the lymphocyte count. Infections caused by the bacterial species *Bordetella pertussis*, the organism that causes the respiratory disease whooping cough, are associated with extraordinary lymphocytosis, with lymphocyte counts between 20,000 and 80,000/μl. The pertussis microorganism releases a factor that somehow stimulates the increase in blood lymphocytes. However, a reactive lymphocytosis of this degree ordinarily is unusual in adults. Viral infections frequently increase the lymphocyte count and induce substantial atypicality to the morphology of the lymphocytes. Processes affecting the number of peripheral blood lymphocytes frequently can cause proliferation of lymphocytes in the lymph nodes and the spleen. Such enlargements of the lymph nodes and spleen are called, respectively, *lymphadenopathy* and *splenomegaly*.

An infection affecting the lymphoid system frequently encountered in clinical medicine is *infectious mononucleosis*. In infectious mononucleosis there is a fever, sore throat, enlargement of the lymph nodes and spleen, and a lymphocytosis with atypical lymphocytes. The signs and symptoms persist for variable lengths of time, from as short as days to as long as months. The term "mononucleosis" is a meaningless archaic holdover from times of equivocation over the cell type increased in the blood. The most common cause of infectious mononucleosis is an infection with a DNA herpes virus that infects B cells, the Epstein-Barr virus (EBV). The atypical lymphocytosis of infectious mononucleosis is a reaction of T cells to the infected B cells. Any and all lymphoid organs can become enlarged in infectious mononucleosis. Although debility is the main clinical problem of infectious mononucleosis, an occasional serious complication is rupture of the enlarged spleen, which is abnormally susceptible to trauma. Sometimes the enlargement and ulceration of the pharyngeal tonsils can be sufficient to interfere with nutrition. In such instances, brief treatment of the patient with corticosteroids can produce remarkable shrinkage of the lymph nodes and amelioration of the symptoms.

Diseases that affect the normal balance of cells of the lymphoid system can occasionally lead to abnormal immune responses. Rare patients with infectious mononucleosis will develop autoantibodies against their own blood cells or other tissues. Very rarely, the proliferation of atypical T cells can be sufficiently intense as to behave like a malignant neoplasm and progresses to kill the patient by infiltrating vital organs. This catastrophe has occurred within families, and the susceptibility to such a devastating course of EBV mononucleosis is transmitted as an X-linked trait, leading to this condition being named the *X-linked lymphoproliferative syndrome*. Although cancerous in its invasive behavior, this disorder is not an expansion of a single cell clone as occurs in the leukemias. EBV infection is strongly associated with a B-cell neoplasm of Africans called Burkitt's lymphoma and with epithelial neoplasms of the nasopharynx. When normal blood lymphoid cells are cultivated in tissue culture, it appears that it is a chronic infection with EBV that confers immortality on the cells, permitting them to persist under culture conditions. For all these reasons, EBV is suspected as an oncogenic (i.e., cancer-causing) virus. The verdict is not in, however, as it is also possible that these tumors are only susceptible to infection with EBV. Nevertheless, there is no doubt but that EBV causes infectious mononucleosis.

The diagnosis of infectious mononucleosis caused by EBV can be suspected by observation of an atypical lymphocytosis in the setting of appropriate clinical signs and symptoms, usually in a young adult. The diagnosis can be established by observing a rise in antibody titers against EBV several weeks after the onset of the illness. This serological test is rarely necessary, however, because of an unusual immunological phenomenon associated with the disease. Within weeks after the onset of signs and symptoms, the patient's serum contains an IgM antibody that reacts with erythrocytes of various animal species. The reason for the production of this antibody, called *heterophile* (meaning "likes other species"), is unclear, but the presence of heterophile antibody is extremely useful for the diagnosis of EBV infectious mononucleosis. The capacity of a patient's serum to agglutinate sheep or horse erythrocytes establishes the presence of heterophile antibodies. Heterophile antibodies appear in other disorders affecting the immune system, such as serum sickness. But the specificity of the presence of a heterophile antibody for infectious mononucleosis can be established by absorption tests. The heterophile found in EBV infectious mononucleosis will bind to cow but not to guinea pig erythrocytes. Therefore, if the patient's serum persists in agglutinating sheep or horse erythrocytes after exposure to guinea pig erythrocytes, and the loss of this agglutination potential occurs after reaction with beef erythrocytes, the heterophile reaction is specific for EBV infectious mononucleosis.

The clinical picture of infectious mononucleosis can arise in other viral infections such as viral hepatitis and infections with cytomegalovirus. Both infections occur typically in persons who have recently received many blood transfusions. The protozoan *Toxoplasma gondii*, an organism that can be acquired from the ingestion of poorly cooked meat, as well as from house cats, can also cause an illness resembling infectious mononucleosis. Unlike EBV infectious mononucleosis, these other infections do not elicit high EBV or heterophile antibody responses. Some bacterial infections also cause a clinical picture resembling infectious mononucleosis. Typhoid fever, secondary spyhilis, and leptospirosis are examples that must be considered in patients with the signs and symptoms of infectious mononucleosis who fail to demonstrate heterophile antibodies after appropriate absorptions.

Patients with diseases affecting lymphoid cells usually present with generalized signs and symptoms, as well as enlargement of many lymphoid organs, the spleen, and peripheral lymph nodes (Fig. 20-1). The lymph nodes may enlarge up to several centimeters in diameter and may become tender and painful. Usually the lymph nodes are freely movable when probed by the examiner's fingers. Some infections have a predilection to enlarge particular lymph nodes. It is very common for cervical lymph nodes to be enlarged in viral diseases of the respiratory tract and in infectious mononucleosis. In rubella virus infections, the preauricular lymph nodes are uniquely enlarged. Generalized lymphadenopathy is also a manifestation of the acquired immune deficiency syndrome (AIDS) or its precursor AIDS-related complex (ARC) (Ch. 21).

Occasionally the physician encounters enlargement of lymph nodes in a single area with little or no obvious evidence of systemic disease. A first consideration should always be whether an infection or a neoplasm exists in the region providing lymphatic drainage to the involved lymph node. In cases of infections and inflammatory conditions associated with lymph gland enlargement, the lymph node may be actually infected (lymphadenitis), or it may be infiltrated or simply reacting to the infection or some other process in the drainage area (lymphadenopathy). It is common for inguinal lymph nodes to be palpable in adults, probably because of subclinical fungal infections affecting the feet. A biopsy of an enlarged reactive lymph node will usually show normal lymph node architecture as well as increased number and size of germinal follicles.

If microorganisms are within the lymph node, they might be visible or possibly can be cultivated. In the case of acute bacterial infection, necrosis and abscess formation with invasion by polymorphonuclear leukocytes will be observed by the pathologist. Infections attributable to tuberculosis or other facultative intracellular parasites can be associated with lymph nodes containing granulomata with or without giant cells. Any infection can lead to reactive enlargement of lymph nodes. Some infections particularly prone to produce lymphadenopathy include anthrax, bubonic plague, tularemia, tuberculosis, and syphilis. Cat scratch fever is a febrile illness associated with reactive enlargement of lymph nodes following a cat scratch in the area draining the lymph node. The cause of this reaction is not definitely known, although there is some evidence that an unusual bacillary organism is responsible.

The enlargement of lymph nodes in an otherwise asymptomatic patient can herald the presence of a malignant neoplasm. This neoplasm can originate from the lymphoid system itself, in which case the disorder is a lymphoma, or reflect invasion of the lymph nodes by an unrelated cancer. Lymph nodes enlarged by the presence of epithelial malignant neoplasms will frequently feel very hard to the touch because of the extensive fibrosis elicited by the malignant cells. If, because of persistence, large size, or rapid enlargement of a lymph node, the physician decides to have the node surgically excised, the pathologist should be alerted in advance. The pathologist will want to prepare some of the tissue in such a way as to allow for the detection of lymphocyte surface markers as described earlier in this chapter (see also Ch. 22). Once the specimen has been fixed in formalin for routine histological examination, it is possible but more difficult to perform marker studies.

SUGGESTED READINGS

Alt, F.W., Blackwell, T.K., & Yancopoulos, G.D. (1987) Development of the primary antibody repertoire. Science *238*:1079–1087.

Cooper, M.D. (1987) B lymphocytes. Normal development and function. N. Engl. J. Med. *317*: 1452–1456.

Kohler, G. (1986) Derivation and diversification of

monoclonal antibodies. Science *233*:1281–1286.

Marrack, P., & Kappler, J. (1987) The T cell receptor. Science *238*:1073–1079.

Nossal, G.J.V. (1987) The basic components of the immune system. N. Engl. J. Med. *316*: 1320–1325.

Young, J.D.E., & Cohn, Z.A. (1986) Cell-mediated killing: A common mechanism? Cell *46*:641.

21

Immunodeficiency and Autoimmunity Caused by Defects of the Lymphoid System

The immense complexity of the lymphoid system renders it highly susceptible to the derangements that impair the immune response. These abnormalities may be hereditary or acquired, transient or permanent, and affect the sensory (afferent) or effector (efferent) limbs of the system. The clinical consequence of lymphoid deficiency may stem primarily from failure to deal adequately with microorganisms (immunodeficiency) or may reflect a loss of control over the ability to discriminate self from nonself and manifest itself as autoimmune disease. Immunodeficiency and autoimmunity may coexist in the same instances. Under certain circumstances, clinicians purposely create lymphoid deficiency. This immunosuppression is done to prevent rejection of transplanted organs or to ameliorate the ravages of autoimmune disorders.

GENERAL FEATURES OF IMMUNODEFICIENCY

In disorders in which antibodies are deficient, the patient suffers from recurrent and severe infection caused by high-grade encapsulated pathogens, such as *Diplococcus pneu-*

moniae, Streptococcus pyogenes, Hemophilus influenzae, and *Neisseria menigitidis*. This susceptibility is the result of impaired opsonization and recognition of these organisms by macrophages. The diagnosis of antibody deficiency is easily established by measuring the serum immunoglobulin concentrations by means of the techniques described in Chapter 17.

If a lymphoid deficiency is primarily a decreased functioning of T cells, the affected person is susceptible to infection with facultative intracellular parasites, such as fungi, viruses, and mycobacteriae. This susceptibility arises from the failure of T cells to arm macrophages to deal with these parasites and from the inability of certain killer T cells to destroy pathogens or pathogen-infected host cells that sustain the microorganisms. Such patients frequently have white patches in the oral cavity, which represent growth of the fungus *Candida albicans*, also called *Monilia* or thrush.

A common virus infection that becomes problematic in the setting of T-cell dysfunction or deficiency is varicella-zoster. Primary exposure to this virus usually causes chickenpox, a self-limited disease characterized by fever and a bullous rash in the normal host. In the

Antibody Deficiency States

Congenital
> X-linked Agammaglobulinemia
> X-linked Hypogammaglobulinemia
> with elevated IgM levels
> Dysgammaglobulinemia
>> Selective IgG subclass deficiency
>> IgM deficiency
>> IgA deficiency
> Ataxia Telangiectasia (IgA hypercatabolism)
> Wiskott-Aldrich Syndrome (defective anti-polysaccharide antibody formation)

Acquired
> Common variable hypogammaglobulinemia
> Neoplasm-associated hypogammaglobulinemia
>> Chronic lymphatic leukemia
>> Thymoma
>> Multiple myeloma
> Protein-losing states
>> Nephrotic syndrome
>> Enteropathy
>> Intestinal—lymphatic fistula
> Radiation, chemotherapy and splenectomy, treatment for Hodgkin's disease

Disorders That Often Lead to Recurrent or Severe Infections from Facultative Intracellular Parasites

Disorders affecting T lymphocytes
> Congenital thymic aplasia
> Cytotoxic antibodies against T lymphocytes
> Hodgkin's disease
> Sarcoid
> Acquired immune deficiency syndrome (AIDS)

Disorders affecting all lymphoid cells
> Severe combined immune deficiency, congenital X-linked, and autosomal recessive variants
> Immunosuppressive therapy
>> Corticosteroids
>> Antimetabolites
>> Ionizing irradiation

Pathogenesis unclear
> Wiskott-Aldrich syndrome (thrombocytopenia, eczema, X-linked)
> Protein-calorie malnutrition
> Mucocutaneous candidiasis

T-cell-deficient person, the infection can become fulminant, leading to fatal pneumonia and encephalitis. After the initial infection in the normal host, the virus becomes dormant but persistent in sensory ganglia of the central nervous system (CNS). It can emerge under some circumstances by migrating down the neurons into the skin in regions innervated by the particular ganglion and can cause a painful bullous eruption in that area called *herpes zoster*, or *shingles*. Although localized herpes zoster can occur in normal persons, it arises frequently in T-cell-deficient patients and can disseminate widely over the body. If it affects the trigeminal nerve tract, it can cause a painful ophthalmitis.

Patients with T-cell deficiency can also fall prey to the ravages of a slow virus that causes multifocal leukoencephalopathy, a widespread cerebral degeneration that results in motor and sensory dysfunctions and dementia.

An additional complication of severe T-cell deficiency or malfunction is the syndrome called *graft-versus-host disease* (GVHD). This condition arises when the immunoincompetent host receives an infusion of foreign T cells. Such an infusion occurs if the patient receives a transfusion of whole blood or bone marrow in an attempt to reconstitute a failed bone marrow, or occasionally it occurs in utero when maternal lymphocytes gain access to the circulation of an immunodeficient fetus. The deficiency of host T-cell function results in an inability to reject the foreign T cells. However, the infused T cells have no such problem and, if viable and present in sufficient quantities, recognize the new host as foreign and proceed to proliferate and try to kill host cells and tissues. The skin, gastrointestinal tract, and liver are prime targets of this onslaught, so that patients with graft-versus-host disease can develop jaundice from liver failure, exfoliative dermatitis, and diarrhea with fluid and electrolyte depletion, and even frank sloughing of the gut mucosa. The practical issue here is that patients with suspected T-cell deficiency should either not receive whole blood or leukocyte transfusions, or else the blood products to be used should be treated first with ionizing radiation, which prevents the T cells from proliferating.

The diagnosis of T-cell deficiency or malfunction can be established by means of skin tests with antigens that ordinarily elicit cell-mediated immune reactions. An intradermal injection of these antigens (e.g., killed *Candida albicans*, killed mumps virus, or a protein of the *Streptococcus* called streptokinase) normally causes an accumulation of lymphocytes and macrophages manifest as an area of induration within a few days. For a skin test to give a positive reaction, the subject must have been previously exposed to the antigen as well as have normal T-cell function.

Both T- and B-cell derangements may exist in some lymphoid-deficiency states. Autoimmunity can express itself by the formation of antibodies against blood cells, leading to autoimmune hemolytic anemia, thrombocytopenia, or leukopenia. Autoantibodies against circulating proteins, such as immunoglobulin molecules, leads to immune complex disease in various forms or organ damage, especially in the joints and kidneys.

racic duct and drain lymphocytes. Rarely, an equivalent situation occurs in the clinical setting, if a fistula develops between the bowel and the thoracic duct. This event, leading to the indiscriminate loss of T and B lymphocytes, can follow abdominal trauma or as a consequence of cancer of the large bowel. It is also a feature of a congenital disorder called *intestinal lymphangiectasia*, in which lymphoid channels become massively dilated and allow lymphocytes and proteins to drain into the bowel lumen. In these disorders, patients usually have a very low blood lymphocyte count. The patients also have peripheral edema, because of the concomitant loss of lymphatic protein, which leads eventually to a state of plasma protein deficiency with a resulting loss of intravascular osmotic pressure.

Medication-Associated Immunosuppression

Certain pharmacological agents used in medicine are uniquely or particularly toxic to lymphoid cells. Corticosteroids, which are more toxic to T cells than B cells, kill lymphocytes after binding to cytoplasmic receptors. Azathioprine, 6-mercaptopurine, and methotrexate are antimetabolites that interfere with the synthesis of DNA. Cyclophosphamide is converted by the liver to alkylating agents, compounds that cross-link base pairs in DNA. These and other drugs used in cancer chemotherapy, especially if combined with ionizing radiation therapy delivered to large regions of the body, reduce the number and function of lymphoid cells and lead to varying degrees of immunosuppression.

DISORDERS OF IMPAIRED B- AND T-CELL FUNCTION

Lymphocyte Depletion

One method used in the laboratory for inducing a profound immunodeficiency state in experimental animals is to cannulate the tho-

Severe Combined Immune Deficiency

Severe combined immune deficiency is a congenital disorder of profound lymphoid cell dysfunction. In its most virulent form, the disease becomes manifest very early in life. Infants with this disorder rapidly lose T-cell function and, later, B-cell function. Patients commonly manifest a failure to gain weight and have a persistent diarrhea. The ordinary susceptibility of infants to infection if markedly increased. If an attempt is made to immunize the patient with live virus, such as those used against polio or smallpox, even these attenuated viruses cause devastating and even fatal infections. The chronic infections of these patients render them anemic. If a well-meaning physician gives such a patient a blood transfusion, catastrophic graft-versus-host disease can occur. Unless maintained in a germfree environment indefinitely, affected patients die of infection. The definitive treatment for the disease is reconstitution of the patient's lymphoid system by infusion of normal lymphoid stem cells from the bone marrow of a histocompatible donor. The stem cells recapitulate the process of development ordinarily occurring in utero, interacting with the thymus and marrow of the recipient and establishing a normal lymphoid immune system.

The inheritance of severe combined immune deficiency is of an autosomal recessive pattern in half the patients and X-linked in the rest. In half the patients showing X-linked inheritance, the disorder can be related to an enzyme deficiency resulting in a metabolic derangement affecting purine metabolism. The lymphoid cells, and in most cases other blood cells of the patients, are deficient in either adenosine deaminase, purine nucleoside phosphorylase, of 5'-nucleotidase. The reactions catalyzed by these enzymes are shown in Figure 21-1. Why these enzyme deficiencies are particularly deleterious to lymphoid cells is unclear. T cells appear more susceptible than B cells, possibly explaining why T-cell abnormalities appear first. Infusions of normal erythrocytes can produce temporary improvements in immune function in patients with severe combined im-

Fig. 21-1. Pathways of purine metabolism affected by enzyme deficiencies associated with genetic severe combined immune deficiency syndromes.

mune deficiency because of absence of adenosine deaminase. The adenosine-deaminase-containing erythrocytes trap and soak up the elevated blood adenosine levels in the patients, thereby acting as an adenosine sink. The transient changes in immune function possibly reflect an abrogation of the presumed toxic effects of the high adenosine concentrations of lymphoid cells.

DISORDERS IN WHICH PRINCIPALLY T-CELL FUNCTION IS IMPAIRED

Any infection caused by one organism, especially when severe, can transiently impede the response of T cells to others. This impairment can be diagnosed by the failure of the patient to mount a cell-mediated immune response against an antigen deposited in the skin. This failure to respond is called *anergy*. Inflammatory states not known to be caused by microorganisms also are associated with T-cell hypofunction. These states include sarcoidosis and other idiopathic granulomatous disorders and malignant neoplasms, especially Hodgkin's disease (see Ch. 25). Severe protein and calorie malnutrition seriously impedes T-cell function. Measles, ordinarily a self-limited viral disease of childhood, has devastated populations living in regions of endemic malnutrition.

In a rare congenital disorder called the *DiGeorge syndrome*, the patient is born without a functioning thymus or parathyroid gland, probably because of an in utero viral infection that impedes development of the third branchial pouch area. The absence of a thymus in fetal and neonatal period prevents the normal development of lymphoid cells into T cells; such patients suffer the consequences of absent cell-mediated immunity. Some patients with this disorder have been treated successfully by transplantation of a fetal thymus.

Acquired Immune Deficiency Syndrome

The acquired immune deficiency syndrome (AIDS) has transformed immunodeficiency from an arcane and rare disorder into a major public health concern. AIDS is thought to result from the destruction of the host's helper (CD4) T lymphocytes by a slow-acting retrovirus known currently as *human immunodeficiency virus, type I (HIV-1)*. The virus enters cells that express the plasma membrane molecule designated CD4, these cells being helper lymphocytes and mononuclear phagocytes. The virus, like other retroviruses, uses a reverse transcriptase enzyme to copy its genetic material, which is RNA, into DNA, and this DNA integrates with the host-cell DNA. There it may remain dormant for some time, but eventually it programs synthesis of infective virions, often in response to stimuli that elicit lymphocyte activation. The viruses then slowly but inexorably spread from cell to cell by budding from the surface of the infected cell and entering an uninfected one. They also infect by promoting syncitium formation between infected and uninfected cells. Virus production results in killing of the host T cell. Over a period of months to years an increasing number of CD4-bearing cells, especially lymphocytes, are destroyed. Given the central role of helper T lymphocytes in cell-mediated immunity, this destruction renders the afflicted host bereft of defense against facultative intracellular parasites. Monocytes and macrophages are less susceptible to destruction, but may carry the virus throughout the body and, in response to viral infection, may elaborate toxic products that destroy normal host tissues. The incubation period between initial infection and disease can be extremely long, up to 10 years, and this long interval led to early optimism that some infected persons might not develop AIDS. With time, however, it has become apparent that infection dooms the host to die eventually of opportunistic infections or other complications summarized below.

Clinical Features

The usual manifestation of AIDS is an infection associated with impaired cellular immunity. Oral moniliasis, cutaneous *Herpes zoster* infections, and gastrointestinal *Clostridium difficile* infestations are common, but particularly important and potentially lethal is lung inflammation caused by the protozoal organism *Pneumocystis carinii*. Cough, fever, and shortness of breath characterize this infection, the treatment of which requires antibiotics and may necessitate ventilatory support. The antibiotics, a combination of trimethoprim and a sulfonamide or pentamidine interfere with folic acid metabolism of the infecting pathogen. Unfortunately, these antibiotics frequently elicit allergic reactions in the patients. Mycobacterial infections are often encountered in AIDS. *Mycobacterium tuberculosis* is containable by effective antituberculous antibiotics, but another mycobacterium, *Avium intracellulare*, ordinarily a saprophyte but devastating to the immunosuppressed AIDS sufferer, has no known effective therapy. *Toxoplasma gondii*, another protozoal pathogen, and fungi such as *Cryptococcus neoformans* can invade the central nervous system of AIDS patients.

Another feature of AIDS is the appearance of unusual cancers. The most characteristic is a neoplasm known as *Kaposi's sarcoma*, a proliferation of blood-filled capillaries that has a red-purple appearance. Kaposi's sarcoma was originally described as an indolent neoplasm of elderly Jewish or Mediterranean men and of immunosuppressed Africans, but in AIDS patients it can be a rapidly growing and lethal disease. A second cancer found in AIDS patients is a virulent neoplasm of B lymphocytes, *diffuse histiocytic lymphoma* (Ch. 26). The disorder can arise in any body organ, but characteristically it presents in the central nervous system of AIDS victims. The propensity of AIDs patients to develop certain cancers is also seen in other forms of immunodeficiency and may be a result of abnormal immune surveillance against cancer cells or of injury to normal cells caused by uncontrolled action of the intact elements of the immune system. Indeed, AIDS patients also have unusual autoimmune disorders, such as immune thrombocytopenia, and reactions to medications as mentioned in the previous paragraph.

Cerebral atrophy leading to dementia and wasting are additional attributes of AIDS. Evidence suggests that the HIV-1 virus infests mononuclear phagocytes in the brain, and that somehow this infection results in the destruction of neuronal tissue. Cerebral toxoplasmosis or cerebral lymphoma must be differentiated from this AIDS-associated encephalopathy. The wasting associated with AIDS may arise from chronic infection with various pathogens or from the elaboration of catabolic substances such as interleukin 1 or tumor-necrosis factor by HIV-infected mononuclear phagocytes. AIDS patients often suffer from chronic diarrhea either due to intestinal parasites such as *Clostridium difficile*, *Cryptospiridium*, or shigellosis or possibly to HIV infection of the gastrointestinal epithelial cells, which contributes to inanition.

The varied manifestations of AIDS has caused it to supplant syphilis as "the great imitator." At the present time the "official" diagnosis of AIDS as established by the Center for Disease Control requires that the patient have suffered from a clear-cut AIDS-related infection or from Kaposi's sarcoma or B-cell lymphoma in the setting of immunodeficiency without there being another explanation for the immunodeficiency. A patient with lymphadenopathy, fever, night sweats, and immunodeficiency, especially if a member of a defined AIDS risk population, in the absence of the "official" criteria is said to have *AIDS-related complex* or *ARC*.

Epidemiology

Epidemiologists hypothesize that the virus originated in rural central Africa and was carried by infected patients to cities. From there it was transported by Africans traveling to Europe and to the Caribbean basin by Haitians who had worked in Zaire. The residence of the virus in blood cells meant that transmission followed the exchange of blood and blood products. Accordingly, passage of AIDS has been documented by whole blood transfusion, by the infusion of certain blood fractions used as replacement therapy for inherited disorders of blood coagulation, and by blood mixing between infected mothers and their fetuses. Another important vector for blood-borne AIDS virus transmission has been contaminated needles used by drug abusers. By far the major mechanism of spread of this disease, however, has been venereal, and the establishment of the virus in homosexual men during the mid-1970s resulted in its widespread dissemination in this population. There are some differences in disease manifestations in the different risk groups. Infected neonates develop symptoms more quickly than adults, and Kaposi's sarcoma is more common in male homosexual victims than in other patients. An important point is that abundant evidence indicates that contact with body fluids of AIDS patients other than blood or genital secretions constitutes little risk of infection. The incidence of AIDS has risen exponentially from a handful in 1980 and is estimated to exceed 270,000 by 1991.

Diagnosis

The discovery of HIV-1 as the probable cause of AIDS and ARC has led to immunological tests for diagnosis of infection, as infected persons generate antibodies to components of the virus. Serological tests for serum antibodies to the AIDS virus are routinely done on blood samples donated for transfusion (Ch. 30). When else to perform this test has been a controversial issue. Presently, physicians may request an antibody test on the serum of patients suffering from signs or symptoms of AIDS, provided that the patient gives consent. Members of risk groups may obtain such tests

at so-called alternate test sites, which also provide counseling should the test be positive.

In the most widely used screening test, known as an *enzyme-linked immunosorbant assay (ELISA)*, a series of wells are coated with viral antigen and test serum samples are added to the wells. If a sample contains antibodies to the viral antigen, they will bind to the antigens on the surface of the well. The well is washed and then reacted with an antibody against immunoglobulins. This "secondary" antibody, which is linked to an enzyme that generates a colored product from a chromogenic substrate, remains in the well only if antibodies to the AIDS antigen are present. After washing, the substrate is added and the amount of product is determined colorimetrically. If the serum sample contained antibody, color formation takes place. One problem with ELISA tests, other variations of which are possible, is that a significant number of false-positive results arise. Therefore, a positive test is followed up by another test in which virus is dissolved in the detergent sodium dodecyl sulfate and the viral components are separated on a gel by electrophoresis. The proteins in the gel are transferred to nitrocellulose paper, which is then reacted with antibodies linked to a color-producing enzyme. This analysis is more rigorous, because proteins migrate in the electric field at a rate inversely proportional to molecular weight. Therefore, detection of antibody-reactive polypeptides of appropriate mobilities increases the rigor of the test. Even this so-called Western blotting technique, however, yields false positives. The problem of false positivity and fear of violation of civil liberties have inhibited the application of these tests from routine screening of healthy people. The armed forces, on the other hand, do screen all volunteers for military service in the United States.

The application of antibody screening has drastically diminished the transmission of AIDS by blood transfusion. In addition, heating of blood concentrates and other purification techniques have decreased the risk for patients with coagulation disorders. Unfortunately, there is a "window" of weeks to months between infection and seroconversion, so some infected blood donations may slip through the screening process in this way. It is also likely that the tests also fail in some instances for technical reasons.

Treatment and Prevention

Aside from the management of opportunistic infections and neoplasms, there is presently little in the way of specific treatment. The AIDS epidemic has intensified efforts to develop specific antiviral therapies. One approach has been to design chemicals that inhibit the reverse transcriptase enzyme of the virus. One such agent, a dideoxynucleoside called azidothymidine or zidovudine (abbreviated AZT), has been shown to decrease the incidence of infections in AIDS patients. Regrettably, the effect of the drug, which is quite expensive, is transient, and some patients experience serious side effects, including bone marrow failure. A theoretical avenue made possible by recombinant DNA technology is to prevent virus dissemination within the body by infusion of soluble CD4 molecules, the cell surface receptors to which the HIV binds to enter cells. Such "bogus" receptors cover the determinants on the free virus that promote cell entry and also prevent cell to cell transfer of the virus by syncitium formation. Efforts to produce a vaccine against HIV are hampered by considerable genetic variation between viral isolates. Moreover, because patients with the disorder have demonstrable humoral and cell-mediated immune reactions to the virus, it is unclear whether vaccination will inhibit the disease. In the absence of effective treatment or a vaccine, *the avoidance of infection* remains the most potent weapon against AIDS. Because transmission by casual contact is rare, purging of infected blood from the transfusion pool, prevention of exposure to contaminated hypodermic needles, and use of condoms to minimize exposure to infected genital fluids are highly effective measures.

DISORDERS OF IMPAIRED B-CELL FUNCTION AND OTHER DISEASES AFFECTING ANTIBODIES

A family of congenital and acquired disorders, the antibody deficiency syndromes, encompass a spectrum of abnormalities ranging from the total absence of B cells to B cells variably incapable of making antibodies. With further research, the antibody deficiency syndromes are being found to be increasingly heterogeneous.

Congenital Diseases

Congenital agammaglobulinemia is X-linked in inheritance. The absence of circulating immunoglobulins results from either the absence or nonfunctioning state of B cells. In X-linked hypogammaglobulinemia, B cells make large quantities of IgM, but not IgG or IgA. The dysgammaglobulinemias are diseases in which there is a selective inability of B cells to generate certain subclasses of IgG.

One of every 500 persons lacks IgA, both in blood and in secretions. These IgA-deficient people lack B cells capable of producing IgA. It is not absolutely certain that such patients are unusually susceptible to infections. However, they are at risk for making antibodies to IgA, should they receive blood transfusions from normal persons and may have serious reactions when given multiple transfusions. Another situation associated with IgA deficiency is a rare genetic disease transmitted as an X-linked disorder, called *ataxia telangiectasia*. In this situation, the reason for low IgA levels is not a lack of IgA-producing B cells, but rather an abnormally exuberant breakdown of the protein. Affected patients have tortuous superficial capillaries, the telangiectasias, visible on the skin of the antecubital fossae and on the sclerae of the eye. They have perversions of cerebellar function and mental retardation, responsible for the ataxia. In addition to IgA deficiency, these patients have various subtle anomalies of immune function, including a propensity to develop autoantibodies and malignancies of the lymphoid system.

Another unusual X-linked inherited disease is *Wiskott-Aldrich syndrome.* Wiskott-Aldrich syndrome appears early in life with eczema, thrombocytopenia, and repeated infections. The immunological bases of these abnormalities are not clear. They reflect a subtle derangement of the lymphoid system, preventing the normal elaboration of certain antibodies against polysaccharides, which may account for the susceptibility to infection. Improper regulation of immune responses allow autoantibodies to develop, explaining in part the thrombocytopenia, a consequence of antiplatelet autoantibodies. This disease has been cured by transplantation of bone marrow.

Antibody deficiency can arise as part of the plasma protein losses incurred in intestinal lymphangiectasia.

Acquired Disorders

At any time in life, an unexplained event can prevent previously normal B cells from maturing properly or from secreting immunoglobulins. This acquired antibody deficiency, called *common variable hypogammaglobulinemia,* is the most frequent cause of immunoglobulin deficiency encountered in practice. Some infected patients go on to develop lymphoid neoplasms.

Conversely, impairment of antibody formation occurs frequently in the setting of certain neoplasms of the lymphoid system. Often patients with chronic lymphatic leukemia or with tumors of the thymus produce subnormal quantities of immunoglobulins. Furthermore, patients with these diseases may develop autoantibodies against normal blood cells. The basis of the immunoglobulin deficiency in this setting is in part a crowding out of normal B cells in lymphoid organs by overgrowth of malignant clones. Alternatively, the production of autoantibodies against normal B cells may ac-

count for the immunoglobulin deficiency. Finally, imbalances in suppressor and helper subsets of T cells caused by the neoplastic process may impair antibody formation.

Another neoplasm associated with impaired antibody production is multiple myeloma, a clonal proliferation of plasma cells described in Chapter 27. This tumor, unlike chronic lymphatic leukemia or most of the lymphoid malignancies, does not primarily involve the lymph nodes or blood, but rather the bone marrow, and is associated with the formation of large amounts of useless immunoglobulins. It is possible that the clonal proliferation of malignant B cells crowds out normal B cells. However, the abnormal immunoglobulins have been shown to stimulate mononuclear phagocytes to suppress immunoglobulin synthesis by normal B lymphocytes.

If a loss of immunoglobulins exceeds production, a state of hypogammaglobulinemia can result. In general, a protein-losing state such as the nephrotic syndrome, wherein plasma protein pours into the urine, or in protein-losing enteropathy, in which the source of plasma protein loss is the gastrointestinal tract, the immunoglobulin deficiency can be sufficiently profound to cause recurrent infections.

An immunodeficiency state of particular importance to the hematologist is a consequence of multiple insults to the immune system affecting both phagocytes and lymphoid cells, that can result from aggressive treatment of a lymphoid neoplasm, Hodgkin's disease. It is often necessary to remove the spleen of patients with Hodgkin's disease for diagnostic purposes. In cases of extensive disease, treatment may require considerable application of ionizing radiation to lymphoid tissue and admixture of systemic chemotherapy that is toxic to lymphoid cells. This therapeutic tour de force, which can actually be curative against the malignancy, wreaks sufficient havoc to the antibody-forming mechanism to prevent the maintenance of normal levels of immunoglobulins against high-grade encapsulated pathogens. The combination of antibody deficiency and the absence of a spleen renders the patient extraordinarily susceptible to infections with encapsulated organisms, such as the *Pneumococcus, Haemophilus influenzae*, or *Streptococcus*, and these infections can be overwhelming and fatal.

TREATMENT OF IMMUNODEFICIENCY DISORDERS AFFECTING ANTIBODIES

Except in those states in which protein losses or catabolism are excessive, replacement therapy with human immunoglobulin preparations is possible. The half time for the clearance of normal immunoglobulin is about 30 days, so that monthly administrations of immunoglobulin are an acceptable treatment of antibody deficiency syndromes. The immunoglobulins are obtained from relatively easy fractionation procedures done on plasma acquired from blood donors. The product, consisting primarily of IgG, is usually called γ-globulin. The major drawbacks of immunoglobulin administration are that immunoglobulin preparations must usually be given by intramuscular injections. The reason for this route of administration is that most commercial immunoglobulin preparations contain aggregates of IgG that can activate complement and produce anaphylactic reactions, if given intravenously. Another problem is that immunodeficient patients often have a propensity to generate autoantibodies and will produce antibodies against the injected immunoglobulin, resulting in its rapid clearance. Therefore, the plasma immunoglobulin levels of patients receiving γ-globulin should be monitored periodically. The use of immunoglobulin in patients with high concentrations of paraproteins but low normal immunoglobulins presents a special problem. The high endogenous immunoglobulin levels cause all immunoglobulins —endogenous or administered—to be catabolized rapidly. Therefore, more frequent immunoglobulin administration is required in this setting, and such treatment may not be practical.

AUTOIMMUNITY

During fetal life, the developing immune system becomes programmed not to react to host antigens. Accordingly, exposure of the fetus even to foreign matter will cause it to fail to react to later contact with that antigen, a state defined as *tolerance*. Instead of a sustained clonal proliferation of specific B or T cells in response to antigens, the induction of tolerance in utero or postnatally by a complex set of factors in which the timing and dose of antigen; failure of cell–cell interaction; pathological cell–cell interaction, such as excessive T-cell suppression; or blockade of crucial receptors by persistent or excessive antigen or by immune complexes result instead in an abortion or depletion of such clones.

Tolerance to autologous tissues is not absolute, however, in that immune responses to self occur. The process that turns off the immune response when the offending antigen is no longer present, for example, is, in a sense an example of *autoimmunity*. The very novelty of the variable portion of antibody molecules or T-cell antigen receptors generated by the recombination of germ-line genes to react with specific antigens causes the immune system to see them as "foreign." Hence, the system produces an immune response to the immune response. The resulting cascade of "antibodies against antibodies" or of cell-mediated immunity against activated T cells is known as an *idiotype network*, from the Greek *idios* meaning "unique." This physiological *idiotype response* can become pathological when the antibody-antibody complexes elicit inflammatory responses. Immune complexes of this sort underlie the pathogenesis of disorders such as cryoglobulinemia and certain kinds of vasculitis (see also Ch. 17).

Another cause of autoimmune disease is when the immune response to infectious agents, especially viruses, elicits immunological reactions to host tissues. This process may be facilitated by the binding of viruses to human lymphocyte antigens (HLA) on cell surfaces, in which case the recognition of the foreign pathogen overlaps self-configurations on the HLA molecules. The connection between the HLA system and autoimmunity is strengthened by the epidemiological association between certain host histocompatibility genotypes and autoimmune disorders. The role of HLA type may be direct as regards the binding of antigens to cell surfaces or indirect, having to do with the innate reactivity of the immune system to all antigens. Other genetic factors clearly are involved in autoimmunity, however, in that certain families express large numbers of autoantibodies that are not definitely associated with histocompatibility type. Additional evidence for an infectious provocation of autoimmunity is the association of autoimmunity with immunodeficiency states—in which the persistence of pathogens may be greater in the host—and its expression following infections, especially in children. Autoimmunity may be highly tissue specific, as, for example, autoimmune thyroiditis, or may be quite generalized, as in systemic lupus erythematosus.

Autoimmunity plays a pathogenetic role in many hematological diseases. Particularly important examples are the immune-mediated cytopenias (autoimmune hemolytic anemia, autoimmune thrombocytopenia, autoimmune neutropenia) and pernicious anemia (autoantibodies to parietal cells or to intrinsic factor).

SUGGESTED READINGS

Burdette, S., & Schwartz, R.S. (1987) Idiotypes and idiotypic networks. N Engl. J. Med. *317*: 219–224.

Edelman, A.S., & Zolla-Pazner, S. (1989) AIDS: a syndrome of immune dysregulation, dysfunction, and deficiency. FASEB J. *3*:22–30.

Fauci, A.S. (1988) The human immunodeficiency virus: Infectivity and mechanisms of pathogenesis. Science *239*:617–622.

1987 Revision of case definition for AIDS for surveillance purposes (1987) MMWR *36*:4S.

Rosen, F.S., Cooper, M.D., & Wedgewood, R.J.P. (1984) The primary immunodeficiencies. N Engl. J. Med. *311*:235–242; 300–309.

Seligman, M. Hitzig, W.H., Eds. (1980) Primary Immunodeficiencies. Elsevier–North–Holland Biomedical Press, New York.

Shilts, R. (1987) *And the Band Played On. Politics, People and the AIDS Epidemic.* St. Martin's Press, New York.

WHO Scientific Group on Immunodeficiency (1979) Immunodeficiency. Clin. Immunol. Immunopathol. *13*:296–359.

Lymphoid Neoplasms: Overview

Lymphoid neoplasms are composed of transformed lymphoid cells that exhibit uncontrolled growth and invasion. Compared with the classification for neoplasms of phagocytic cells, that for lymphoid neoplasms is much more complex. This complexity arises from the great biological diversity of lymphoid cells that is not readily apparent from their morphology. The current understanding of the biology of lymphoid cells is becoming increasingly helpful in the diagnosis and treatment of lymphoid neoplasms. However, the classification of lymphoid neoplasms is still often based on more archaic anatomical and histological considerations.

The cause of leukocyte neoplasia is unknown. Mutations in the genetic material of susceptible lymphoid cells may lead to the proliferation of malignant clones. As in other forms of neoplasia, mutagenic agents such as ionizing radiation, chemicals, and viruses are possible causes of this hypothetical genetic change, although cells of the lymphoid system appear to be less susceptible to the carcinogenic influences of ionizing radiation than those of the phagocyte system. On the other hand, there is more evidence linking viruses with lymphoid neoplasia in animals and in humans. Epstein-Barr virus (EBV) infection causes the atypical lymphocytes of infectious mononucleosis and is associated with some cases of the neoplastic cells of one specific human lymphoid tumor (Burkitt's lymphoma). Recent work has provided strong evidence that a retrovirus is the cause of one variant of a human T-cell leukemia that is endemic in southern Japan and in the Caribbean basin. Nevertheless, a causal relationship between viruses and most lymphoid neoplasms in humans is far from established.

Another condition associated with the development of lymphoid neoplasia, usually of one particular type, is immunodeficiency, for example, the frequent occurrence of lymphoid neoplasms in patients with the congenital disorder *telangiectasia*. Occasionally, congenital or acquired antibody deficiency states precede the development of this lymphoid neoplasm. Patients with AIDS or receiving immunosuppressive treatment to prevent the rejection of engrafted organs, usually the kidney, have been observed to have a relatively high incidence of this type of lymphoid neoplasms. Because immunodeficiency and immunosuppression dispose to recurrent or chronic infections, one may speculate that it is the infection rather than the immunodeficiency per se that is most closely related to the development of the lymphoid malignancy. For example, there is an epidemiological relationship between chronic malarial infestation in the development of Burkitt's lymphoma. The injection of pristane into the peritoneal cavity of a certain strain of mice causes a large proportion of these mice to develop a malignant neoplasm of B cells. However, the carcinogenic effect of the oil is limited to that particular genetic strain. Therefore, the effect of inflammation or infection in producing lymphoid malignancy is dependent on a particular feature of the host that is genetically programmed, possibly a subtle form of immunodeficiency or an imbalance in the numbers or functions of lymphoid cells.

The evidence for such a relationship between imbalances in the immune system and the development of lymphoid neoplasms is the epidemiological association between certain autoimmune disorders and lymphoid neoplasms. It has been reported that patients with lymphoid malignancies have increased numbers of cases of autoimmune disorders, such as systemic lupus erythematosus (SLE), in their blood relations. Furthermore, certain lymphoid neoplasms develop in patients with some diseases of an autoimmune type. One example is Sjögren's syndrome, which is characterized by salivary and lacrimal gland impairment, caused by the invasion of these glands by lymphocytes. Another example is celiac disease, in which there is a degeneration of the epithelial lining of the small intestine and lymphoid cell infiltrates in the intestinal submucosa.

As described in Chapter 19, a unifying principle behind the multiple routes to neoplasia is the abnormal expression of cellular oncogenes or the incorporation of viral oncogenes into mammalian cells. Oncogenes have been identified in a variety of animal and human lymphoid neoplasms, and some possible mechanisms of their expression have been identified. Most interestingly, some of the cellular oncogenes of lymphoid cells reside in regions of the genome that undergo rearrangement in the course of normal lymphoid cell maturation, suggesting how chronic immune stimulation might predispose to lymphoid neoplasia.

In certain disorders characterized by the proliferation and invasion of tissues by lymphoid cells, it has not been possible to identify the existence of a malignant clone. Hodgkin's disease, described in Chapter 25, is one example. Another is the unusual situation described in

Chapter 20, in which patients with infectious mononucleosis die from an apparently malignant proliferation of lymphoid cells. Still another example is angioimmunoblastic adenopathy, a disorder characterized by lymphadenopathy. Patients have a systemic disease characterized by manifestations of inflammation, including polymorphonuclear leukocytosis, monocytosis, elevation in the concentration of the plasma acute-phase reactants, and immunoglobulins, with resulting rouleau formation and high erythrocyte sedimentation rates. Many of these patients have associated autoimmune phenomena, such as rheumatoid arthritis, immune complex inflammatory disease, or autoimmune blood cell destruction. The lymph node enlargement is characteristic in that the number of cells ordinarily found in lymph nodes increases, accompanied by a proliferation of capillaries that branch at perpendicular angles. This histology is what gives this disease the name *angioimmunoblastic adenopathy*. In some cases, angioimmunoblastic adenopathy occurs in patients who have been receiving various types of medication, suggesting a reactive response. The natural history of angioimmunoblastic adenopathy is variable. Some patients undergo spontaneous remissions, whereas others succumb to progressive debilitation, eventually leading to death. Destructive organ infiltration by the lymphoid process may be a feature in this relentless course. There is no evidence that treatment affects the outcome of angioimmunoblastic adenopathy.

ANATOMY

If the expression of the malignant lymphoid proliferation takes place predominantly in the bone marrow and peripheral blood, the disorder is defined as a lymphatic leukemia. *Acute lymphatic leukemia (ALL)* describes an aggressive and rapidly destructive process; *chronic lymphatic leukemia (CLL)* is a relatively indolent disorder.

The term *lymphoma* encompasses a family of diseases in which the primary expression of the malignant process is in the tissues, usually in the lymph nodes, spleen, and other lymphoid organs, but occasionally in extralymphatic tissue sites. For lymphomas, there is a staging system for analyzing the extent of involvement of the body by the malignant process (Table 22-1). This staging system is particularly useful in the evaluation of patients with Hodgkin's disease. Stage I refers to involvement of a single region of lymph nodes, for example, a group of cervical lymph nodes, the left or right axillary lymph nodes, or the left or right inguinal lymph nodes. Stage II defines involvement of two or more regions of lymph nodes, but restricts the involvement to one or the other side of the diaphragm. For example, a stage II lymphoma might involve the right or left axillary and right or left cervical lymph nodes on one side of the body, or mediastinal and cervical lymph nodes. Stage III lymphoma is present when two or more lymph node-bearing regions are involved on both sides of the diaphragm. Involvement of para-aortic and mediastinal lymph nodes would be an example of a stage III lesion. For stages I through III, the subscript S designates that the spleen is involved. The subscript E denotes extension of the disease from the lymph node into contiguous tissues. For example, involvement of the parenchyma of the lung by direct extension of disease arising in mediastinal lymph nodes with involvement of cervical lymph nodes would represent stage II$_E$. Disease encompassing the mediastinum, the para-aortic region, and the spleen would be classified as Stage III$_S$. Stage IV represents disseminated lymphoma, possibly involving the liver, the bone marrow, or other organs.

The initial evaluation of the extent of lymphoma is done by means of physical examination of the patient and by radiographic examinations routinely used in clinical practice. This approach is called *clinical staging*. To evaluate the extent of disease in the abdomen, it is sometimes necessary and desirable to subject the patient to an exploratory laparotomy or to use an endoscopic procedure called a *laparoscopy*, in which an endoscope is inserted into the peritoneal cavity. This more invasive approach is called *pathological staging*. The usefulness of this staging classification and the necessity for precise evaluation of the extent of disease depend on the type of lymphoma and the age and condition of the patient.

Lymphomas are often first recognized by the painless enlargement of one or more of the peripheral lymph nodes. Alternatively, the enlargement of internal lymph nodes or growth of lymphoma in an extralymphatic location such as the intestine, bone, or nasopharynx causes symptoms by encroaching on internal organs. Compression of the tracheobronchial tree by lymphoma can produce respiratory difficulties, such as cough, wheezing, or dyspnea. More widespread growth of the neoplasm can obstruct lymphatic drainage in the chest, resulting in pleural effusions with dyspnea. The narrowing of the superior vena cava or other major veins returning to the heart can lead to superior vena cava syndrome. In this condition there is flushing and edema of the face. Because of the generalized distribution of lymphoid tissue in the body, practically any organ system can become impaired should lymphoma arise in or near it.

Table 22-1. Staging: Extent of Disease[a]

Stage	Definition
I	Involvement of a single lymph node region
II	Involvement of two or more lymph node regions on the same side of the diaphragm (II), which may be accompanied by localized involvement of an extralymphatic organ or site (II$_E$)
III	Involvement of lymph node regions on both sides of the diaphragm (III), which may also be accompanied by involvement of the spleen (III$_S$) or by localized involvement of an extralymphatic organ or site (III$_E$)
IV	Diffuse or disseminated involvement of one or more extralymphatic organs or tissues, with or without associated lymph node involvement

[a] The presence or absence of fever, night sweats, and/or unexplained loss of 10 percent or more of body weight in the preceding 6 months is denoted by the suffix letters B and A, respectively.

HISTOLOGY

Hematologists and pathologists have attempted to classify lymphoid neoplasms according to the histological appearance of cells obtained from the blood, bone marrow, or lymphoid organs. In this pursuit, cell size, cell-staining characteristics, nuclear shape, and the appearance of cells forming nodules that resemble lymphoid follicles or diffuse sheets have all been taken into account. The morphology of lymphoid neoplasms has correlated somewhat with their biological behavior, thereby providing a relatively useful classification for the clinician. The microscopic appearance of lymphoid neoplasms is described in the chapters that follow.

IMMUNOBIOLOGY

In recent years, it has become possible to supplement the histological analysis of lymphoid neoplasms with the type of marker analysis that defines the lineage and stage of maturation of lymphoid cells (Fig. 22-1). This approach has permitted definition of the likely cell of origin of many lymphoid neoplasms, and in some cases it has sorted out malignancies that appeared very similar on histological examination but that were very different in clinical behavior. Unfortunately, some lymphoid neoplasms still escape definition by currently available techniques.

The development of monoclonal antibodies reacting with cell surface antigens characteristic for B cells and T cells for particular stages of maturation of lymphoid cells and in some cases indicative of clonality of the cells has been an important step in advancing the classification of lymphoid neoplasms (see Ch. 20). It is commonplace, therefore, for samples of peripheral white blood cells or of gently dispersed lymph nodes or tumor masses to be reacted with a panel of monoclonal antibodies such as the ones listed in Table 20-1 and then analyzed by immunofluorescence microscopy or by flow cytometry in a fluorescence-activated cell sorter. The latter technique has the advantage of automation and the ability through application of different fluorophores and wavelengths to detect simultaneously the reactivity of several different antibodies. It can also determine cell size by the extent to which the cell scatters incident light and document nuclear ploidy from reactivity of the cells with fluorescent DNA-binding dyes. The application of a panel of varying specificity of antibodies helps add confidence to straightforward diagnostic cases and may help clarify more difficult instances. This approach was initially especially useful for the diagnosis and classification of B-cell neoplasms, as these are the most frequent lymphoid malignancies. The ability, for example, to detect surface expression of immunoglobulins of one or another (lambda or kappa) light chain class by monoclonal antibody reactivity is a simple diagnostic test for clonality of a B-cell population. Although individual B lymphocytes produce either lambda or kappa light chains, a mixture of normal B lymphocytes expresses both types of light chain, whereas a clone of B cells will show one or the other exclusively. The monoclonal antibodies reactive with T cells are useful for identifying a neoplasm as being of T-cell origin as well as helping to pinpoint its maturational stage. They do not, however, prove clonality of the T-cell proliferation.

A refinement in the classification of B-cell neoplasms and a handle on the clonality of T-cell tumors has arisen from molecular genetics, specifically from the ability to detect clonal populations of cells with rearranged genes. As explained in Chapter 20, B and T cells establish a repertoire of immunoglobulins and T-cell antigen receptors, respectively, by putting mRNA-translating parts of these molecules together in different combinations. Because each cell expresses a particular rearranged gene, samples of normal B cells and T cells represent populations with multiple gene rearrangements. A single clone of B cells, however, demonstrates only a unique pattern of immunoglobulin gene rearrangements, as

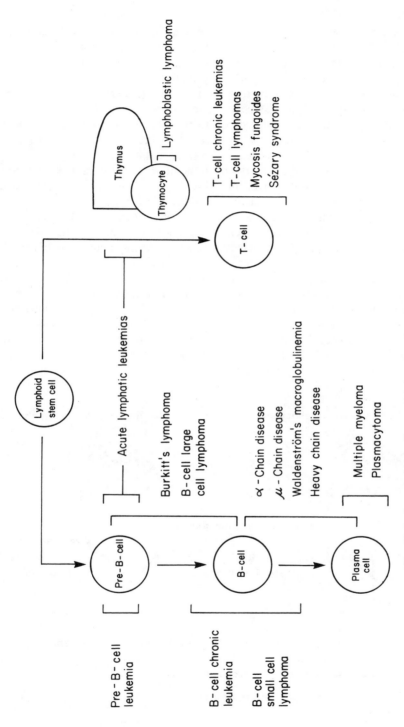

Fig. 22-1. Lymphoid neoplasms: Origins according to immunological differentiation.

detected by the technique known as *Southern blotting* (named for its originator, E. M. Southern) (Fig. 22-2).

DNA is isolated from the cells to be tested and partially digested into fragments by bacterial *restriction enzymes* that recognize particular nucleotide base sequences. The fragments are then subjected to electrophoresis through a porous gel that separates them according to length, the shorter segments moving faster in the electrical field. The gel is then overlaid with nitrocellulose paper, and fluid convection is used to transfer the DNA fragments in the gel onto the filter to which they adhere in a position replicating where they traveled in the gel. Radioactively labeled genomic or cDNA probes encoding a region of the gene of interest, for example, the J region of the T-cell receptor DNA or the J region of the immunoglobulin gene, bind to the particular DNA fragments on the paper that have the appropriate complementary sequences. The paper is apposed to an x-ray film, and the location of these complexes on the paper is then detected by radioautography. In most lymphoid cell preparations the probes will react slightly with fragments containing unrearranged germ-line genes. The variation in restriction enzyme targets in normal cell populations presents so many different-sized reactive fragments that the probes do not bind with sufficient density to be detected. In clonal cell populations, on the other hand, the probe recognizes the fragment containing the single rearranged sequence in addition to the germ-line sequence-containing fragment, and an additional band appears on the autoradiogram.

Chapter 19 explained how clonal chromosomal rearrangements are the rule in the malignancies affecting phagocytic lineage cells. This is also the case for lymphoid neoplasms. In these disorders, the chromosomal rearrangements frequently involve segments including the loci encoding immunoglobulin heavy or light chains or the subunits of the T-cell receptor. As in the case of the phagocytic cell neoplasms, the rearrangements may relocate these segments into conjunction with onco-

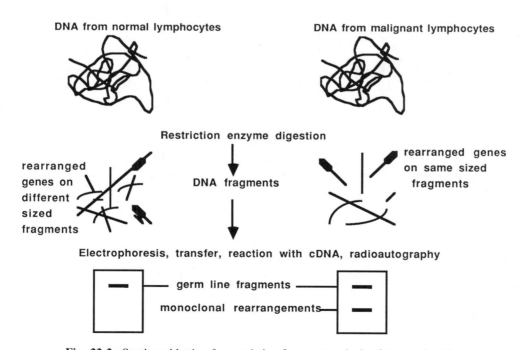

Fig. 22-2. Southern blotting for restriction fragment analysis of tumor clonality.

genes such as *c-myc*, and overproduction of the *c-myc* gene product accompanies the malignant transformation. In summary, then, surface antigens, gene rearrangements, and chromosomal aberrations complement histological, anatomical, and clinical classification of the lymphoid malignancies.

Why is the classification of lymphoid neoplasms so important? Lymphoid neoplasms are a heterogeneous group of diseases having variable rates of progression. The diseases vary in responsiveness to different treatments. Some are more responsive than others, and a few have a potential for cure. Therefore, knowledge of when to treat a given disease with what modalities, and how vigorously, is of profound practical importance. We often lack the information on which to make decisions pertinent to these points. Therefore it is hoped that a more precise classification of lymphoid neoplasms will relieve the frustrations that beset our current abilities to predict the natural history of lymphoid tumors and to treat them.

Meantime it is necessary to use anatomical, histological, and immunological approaches. Consult Figure 22-1 when reading Chapters 24 through 27, which describe the various lymphoid neoplasms.

SUGGESTED READINGS

DeVita, V.T., Jr., Jaffe, E.S., & Hellman, S. (1985) Hodgkin's disease and the non-Hodgkin's lymphomas. p. 1623. In *Cancer, Principles and Practice of Oncology*, 2nd Ed. JB Lippincott, Philadelphia.

Foon, K.A., & Todd, R.F. III (1986) Immunologic classification of leukemia and lymphoma. Blood 68:1.

Showe, L.C., & Croce, C.M. (1987) The role of chromosomal translocations in B- and T-cell neoplasia. Ann Rev Immunol 5:253.

Waldmann, T., Korsmeyer, S.J., & Bakhshi, A. (1985) Molecular genetic analysis of human lymphoid neoplasma. Ann Intern Med *102*:497.

Acute Lymphatic Leukemia

GENERAL FEATURES

Acute lymphatic leukemia is the expansion of a clone of malignant cells, which if left untreated, rapidly leads to death. Acute lymphocytic leukemia initially arises in the bone marrow, but it progresses to involve the blood and peripheral tissues. The morphology of the bone marrow in acute lymphatic leukemia is characterized by a monotonous infiltrate of lymphoid cells called *lymphoblasts*. Like typical lymphocytes, the lymphoid blasts in acute lymphatic leukemia tend to have a high nuclear: cytoplasm ratio, and the nuclei have coarse chromatin and indistinct nucleoli. The cells may vary in size from that of typical lymphocytes to cells three to four times that volume. The cytoplasm ordinarily has no granules (Fig. 23-1).

In nearly all cases of acute lymphatic leukemia, the cells contain the thymocyte enzyme terminal deoxyribonucleotide transferase (Tdt) and, to a variable extent, express other markers indicating different expressions of lymphoid differentiation. Two-thirds of affected patients have cells bearing an antigen on the outer surface of the membrane that is unique to lymphoid cells of this disease. This antigen is called the *common acute lymphocytic leukemia antigen* (or *CALLA*). Lymphoid cells bearing this antigen tend to be null cells, that is, they have no surface markers for T cells or for B cells. Nevertheless, despite lacking immunological markers of B cells and expressing a thymocyte enzyme, the malignant cells of "common" acute lymphatic leukemia show immunoglobulin gene rearrangements characteristic of B cells at a very early (pre-B) stage of development.

In about 15 percent of cases of acute lymphatic leukemia, the lymphoid blasts bear surface markers characteristic of T cells. In a very few cases, the cells contain cytoplasmic immunoglobulin, a feature of more mature pre-B cells than the phenotype in "common" acute lymphatic leukemia. Also, in a small number of cases, the lymphoid blasts may also have surface immunoglobulin and complement receptors, surface markers distinct for B cells. In acute lymphocytic leukemia of B-cell type, the neoplastic cells have a characteristic chromosomal abnormality in which there is a translocation of genetic material between chromosomes 8 and 14. The division of cases of acute lymphatic leukemia into immunobiological categories has implications for prognosis of the disease and its responses to treatment. The "common" pre-B cell variety of the disease has the best prognosis, the more mature pre-B cell variety has the worst prognosis, and the T-cell variety has an intermediate prognosis.

Acute lymphatic leukemia is the principal neoplasm of children aged 2 to 8. There is a distinct biological difference between child-

Fig. 23-1. Microscopic appearance of acute lymphatic leukemia cells.

acute lymphatic leukemia in which the symptoms in the bones preceded the development of overt bone marrow failure manifested by reduction in the peripheral blood counts. Invasion of other organs by the leukemic process generally occurs first in organs contiguous with the blood and lymphatic system, the lymph nodes, spleen, and liver. However, any tissues are susceptible to invasion, including the central nervous system. In cases of acute lymphatic leukemia in which the blast cells bear T-cell markers, masses of leukemic infiltration are often observed in the mediastinum. This phenomenon possibly represents a homing propensity by the malignant T cells toward the thymus gland.

TREATMENT OF ACUTE LYMPHOCYTIC LEUKEMIA

Chemotherapy is the primary treatment for this disease. Therapy is directed toward complete eradication of the leukemic cells, which is attempted by means of cytotoxic drugs. The principles of induction of a remission in addition to the maintenance of that remission are similar to treatment described for acute non-lymphocytic leukemia (Ch. 19). In practice, however, the approach to therapy and the expected results, especially in childhood acute lymphocytic leukemia, differ somewhat from the approach to acute nonlymphocytic leukemia.

The leukemic blast cells of most cases of acute lymphatic leukemia are very susceptible to killing by cytotoxic drugs, especially by corticosteroids, reflecting the sensitivity of lymphoid cells to this agent. Indeed, a combination of the corticosteroid prednisone and the drug vincristine, which prevents the assembly of microtubules, is sufficient to induce a complete remission in most cases of acute lymphatic leukemia. As neither of these drugs is particularly toxic to other bone marrow cells, it is theoretically possible to induce a remission in acute lymphatic leukemia without causing the patient to endure the dangerous 3-week or so period of complete bone marrow failure

hood and adult lymphatic leukemia with respect to the outcome of treatment. The prognosis for children is much better than for adults.

EFFECTS OF ACUTE LYMPHATIC LEUKEMIA ON THE HOST

As in acute nonlymphocytic leukemia, the initial and most important manifestation of acute lymphatic leukemia is bone marrow failure. Suppression of normal bone marrow elements leads to anemia, thrombocytopenia, and neutropenia, which predispose to weakness and pallor, bleeding, and serious bacterial infections, respectively. Occasionally the bone marrow infiltration with the neoplasm can cause thinning of the bones and bone pain. The latter symptom has sometimes resulted in an incorrect diagnosis of arthritis in cases of that patients with acute nonlymphocytic leukemia must undergo during remission induction. Although mature pre-B cell markers, high leukemic blast concentration in the blood, infiltration of organs with blasts, and male sex suggest a worse prognosis, it is not currently possible to identify with certainty which patients will respond satisfactorily to a mild regimen. It is therefore necessary to subject nearly all patients to more vigorous treatment, and therefore to additional side effects.

As is the case with acute nonlymphocytic leukemias, the evolution of therapy of acute lymphatic leukemia involves tests of different regimens for *induction* of a remission, *consolidation* of the remission, *maintenance* therapy, and determination of the optimal *duration* of treatment. Supportive care for complications of the disease and of the treatment plays an important role in the overall management of the patient.

In the development of treatment of children with acute lymphatic leukemia, the incidence of complete remissions became sufficiently frequent and duration sufficiently long that it was possible to discern that some relapses resulted from the persistence of leukemic cells in certain sanctuaries, such as the central nervous system. It was found that treatment of the brain and spinal cord either with radiation alone or in combination with chemotherapy delivered to the cerebrospinal fluid by the administration of drugs through a needle into the lumbar cistern could prevent such relapses in most cases. The use of maintenance therapy with drugs other than those employed to induce remissions further reduced the incidence of relapse. This approach to treatment permitted well over 50 percent of children with acute lymphatic leukemia to enjoy sufficiently long, complete remissions as to use the term "cure." Considering that only 20 years ago a diagnosis of acute lymphatic leukemia in children was virtually a death sentence, the degree of success in treatment of acute lymphatic leukemia was spectacular. However, a significant fraction of children and nearly all adults with acute lymphatic leukemia still suffer relapse when treated with the regimens found so successful in other children. This problem has led hematologists to apply more aggressive chemotherapy regimens against acute lymphatic leukemia, more akin to those used in acute nonlymphocytic leukemia. The problem with this approach is that the short-term bone marrow and long-term immunosuppressive effects of the chemotherapy can erode some of the possible beneficial effects of increased tumoricidal potentials of more drugs. It is hoped that a more precise cytological classification of acute lymphatic leukemia will succeed in sorting out those patients who require more aggressive treatment from those who do not. At present, it is only possible to say that the neoplasms bearing T-cell, B-cell, or pre-B-cell characteristics are clearly less favorable than the common null cell types of acute lymphatic leukemia.

Adults with acute lymphatic leukemia do not fare as well as most children between the ages of 2 and 8. Although a high proportion of complete remission can be achieved in adults with acute lymphatic leukemia, the inevitability of eventual relapse is high, with only a small fraction of patients enjoying complete remissions that last more than a couple of years. Therefore, bone marrow transplantation is being assessed as therapy for young adult patients with acute lymphatic leukemia following the induction of a complete remission. The question as to why the "childhood" variant of acute lymphatic leukemia is so much more amenable to cure by chemotherapy is of great practical importance to hematologists.

SUGGESTED READINGS

Rivera, G.K., & Mauer, A.M. (1987) Controversies in the management of childhood acute lymphoblastic leukemia: Treatment intensification, CNS leukemia, and prognostic factors. Semin Hematol *24*:12.

Sallan, S.E., & Weinstein, H.J. (1987) Childhood acute leukemia. p. 1028. In Hematology of Infancy and Childhood. Nathan, D.G., Oski, F., Eds. WB Saunders, Philadelphia.

The Chronic
Lymphatic Leukemias

The chronic lymphatic leukemias are a family of neoplasms characterized by the proliferation of a clone of lymphoid cells that circulates in the blood and infiltrates the bone marrow and, to a variable extent, other tissues. In contrast to what occurs in acute lymphatic leukemia, the deleterious effects of malignancy on the organism develop slowly or not at all.

GENERAL FEATURES

The diagnosis of *chronic lymphatic leukemia* is very likely when the blood of an adult, usually a man, contains more than 15,000 lymphocytes/µl, or when more than 40 percent of the nucleated cells in the bone marrow are lymphocytes. These lymphocytes may be typical or atypical, but ordinarily they are not as bizarre as the blasts seen in acute lymphatic leukemia. The lymphocyte count in the blood may be extremely high, exceeding 100,000 cells/µl.

Most cases of chronic lymphatic leukemia represent clonal proliferations of relatively mature-looking B cells. Like normal B cells, the malignant cells have complement receptors and immunoglobulins on the external surfaces of their plasma membranes. The clonal nature of the proliferation can be demonstrated by measurement of glucose 6-phosphate dehydrogenase isoenzymes, as described for acute non-

lymphocytic leukemia (Ch. 19), and by the fact that the surface immunoglobulin on the malignant B cells is of only one light chain class, for example, ϰ or λ. The cells ordinarily have surface immunoglobulins with heavy chains of both the µ and δ classes, that is, the surface immunoglobulins are of the IgM and IgD classes, as is the case for normal B cells. The leukemic B lymphocytes differ quantitatively from normal B cells in that the former express less immunoglobulin on their membranes than the latter.

As expected for a clonally expanded B-cell line, leukemic cells from patients with B-cell chronic lymphatic leukemia have clonally rearranged immunoglobulin heavy or light chain genes. In addition, the B cell chronic lymphatic leukemia cells may have cytogenetic abnormalities, the most frequent finding being trisomy 12. Serological evidence of previous exposure to the human leukemogenic retrovirus HTLV-I was unexpectedly high in patients with chronic lymphatic leukemia in an area endemic for the virus. Additional laboratory studies revealed that the leukemic cells produced antibodies reacting with viral envelope glycoproteins. This observation suggested that this virus may have a cofactor role in the causation of chronic lymphatic leukemia.

The leukemic B cells also perform less well than normal cells in tests of B-cell function such as proliferation in response to mitogens or in induction of immunoglobulin synthesis. B-cell chronic lymphatic leukemia cells express, in addition to surface immunoglobulin molecules, receptors for IgG (Fc receptors), C3 receptors, the histocompatibility antigen HLA-DR (Ia), a variety of B-cell antigens (CD19, CD20, CD21), and, curiously, a T-cell antigen (CD5). B-cell chronic lymphatic leukemia cells may also express chromosomal abnormalities of which trisomy 12 is the most common. The low proliferative activity of the leukemic B cell in this disease makes detection of chromosomal aberration difficult.

In a minority of cases of chronic lymphatic leukemia, the lymphoid cells in the blood have T-cell markers, and these may exhibit suppressor or helper functions. T-cell chronic lymphatic leukemia cells have clonally rearranged T-cell receptor genes and may also have cytogenetic abnormalities, the most usual being an inversion of chromosome 14, inv(14) (q11q13).

EFFECTS OF CHRONIC LYMPHATIC LEUKEMIA ON THE PATIENT

Chronic lymphatic leukemia is often a benign disease that tends to affect elderly men, who may die of other causes and infrequently need specific treatment for the disorder. However, a number of possible manifestations of the disease can affect the well-being of the patient.

Organ Infiltration

The lymph nodes and the spleen are most susceptible to enlargement because of infiltration by chronic lymphatic leukemia cells. When the lymph nodes, bone marrow, and spleen become intensely infiltrated, chronic lymphatic leukemia may become relatively indistinguishable from the disorder called *diffuse well-differentiated lymphocytic lymphoma*, in that the architecture of these organs is replaced with sheets of small lymphocytes. However, the concentration of surface immunoglobulin is higher in lymphocytes of patients with diffuse well-differentiated lymphoma than in the cells of patients with chronic lymphatic leukemia. Late in the evolution of chronic lymphatic leukemia or in atypical cases or variants of chronic lymphatic leukemia, infiltrations of other organs, including the lung, kidneys, and skin, can occur. The enlargement of lymph nodes and the spleen can become sufficient to cause pain or compromised function of contiguous organs, and proliferation of leukemic cells in the bone marrow can result in anemia or thrombocytopenia.

Prolymphocytic leukemia is a variant of B-cell chronic lymphatic leukemia. The cells are larger and more immature in appearance than the usual B-cell chronic lymphatic leukemia cells and have prominent nucleoli. The cells tend to have more surface immunoglobulin and less T1 antigen. The morphology and surface phenotype of prolymphocytic leukemia is associated with higher leukemic cell counts and more pronounced splenomegaly. Prolymphocytic leukemia may therefore represent a progression to greater malignancy of B-cell chronic lymphatic leukemia.

Another variant of classic chronic lymphatic leukemia is marked by malignant cells having a propensity to invade the skin. In the *Sézary syndrome* diffuse infiltration of the skin occurs, leading to generalized reddening and thickening and scaling (erythroderma). Cells in the Sézary syndrome have characteristic convoluted nuclei, unusual in classic B-cell chronic lymphatic leukemia (Fig. 24-1). These *Sézary cells*, as they are called, have T-cell markers and T-cell functions. They lack terminal deoxyribonucleotide transferase, indicating a more mature cell structure than that of acute lymphatic leukemia. The first virus implicated in the etiology of human lymphoid neoplasia was isolated from a patient with Sézary syndrome. This previously unrecognized virus is a C-type retrovirus now named *human T-cell leukemia virus* type I (or HTLV-I). Following further study it has become evident that the as-

Fig. 24-1. Appearance of Sézary cell (**A**), lymphosarcoma cell (**B**), and hairy cell (**C**).

sociation of this virus with the Sézary syndrome is unusual, but that the virus is probably the cause of another T-cell neoplasm described in Chapter 26.

Just as diffuse well-differentiated lymphoma is analogous to chronic lymphatic leukemia, there is a form of T-cell lymphoma that invades the skin but does not express a blood lymphocytosis. This disease, called *mycosis fungoides*, presents as patches of scaly nodular and ulcerative lesions on the skin. The skin lesions have a purplish hue indicative of inva-

sion by cells in addition to the inflammatory process. Both mycosis fungoides and Sézary syndrome can eventually evolve to invade the lymphoid organs and other tissues.

Late in evolution, the cells observed in the chronic leukemias can become more primitive in appearance, acquiring the features of cells seen in more aggressive lymphoid neoplasms that grow rapidly and invade widely. Together with the metamorphosis in morphology, the behavior of the disease becomes increasingly malignant, and rapid and extensive organ invasion follows. When chronic lymphatic leukemia progresses to a large cell lymphoma, the condition is called *Richter's syndrome*.

Conversely, lymphoid neoplasms initially involving lymph nodes and other tissues, the lymphomas, can express malignant cells in the blood. In such cases, atypical lymphocytes may have an indentation extending two-thirds across the center of the nucleus; these cells are termed *lymphosarcoma cells* (Fig. 24-1), and the entity is called *lymphosarcoma cell leukemia*.

As tests for detecting monoclonal surface immunoglobulin on lymphocytes have become more sensitive, it has been possible to show that many patients with B-cell neoplasms primarily involving lymph nodes, that is, lymphomas, have at least some malignant cells in the circulation. In the unusual cases of chronic lymphatic leukemia in which the cells bear T-cell markers, infiltration of the skin and masses surrounding the thymus may be encountered more frequently than in patients with typical B-cell chronic lymphatic leukemia.

Advanced chronic lymphatic leukemia or its variants can cause anemia, thrombocytopenia, and occasionally granulocytopenia because of replacement of the bone marrow by the malignant infiltrate. The deficiency of normal peripheral blood cells may be exacerbated by enlargement of the spleen, which sequesters and clears the erythrocytes, granulocytes, and platelets from the blood. In some cases, this clearance is accelerated because of the elaboration of autoantibodies against the normal blood cells.

Immunodeficiency and Autoimmunity

Most patients with typical B-cell chronic lymphatic leukemia have reduced levels of serum immunoglobulin. The cause of this reduction is partly a reflection of the failure of the chronic lymphatic leukemia clone to differentiate into normal plasma cells capable of secreting antibodies. Such patients benefit from immunoglobulin replacement therapy.

A general imbalance in lymphoid cells may also lead to an excess of suppressor activity. In any case, some patients have a sufficient hypogammaglobulinemia to become susceptible to infection with encapsulated bacteria.

The derangements in lymphoid cell balance incurred by the lymphoid proliferation can lead to elaboration of autoantibodies against normal blood cells and other host tissues. Therefore, 10 to 20 percent of patients with B-cell chronic lymphatic leukemia will have autoimmune hemolytic anemia, autoimmune thrombocytopenia, or rheumatoid arthritis.

Paraprotein Production

In most cases of typical B-cell chronic lymphatic leukemia, the malignant cells have small amounts of surface immunoglobulin and are incapable of differentiation into plasma cells. In a small percentage of cases of chronic lymphatic leukemia, patients may express a monoclonal gammopathy, usually with an M component of the IgM class. Monoclonal gammopathies associated with lymphoid neoplasms are described in more detail below and in Chapter 17.

HAIRY CELL LEUKEMIA

An uncommon chronic lymphatic neoplasm is characterized by the proliferation of cells having long cytoplasmic projections (Fig. 24-1). These cells are called hairy cells. The proliferation of cells primarily occurs within the spleen and bone marrow, causing bone marrow failure and sequestration and clearance of normal blood by the enlarged spleen. The major manifestation of the disease is therefore pancytopenia. Only in one-half of cases are significant numbers of hairy cells seen in the blood. The nature of the malignant cell in this disorder has been in dispute, but the occasional finding of monoclonal surface immunoglobulin on the cells strongly suggests that these cells are of lymphoid origin. The leukemia cells contain an enzyme that hydrolyzes phosphate esters at an acid pH, an acid phosphatase, that is resistant to inhibition by sodium tartrate. This tartrate-resistant acid phosphatase can be detected by a histochemical procedure; its presence is strongly suggestive of the diagnosis.

Hairy cell leukemia is interesting because it can respond well to a variety of therapies. Some patients with spleens enlarged by leukemic infiltration react to splenectomy with a marked and prolonged rise in peripheral blood counts and a fall in the number of circulating hairy cells. Treatment of many patients with the adenosine deaminase inhibitor deoxycoformycin results in complete and sustained remissions, as does therapy with recombinant α-interferon. The mechanism of action of α-interferon in this instance is not clear, that is, whether it has a direct cytotoxic effect on the hairy cells, enhances host immunologic reactions against the hairy cells, or promotes the differentiation of the hairy cells.

TREATMENT OF CHRONIC LYMPHATIC LEUKEMIA

B-cell chronic lymphatic leukemia may progress slowly or not at all; Because most patients are elderly, they often die of other causes. When treatment is needed, it is because of the complications of more aggressive evolution of the disease enumerated above, that is, significant organ impairment or the ravages of immune dysfunction.

Because of the basic benignity of chronic lymphatic leukemia, treatment, when needed, can often be mild, consisting of radiation of enlarged or impaired organs or small doses of chemotherapy with alkylating agents. Aggressive phases of chronic lymphatic leukemia characterized by marked splenic enlargements, pancytopenia, painful enlargement of lymph nodes, fever, or weight loss may require more and higher doses of drugs. Treatment of the disease can diminish or abolish paraproteins or the autoimmune disorders associated with it.

SUGGESTED READINGS

Gale, R.P., & Foon, K.A. (1987) Biology of chronic lymphocytic leukemia. Semin Hematol *24*:202.

Golomb, H.J., & Ratain, M.J. (1987) Recent advances in the treatment of hairy-cell leukemia. N Engl J Med *316*:870.

Lee, J.S., Dixon, D.O., Kantarjian, H.M., et al. (1987) Prognosis of chronic lymphocytic leukemia: A multivariate regression analysis of 325 untreated patients. Blood *69*:929.

Mann, D.L., De Santis, P., Mark, G., et al. (1987) HTLV-I-associated B-cell CLL: Indirect role for retrovirus in leukemogenesis. Science *236*:1103.

25

Hodgkin's Lymphoma

When in 1832, Thomas Hodgkin published a paper entitled "On Some Morbid Appearances of the Absorbent Glands and Spleen," he was reporting the first description of malignant lymphoma. Today Hodgkin's disease, or Hodgkin's lymphoma, is viewed as a malignant disorder affecting lymphoid tissue, the morphological appearance of which can be quite variable, but which has one consistent feature: the presence of a large cell with two nuclei called the Reed-Sternberg cell, after its initial describers. Hodgkin's disease was also the first lymphoid neoplasm to be cured, first by radiation therapy and subsequently by combination chemotherapy.

Hodgkin's disease ordinarily presents as a painless enlargement of one or more of the lymph node regions. In distinct contrast to the non-Hodgkin's lymphoma, which are generally widely disseminated at the time of diagnosis, Hodgkin's disease is often localized and may spread slowly through the lymphatic channels to contiguous lymph node regions. The indolent and contiguous route of spread of many cases of Hodgkin's disease has implications for therapy. If the disorder is untreated or if treatment fails, Hodgkin's disease eventually spreads widely and invades normal organs, killing the patient by interfering with the functioning of these organs.

The constant finding of Reed-Sternberg cells renders attractive the idea that these cells represent the malignant proliferation underlying Hodgkin's disease. The large size and bizarre appearance of these cells (Fig. 25-1) are consistent with malignant neoplasia. However, neither a clonal origin nor the cellular lineage of Reed-Sternberg cells has been established. In some respects, Hodgkin's disease behaves as if it were an infection or inflammatory disease. The lymph node architecture becomes replaced by normal inflammatory cells; these cells ordinarily outnumber the Reed-Sternberg cells. Furthermore, patients with Hodgkin's disease frequently manifest signs and symptoms associated with inflammation, such as fever, weight loss, polyclonal hypergammaglobulinemia, changes in acute phase reactant proteins, monocytosis, eosinophilia, and soaking night sweats.

When describing a patient with Hodgkin's disease, the staging system of lymphoma also takes into account whether a patient has systemic symptoms that can be ascribed to neoplasm. The symptoms are (1) an unexplained loss of more than 10 percent in body weight, (2) soaking night sweats, and (3) fever. The absence of these features designates a patient as stage A (e.g., Stage IA or IIA), presence of the symptoms indicates stage B (e.g., IIIB or IVB). An unusual systemic manifestation of Hodgkin's disease is periodic fever that is present for some days, remits, and then returns. This symptom has been named *Pel-Ebstein fever* after the physician who first described it. Some patients diagnosed as having Hodgkin's disease complain of pain in affected lymph nodes after ingesting alcohol. Hodg-

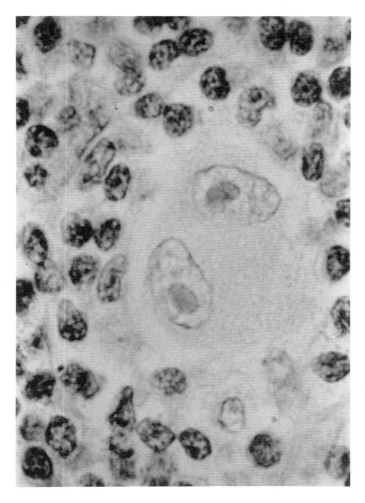

Fig. 25-1. Reed-Sternberg cell.

kin's disease patients may occasionally suffer from severe, generalized itching of the skin. As is the case for many inflammatory conditions and some neoplasms, patients with Hodgkin's disease may express anergy.

The histology of Hodgkin's disease is classified according to the cells surrounding the Reed-Sternberg cells. A uniform infiltrate of normal-appearing typical lymphocytes in the presence of Reed-Sternberg cells defines what is called *lymphocyte predominant* Hodgkin's disease. If the surrounding infiltrate consists of macrophages, lymphocytes, and eosinophils, the entity is called *mixed cellularity* Hodgkin's disease. *Nodular sclerosis* Hodgkin's disease is said to be present when the lymph node contains large bands of collagen. The Reed-Sternberg cells reside in lacunae evident throughout the fibrotic matrix. Lymphocyte predominance, mixed cellularity, and nodular sclerosis are the histologies usually found in young adults, the age population in which Hodgkin's disease most frequently occurs.

A second peak of incidence of Hodgkin's disease occurs in elderly persons. These patients frequently manifest a histological pattern composed of large numbers of extremely bizarre Reed-Sternberg cells and a minimal inflammatory infiltrate. This category of Hodgkin's disease is called *lymphocyte-depleted* Hodgkin's disease.

To some extent, the histological pattern predicts the pace of the disease and response to treatment. Lymphocyte-predominant Hodgkin's disease has the most favorable prognosis, whereas lymphocyte-depleted Hodgkin's disease is most virulent and least responsive to therapy. The histological pattern does not influence treatment. The nodular sclerosis pattern is most often seen in the younger age group of patients affected. Lymphocyte depletion Hodgkin's disease is most often seen in elderly patients with advanced stages of disease.

DIAGNOSIS AND MANAGEMENT

The progressive enlargement of one or more lymph nodes that cannot be explained by a localized or generalized infection requires that the lymph node be excised surgically and examined by a pathologist. Whenever possible, the lymph node of choice for pathological examination should not be an inguinal lymph node, because these lymph glands are so often involved in a reaction to chronic fungal infections of the feet. If a pathologist arrives at a diagnosis of Hodgkin's disease because of the histological pattern of the lymph node, the clinician has the responsibility to evaluate the extent of involvement of the disease, the procedure defined as staging. Staging is especially important in Hodgkin's disease because it determines the approach to treatment. The system of staging for Hodgkin's disease follows the numerical outline described in Table 22-1.

Considerable staging can be obtained by a careful physical examination and simple laboratory information, such as x-ray films of the chest. These techniques enable the physician to identify superficial lymph node involvement, the presenting sign of Hodgkin's disease in by far most cases, to determine whether mediastinal lymph nodes are involved and, if so, whether the disease has extended to involve the lung parenchyma. More elaborate tests

such as computed tomography, magnetic resonance imaging, and radioactive gallium scanning are required to evaluate whether the disease involves lymphoid tissue in the abdomen as well.

The test most frequently employed, however, is the lymphangiogram. Radiopaque contrast material is injected into the lymphatics of the foot in the webbing between the first and second toes. The dye courses up the lymphatic channels of the legs, enters the pelvic system, converges in the channel surrounding the aorta, then into the mediastinum, and eventually into the thoracic duct. A series of x-ray films of the pelvis and abdomen taken over a period of hours reveals in the normal case opacification of lymph nodes encountered by the path of the contrast dye. Lymph nodes showing tumor involvement are recognized by enlargement and by regions within them that do not opacify with the dye. Aberrant flow of the dye is also observed, an indication of obstruction of the lymphatic channel by the Hodgkin's disease. However, to establish with a greater degree of certainty whether abdominal lymph nodes are involved and in order to determine whether Hodgkin's disease has invaded the spleen, it is sometimes necessary to resort to an exploratory laporatomy. During the operation, the surgeon palpates the para-aortic and pelvic lymph node regions and removes any palpable lymph nodes for purposes of biopsy. The surgeon then excises the spleen and may also remove a sample of liver for histological examination. The spleen is then cut into multiple sections and examined by the pathologist for gross and microscopic foci of Hodgkin's disease.

What is the rationale for such elaborate and occasionally invasive staging procedures? The neoplastic proliferation that characterizes Hodgkin's disease can be eradicated by means of sufficient doses of ionizing radiation. Furthermore, when localized, the disease spreads by regional extension to adjacent lymph node regions. Therefore, radiation directed at involved lymph nodes and others surrounding it can cure the localized Hodgkin's disease in a large proportion of cases. For example, for Hodgkin's disease arising in cervical lymph nodes and shown by the staging procedures not to involve the abdomen or mediastinum, radiation would customarily be delivered to both sides of the neck, the axillae, and the mediastinum. This radiation field, called an upper mantle (Fig. 25-2) would serve to treat the obvious disease and the regions to which it most likely would have spread. Even when Hodgkin's disease is more widespread, for example, in Stage II or III disease, more extended radiation fields involving the upper mantle and the para-aortic and pelvic nodal regions are sufficient to be curative in a substantial number of cases.

In addition to being susceptible to radiation, Hodgkin's disease will melt away dramatically, and often permanently, in response to a variety of chemotherapeutic agents (see Ch. 31). Combinations of such drugs can induce complete remissions, and even cures, in more than one-half the patients whose disease recurs after radiation therapy. They can also be used with curative outcome in patients in whom the disease is too widespread, for example, in stage IV, for radiation to be useful, and they can be used repeatedly to salvage patients whose disease has relapsed.

In light of the foregoing, one may well ask why it is necessary to resort to complex and worrisome staging procedures. Why not simply deliver radiation to all node-bearing areas and treat with chemotherapy? The answer to this question lies in the toxicity of the treatment, which is proportional to the amount of treatment given. The side effects of anticancer therapy are described in Chapter 31. However, the most problematic complications of the treatment of Hodgkin's disease are derangements in immunological function and leukemogenesis. The susceptibility to infection with high-grade encapsulated organisms of patients subjected to staging splenectomy and a combination of chemotherapy and radiation for Hodgkin's disease is well known. Both ionizing radiation and anticancer drugs, especially alkylating agents, have the capacity to induce leukemia. The incidence of acute leukemia, usually of the acute nonlymphocytic type, is disturbingly high in patients treated for Hodgkin's disease with both radiation and chemotherapy. The leukemia and other neoplasms, for that matter, can arise within a few years after completion of treatment for Hodgkin's disease. Less lethal, but unpleasant, complications of treatment include infertility and hypothyroidism.

It can be appreciated, therefore, that the clinician is faced with some difficult decisions concerning just how much treatment to deliver to a patient with stage III Hodgkin's disease or with bulky stage I or II disease. Mediastinal disease is defined as 'bulky' if the tumor mass occupies more than a third of the thoracic volume. Moderately localized radiation is clearly adequate for stage I and II disease, chemotherapy is obviously required for stage IV lesions. The treatment guidelines ordinarily dictated by the anatomical extent of Hodgkin's disease may be modified by the histological pattern of a given case. Mixed cellularity or nodular sclerosis morphologies are considered more aggressive than lymphocyte-predominant. Precisely definable treatment recommendations are not available for all situations and are modified as more experience is obtained with different combinations of treatment. In any case, it can be appreciated that it is imperative to obtain as precise a staging as possible in each case, in order to determine the course of therapy.

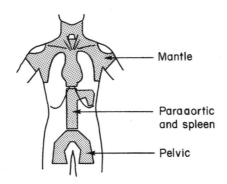

Fig. 25-2. Radiation fields.

SUGGESTED READINGS

Bonadonna, G., Valagusa, P., & Santoro, A. (1986) Alternating non-cross-resistant combination chemotherapy or MOPP in stage IV Hodgkin's disease. A report of 8-year results. Ann. Intern. Med. *104*:739.

Bookman, M.A., & Longo, D.L. (1986) Concomitant illness in patients treated for Hodgkin's disease. Cancer Treat. Rev. *13*:77.

Buzaid, A.C., Lippman, S.M., & Miller, T.P. (1987) Salvage therapy of advanced Hodgkin's disease. Critical appraisal of curative potential. Am. J. Med. *83*:523–532.

Kaplan, H.S. (1972) Hodgkin's Disease. Harvard University Press, Cambridge, MA.

Longo, D.L., Young, R.C., Wesley, M., et al. (1986) Twenty years of MOPP therapy for Hodgkin's disease. J. Clin. Oncol. *4*:1295.

26

Non-Hodgkin's Lymphoma

Non-Hodgkin's lymphoma is the clonal proliferation of morphologically typical or atypical lymphoid cells in lymphoid organs and other tissues.

The classification of these disorders is difficult because anatomical, histological, and immunological characterizations do not always pigeonhole these disorders into clinically useful terms. The dominant approach today is to define non-Hodgkin's lymphoma according to its histological appearance and its clinical features and, whenever possible, to supplement this information by identifying the type of lymphocyte involved in terms of its immunological phenotype (e.g., B cell or T cell).

In examining lymph node biopsy specimens, the pathologist looks for effacement of the normal architecture of the lymph node by a monotonous infiltrate of cells. The cell size is noted, and the lymphoma is broadly grouped into a *small cell* or *large cell* class. When the cells of the lymphoid neoplasm are very large and have vacuolated nuclei with multiple large nucleoli, the lesion is said to be a large cell or histiocytic lymphoma. The term *histiocytic* is outdated, because it was formerly applied to what we now know to be macrophages. Nowadays, macrophages are not called histiocytes and, more importantly, the neoplastic cells of by far most of these diseases are of lymphoid, not macrophage, origin.

The pathologist notes whether the cells have a tendency to form nodules reminiscent of germinal follicles in the normal lymph nodes or the white pulp of the spleen; if this is the case, the lesion is called *nodular* or *follicular* lymphoma. If the cells do not arrange to form such nodules, the pattern is described as *diffuse* lymphoma. The pathologist further describes the morphology of the neoplasm in terms of its differentiation. When the neoplastic cells look somewhat like typical small lymphocytes, the pathologist refers to them as *well-differentiated* lymphocytic cells. When the morphology of the lymphocytes departs from this basic description, the lesion is said to be *poorly differentiated*. The nuclei of the lymphocytes of some lymphomas have predominant infoldings and cleavages, and the descriptive terms *cleaved* or *uncleaved* may accompany the diagnosis.

Most non-Hodgkin's lymphomas are B-cell malignancies. This conclusion is based on the detection of homogeneous immunoglobulin on the outer surface of the membranes of the neoplastic cells, and these immunoglobulins bear either all λ or all $\varkappa$ light chains. The surface immunoglobulin is usually of the IgM and IgG classes. The staining of surface immunoglobulins is greater on cells of the lymphomas than it is on the cells found in chronic lymphocytic leukemia. As described in Chapter 22, B-cell lymphomas express clonal immunoglobulin gene rearrangements.

Over the years, several systems for classifying non-Hodgkin's lymphoma have been proposed, and some bear the names of their founding pathologists, such as Rappaport or

Table 26-1. Classification Schemes for Non-Hodgkin's Lymphoma Cell Types

Working Formulation	Lukes/Collins Classification	Rappaport Classification
Low Grade Lymphomas		
Small lymphocytic	Small lymphocytic	Diffuse well differentiated
Follicular small cleaved	Small cleaved follicular center cell	Nodular poorly differentiated
Follicular, mixed small and large cleaved	Small and large cleaved follicular center cell	Nodular mixed
Intermediate Grade Lymphomas		
Follicular large	Large/small cleaved follicular	Nodular histiocytic
Diffuse small cleaved	Small, cleaved, diffuse follicular center	Diffuse poorly differentiated
Diffuse mixed small and large	Small, large, cleaved, noncleaved, follicular center, diffuse	Diffuse mixed
Diffuse large	Large, cleaved, noncleaved, follicular center diffuse	Diffuse histiocytic
High Grade Lymphomas		
Large, immunoblastic	Immunoblastic sarcoma	Diffuse histiocytic
Lymphoblastic	Convoluted T cell	Lymphoblastic
Small, noncleaved	Small, noncleaved follicular center	Diffuse undifferentiated Burkitt's
Small, noncleaved	Small, noncleaved follicular center	Diffuse undifferentiated non-Burkitt's

Lukes and Collins. To varying degrees, the classifications use the morphologic characteristics such as cell size, differentiation, and nuclear cleavage described above. This chapter follows a classification arising from a U.S. National Cancer Institute panel called the *Working Formulation for Clinical Usage*. A comparison of this approach with the older systems appears in Table 26-1. In general, the degree of malignancy, defined as rapidity of growth and lethality, also termed *grade*, increases from the top to the bottom of the table.

LOW GRADE NON-HODGKIN'S LYMPHOMAS

The neoplastic cells of these diseases either have the morphology of small "mature" lymphocytes or else tend to aggregate into nodules resembling the follicles of lymph nodes. The nodule-forming tumors presumably originated in normal germinal follicles, whereas the diffuse lesions may arise from B lymphocytes residing in the medullary regions of lymph nodes. The surface markers of the small lymphocytic variety of disease resemble those found on B-cell chronic lymphatic leukemia cells, namely weak expression of surface immunoglobulin, C3 and Fc receptors; Ia antigen; B-cell antigens CD19, 20, and 21; and the T-cell marker CD5. The other two variants of low grade non-Hodgkin's lymphoma express larger amounts of surface immunoglobulin as well as Ia, CD19, and CD20 antigens. Unlike the small lymphocytic type, however, the common acute lymphoblastic leukemia antigen (CALLA) is usually expressed and CD5 is not.

Chromosomal anomalies are frequent in low grade lymphomas. One of the most common is a t(14;18) [q32q21] translocation. Because the gene encoding the immunoglobulin heavy chain resides in the affected region of chromosome 14, it is presumed that the neoplastic transformation is somehow associated with the rearrangements occurring in this gene during normal B-cell development. In the translocation a locus known as *bcl-2* moves into the Ig heavy chain locus, and the gene product of *bcl-2* is produced in larger amounts in neoplastic B cells than in normal mature B cells. For this reason it is presumed that *bcl-2* is an onco-gene.

Although the low grade lymphocytic lymphomas, like Hodgkin's disease, tend to arise in lymph nodes and can be slow in growth, they differ from Hodgkin's disease in that they are nearly disseminated at the time of diagnosis. In other words, staging workup procedures will frequently detect disease in areas beyond the region of initial presentation; it means that cure will usually not be achieved by means of localized radiation.

INTERMEDIATE GRADE NON-HODGKIN'S LYMPHOMAS

Follicular large cell tumors express many of the markers associated with the low grade neoplasms, although surface immunoglobulin is found in only 65 percent of cases. The diffuse small cleaved cell variant resembles the follicular counterpart in having large amounts of surface immunoglobulins, Ia, CD19, CD20, and CD21 antigens. The diffuse mixed and diffuse large cells tumors are more heterogenous. Ninety percent of the diffuse large cell neoplasms bear some B-cell markers, but in various combinations. In addition, 10 percent have only T-cell markers. These lymphomas progress more rapidly than the low grade neoplasms.

HIGH GRADE NON-HODGKIN'S LYMPHOMAS

The large cell immunoblastic lymphomas are a partial exception to the rule that the non-Hodgkin's lymphomas are usually disseminated at the time of presentation. Up to 40 percent of these tumors may be localized at initial diagnosis; they are also the type most frequently found outside of lymph nodes, such as in the bones, central nervous system, and the gastrointestinal tract. This is also the lymphoma type that most often arises in patients who are immunosuppressed, for instance in patients with AIDS or who are pharmacologically immunocompromised following organ transplantation.

The T-cell immunoblastic lymphomas are distinguishable from the lymphoblastic variety that in its markers and clinical behavior more closely resembles the T-cell acute lymphatic leukemias. The cells express terminal deoxynucleotidyltransferase activity and a variety of T-cell markers, although the marker phenotype tends to be more mature than that found in T-cell acute lymphatic leukemia and CALLA is only found in 40 percent of cases. The lymphoblastic lymphoma also mimics T-cell acute leukemia in presenting as mediastinal adenopathy.

The disorders grouped in the Working Formulation as "small noncleaved lymphomas" are among the most aggressive and the most interesting. The tumors are proliferations of relatively small cells with round or oval nuclei and multiple prominent nucleoli. Macrophages are often seen within the monotonous background of malignant cells, giving the overall histologic picture an appearance described as a starry sky when seen at low power. The cells have monoclonal immunoglobulin, usually of the IgM type, on their surfaces, indicating a B-cell origin. It has been speculated that these cells arise from the sites possibly of cells ordinarily found in germinal centers of normal lymph nodes. This disease was first described by the British surgeon Dennis Burkitt as a tumor of the jaw of African children living in areas endemic for malaria. This association between malaria and the lymphoma led Burkitt to suspect an infectious basis for the pathogenesis of the disorder. This speculation became more intriguing when it was learned that the affected children had very high titers of antibody in their serum against Epstein-Barr virus (EBV), which, it will be recalled, infests B cells as the causative agent of infectious mononucleosis. This association led to the speculation that Burkitt's lymphoma was the result of chronic immunologic stimulation by malarial infection coupled with transforming effects of the EBV infection.

This lymphoma is encountered infrequently in parts of the world other than the endemic region in Africa. The nonendemic disease is histologically identical to the African variant, but occurs in somewhat older children and young adults and usually presents in the abdominal lymph nodes rather than in the jaw. Moreover, the association between high EBV antibody titers is less constant. Burkitt's lymphoma is an extremely rapidly growing neoplasm; left untreated, it is fulminant and fatal. However, as amplified below, it is sometimes gratifyingly responsive to therapy.

The differences between the so-called endemic (African) and sporadic varieties of this disease are reflected in molecular terms. First, the tumor cells in the African disease almost invariably express C3 receptors, whereas the cells of the sporadic type do not. At the genetic level, both varieties have a t[8,14] translocation in which the *c-myc* oncogene on chromosome 8 usually relocates to the heavy chain immunoglobulin locus on chromosome 14. This dislocation of *c-myc* results in its overexpression, strongly implicating this oncogene in the pathogenesis of the malignant process. In a minority (20 percent) of cases *c-myc* moves to the $\varkappa$ or λ light chain loci on chromosomes 2 or 22, respectively, instead of (t[2;8] and t[8;22]). Although there is heterogeneity in the position of the break in chromosome 8 associated with these translocations, the general organization of the breaks is characteristic for either the endemic or sporadic types of the disease. In the endemic variety of this lymphoma, the so-called class III break point on chromosome 8 is quite distant from the coding region of the *c-myc* locus; in the sporadic variety, the break point is either within (class I) or just upstream (class II) of the *c-myc* locus. In the class I and II breaks, it is the disruption of the *c-myc* gene per se that prevents a regulatory part of the gene from controlling its expression. In the class III rearrangement, enhancing elements in the immunoglobulin gene may drive the transcription of the *c-myc* gene.

HUMAN T-CELL LEUKEMIA/LYMPHOMA VIRUS LYMPHOMA

This disease is endemic in southern Japan and in the Caribbean area, although sporadic cases arise elsewhere. The malignant cells are found in enlarged lymph nodes and circulate in large numbers in the blood, explaining the designation leukemia/lymphoma. An additional characteristic of this neoplasm is a propensity to produce lytic bone lesions and hypercalcemia. The tumor is very malignant and fairly unresponsive to treatment.

The cells are histologically of the large-cell or "histiocytic" type and are diffusely oriented in lymph nodes. Immunologically they are T cells of the helper cell subset.

It is this condition in which the evidence for a viral cause of human lymphoid neoplasia is strongest. Proviral DNA sequences of the human T-cell leukemia virus (HTLV-I) have been identified in the malignant T cells. Antibodies against proteins of this virus are found in the serum of patients and in the serum of persons in endemic areas. Most importantly, the virus causes the malignant transformation of cultured human T cells.

Effects of Lymphomas on the Patient

Organ Infiltration

The well-differentiated lymphomas tend to arise in lymph nodes and to be low in evolution. Like chronic lymphatic leukemia, initially they may cause relatively little problem for the patient. Difficulties, when they occur, sometimes not for 5 to 10 years after onset of obvious disease, arise from painful enlargement of the lymph nodes and spleen or from impingement of these enlarged organs and other structures or from extension of the process directly into other organs. When the bone marrow is extensively involved, bone marrow failure can be a major difficulty. These complications emerge earlier in the poorly differentiated lymphocytic lymphomas, consistent with the more aggressive evolution of these neoplasms. Some of the lymphomas have particular predispositions to arise in certain organs. African Burkitt's lymphoma presents as tumor of the jaw, whereas the American variant more commonly involves the abdomen. Large cell lymphoma has a greater tendency than lymphocytic lymphoma to originate in extranodal tissues.

association with adbominal or, less frequently, respiratory lymphoid proliferation, which varies in degree of differentiation and malignant appearance. The intestinal involvement causes gastrointestinal symptoms and a malabsorption syndrome. This disorder is most frequently observed in young persons residing in the Mediterranean area and the Near East. Secretion of μ heavy chains occurs very rarely and is associated with chronic lymphatic leukemia.

Paraprotein Elaboration

Some well-differentiated B-cell lymphomas in the spectrum ranging from chronic lymphatic leukemia to diffuse well-differentiated lymphocytic lymphoma will express sufficient maturation toward the plasma cell to secrete monoclonal immunoglobulins. The cells sometimes, but not invariably, may have features resembling mature plasma cells. These plasmacytoid lymphocytes have a round, eccentric nucleus with clumps of chromatin around their periphery. The predominant immunoglobulin secreted is IgM; when significant quantities of IgM accumulate in the serum, the disease is designated *Waldenström's macroglobulinemia*. If there is a significant accumulation of excess IgM, the hyperviscosity syndrome described in Chapter 17 can arise. A principal clinical problem of patients with Waldenström's macroglobulinemia can be the presence of the IgM paraprotein, requiring treatment with plasmapheresis if the underlying neoplasm is not responsive to chemotherapy.

Some lymphoid neoplasms may generate immunoglobulin heavy chains of the γ, α, or μ class or fragments thereof without producing light chains. The neoplasms secreting λ heavy chains usually occur in elderly men and often involve nasopharyngeal lymph nodes, the liver, and the spleen. The infiltration of lymphoid tissue in the oropharynx causes a swelling of the uvula. This disease is called λ heavy chain disease. α Heavy chain disease occurs in

Management of Non-Hodgkin's Lymphoma

Knowing when and how much to treat the patient with non-Hodgkin's lymphoma remains a major challenge for clinicians. The low grade lymphomas, like chronic lymphatic leukemia, may require relatively little treatment for long periods of time, as they cause little difficulty for the patient. The non-Hodgkin's lymphomas are initially very sensitive to ionizing radiation and a variety of cytotoxic drugs, including corticosteroids, alkylating agents, antitubulins, anthracyclines, antimetabolites, and others described in Chapter 31. In contrast to the situation in Hodgkin's disease, however, the drugs do not seem to cure the disease or, for that matter in the very benign variants of non-Hodgkin's lymphoma, even clearly alter the natural history of the diseases, which may permit the patient to live for 10 or more years (but see below). Therefore, because of the short- and long-term toxicities of the chemotherapy and radiation therapy, the standard approach has been to subject patients with indolent varieties of non-Hodgkin's lymphoma to as little treatment as possible. If the lymphoma is a paraprotein-secreting B-cell neoplasm causing the hyperviscosity syndrome or other complications, chemotherapy can be helpful in reducing the accumulation of the abnormal protein. Any time that the disease begins to interfere with vital functions, such as respiration, immediate treatment is, of course, required.

Patients with intermediate and high grade lymphomas often require treatment at the time of diagnosis; treatment can definitely affect the natural history of the more aggressive forms of this disease. As with the low grade lymphomas, standard chemotherapy or radiation therapy does not appear to "cure" patients with many variants of the high grade lymphomas, although combinations of antitumor drugs can produce durable complete remissions in a majority of cases.

The large cell, mixed large and small cell and the small noncleaved cell lymphomas are very responsive to chemotherapy; in a significant proportion of cases, complete remissions of sufficient duration to justify the term "cure" can be achieved. Presumably this favorable outcome occurs in part because highly malignant neoplasms may have a large fraction of dividing cells that are particularly sensitive to the treatment. If the treatment is not completely successful, the disease progresses. At present, researchers are testing the hypothesis that extremely aggressive antitumor therapy directed at the lymphomas thought to be "incurable," such as the lymphoblastic, small cell intermediate grade, and even the low grade small cell lymphomas might in fact lead to cures. The strategies often employ allogeneic or au-

tologous bone marrow transplantation (Ch. 32) as part of the treatment approach, which trades off the risk of treatment toxicity (including death) against the hope of long-term cure. Because of the indolent natural history of the low grade lymphomas, it will take a long time to assess the value of this experimental treatment.

SUGGESTED READINGS

Blayney, D.W., Jaffe, E.S., Fisher, R.S., et al. (1983) The human T-cell leukemia/lymphoma virus, lymphoma; lytic bone lesions, and hypercalcemia. Ann Intern Med 98:144.

Fifth International Workshop on Chromosomes in Leukemia-Lymphoma (1987) Correlation of chromosome abnormalities with histologic and immunologic characteristics in non-Hodgkin's lymphoma and adult T cell leukemia-lymphoma. Blood 70:1564.

Koduru, P.R., Filippa, D.A., & Richardson, M.E. (1987) Cytogenetic and histologic correlations in malignant lymphoma. Blood 69:97.

Leder, P., Battey, J., & Lenoir, G. (1983) Translocations among antibody genes in human cancer. Science 222:765.

The non-Hodgkin's lymphoma pathologic classification project (1982) National Cancer Institute sponsored study of classifications of non-Hodgkin's lymphomas: Summary and descriptions of a working formulation for clinical usage. Cancer 49:2112.

Plasma Cell Neoplasms

Plasma cell neoplasma are B-cell tumors in which the predominant neoplastic cell has the morphology of plasma cells. Although plasma cell tumors are lymphoid neoplasms, and plasma cells ordinarily exist in lymph nodes and other lymphoid organs, plasma cell cancer is principally a spectrum of diseases of the bone marrow. The spectrum ranges from an indolent plasma cell proliferation detectable only by its secreted product monoclonal immunoglobulins or fragments thereof, a condition termed *monoclonal gammopathy of uncertain significance*, to a progressive lethal disorder called *multiple myeloma*. Occasionally plasma cell tumors arise in extraosseous nonlymphoid tissues; only very rarely do they involve the peripheral blood as a plasma cell leukemia. About half the cases of plasma cell neoplasms have chromosome abnormalities, including trisomy 3, 5, 9, and 15 and monosomy 13 and 16.

MULTIPLE MYELOMA

Multiple myeloma is a neoplastic monoclonal expansion of plasma cells. In 99 percent of cases, the malignant cells secrete either immunoglobulins or isolated light chains; in either case, the light chains are either of the $\varkappa$ or λ type. The paraprotein is detectable as a serum or urine M component. Two-thirds of multiple myelomas secrete IgG; a third, IgA. Multiple myeloma is a disease of middle-aged

adults; the population it affects is generally younger than that affected by the paraprotein-secreting non-Hodgkin's lymphomas. It has a higher incidence in blacks than in whites.

Effects of Multiple Myeloma on the Patient

Destruction of Bone and Bone Marrow Failure

Growth of the malignant plasma cells throughout the bone marrow of multiple bones causes pancytopenia. In contrast to the acute leukemias, multiple myeloma frequently causes local and generalized bone destruction evident on radiographs of the skeleton as diffuse osteopenia or as multiple lytic lesions. An x-ray film of the skull in disseminated multiple myeloma frequently exhibits what look like multiple bullet holes in the calvarium. The bone erosion may cause the patient to suffer from back and chest pain, which becomes excruciating when the weakened bones fracture, especially the vertebrae and femurs. Vertebral fractures can lead to spinal compression and severe neurological damage. The mechanism of bone destruction appears to be elaboration by the malignant plasma cells of novel bone resorbing molecules originally named osteoclast activating factors (OAF). Some of these factors may be lymphokines such as tumor necrosis factor.

Immunodeficiency

The bone marrow failure of multiple myeloma causes neutropenia, which predisposes the patient to infections with low grade pathogens. The impairment of normal immunoglobulin production in multiple myeloma, resulting from either crowding out or suppression of normal B cells, predisposes the multiple myeloma patient to infection with high grade encapsulated pathogens as well. Not surprisingly, bacterial infections are a frequent complication of multiple myeloma.

Renal and Metabolic Derangements

The paraprotein of multiple myeloma—particularly where the neoplasm secretes light chains that enter the urine (Bence Jones proteinuria) either directly or indirectly because of the accumulation of amyloid—can damage the kidneys, leading to uremia and renal tubular acidosis (Ch. 17). Susceptibility of patients with multiple myeloma to infection may also lead to renal damage as a result of infections in the kidney. The renal failure in and of itself can cause metabolic and serum electrolyte abnormalities, such as hypercalcemia and hyperuricemia. The destruction of bone leads to hypercalcemia; this condition is exacerbated when the patient becomes immobilized because of pain, as well as when the patient has significant renal failure. Because hypercalcemia itself can damage the renal tubules, a vicious circle ensues. Uremia impairs platelet function and red blood cell formation. Thus the renal complications of multiple myeloma can exacerbate the effects of bone marrow failure in causing anemia and hemorrhage.

A minority of myeloma paraproteins are associated with effects related to specific binding to antigens. Most often, the antigen is a normal immunoglobulin variable domain, in which case the paraprotein can be considered anti-idiotypic (see Ch. 21). Cases have been described in which the myeloma protein reacted with riboflavin, resulting in yellowing of the skin, or with peripheral nerve myelin, causing neuropathy.

PLASMACYTOMA AND "INDOLENT" OR "SMOLDERING" MYELOMA

In a small percentage of cases, the plasma cell neoplasma are detected as limited or slowly growing progressive diseases. Local plasma cell tumors of the bone or elsewhere can present as masses contiguous to a bone or in an area of local bone pain. The level of serum immunoglobulins is usually normal in such cases, and M components are minimal or absent. In some instances, the presence of a disseminated plasma cell neoplasm may be discovered in an otherwise asymptomatic patient by the finding of an M component on serum protein immunoelectrophoresis. Such a disorder might evolve into frank symptomatic multiple myeloma, but occasionally it remains unchanged for many years.

Diagnosis of Plasma Cell Neoplasms

Suspicion of a diagnosis of frank multiple myeloma is raised by the symptoms of bone pain, pallor, and possible bacterial infections in a middle-aged or elderly person. The findings of anemia, rouleau formation, proteinuria, hypercalcemia, uremia, lytic bone lesions, and pathological fractures are highly suggestive of the diagnosis.

Distinguishing overt multiple myeloma from monoclonal gammopathy of uncertain significance can be difficult. Table 27-1 lists major and minor criteria of multiple myeloma: One major and one minor criterion or three minor criteria, one of which must be increased plasma cells in the bone marrow and a monoclonal globulin spike, establish a diagnosis of

Table 27-1. Diagnostic Criteria

Major
1. Tissue plasmacytoma
2. > 30% plasma cells in bone marrow
3. > 3.5g/dl IgG or > 2 g/dl IgA monoclonal M components; > 1g/24-h excretion of λ or ϰ light chains in the urine

Minor
A. 10–30% plasma cells in bone marrow
B. Monoclonal M component or urinary light chain excretion at lower levels
C. Skeletal lytic lesions
D. Serum (normal polyclonal) IgM < 50 mg/dl, IgA < 100 mg/dl, IgG < 600 mg/dl

multiple myeloma. In isolated plasmacytomas or indolent multiple myeloma, the paraprotein may be present, but the bone marrow sample can be normal.

Treatment of Plasma Cell Neoplasma

Indolent multiple myeloma or monoclonal gammopathy of uncertain significance requires no treatment. Isolated plasmacytomas can be treated successfully with localized radiation, and new lesions may not appear at all or not until much later.

In contrast, multiple myeloma presents a therapeutic challenge to the physician. Treatment is directed against the diffuse disease, against local lesions that are troublesome, and toward supportive medical care.

Only chemotherapy can produce remissions in disseminated multiple myeloma. A standard chemotherapeutic regimen for this disorder is a combination of phenylalanine mustard, an alkylating agent, and a corticosteroid. More than one-half the patients will enjoy complete remission and many others a partial remission lasting months to even years. Remission is indicated by partial or complete healing of bone lesions, by improvement in anemia and other manifestations of bone marrow failure, and by diminution or disappearance of the paraprotein. The last-named is an especially useful marker for evaluating the effectiveness of treatment and for heralding the onset of relapse.

When chemotherapy is not effective, radiation can be helpful to reduce tumor masses in painful bone lesions and in palliating pathological fractures. General medical measures such as red cell transfusions for anemia, antibiotics for infection, and maintenance of adequate hydration to maximize renal function are important. In patients in whom renal damage is severe or permanent, but in whom chemotherapy is expected to yield a reasonable life expectancy, manifestations of kidney failure can be controlled by means of dialysis therapy.

Hypercalcemia can be an especially troubling complication of multiple myeloma, especially because it causes obtundation and even coma and because it predisposes to and exacerbates renal disease. The management of hypercalcemia begins with hydration and diuretics, which may enhance calcium excretion sufficiently to control the metabolic problem. More resistant hypercalcemia may respond to corticosteroids and the hypocalcemia-producing hormone calcitonin or the antitumor antibiotic mithramycin, which may act by inhibiting osteoclast function. Mithramycin, however, must be used cautiously because it causes thrombocytopenia.

SUGGESTED READING

Farhangi, M. Ed. (1986) Plasma cell myeloma and myeloma proteins. Semin Oncol. *13*:1–382.

Stem Cells and
Stem Cell Disorders

Before the sixth week of gestation of the human embryo, blood cells appear in the yolk sac. Thereafter, the liver becomes the site of blood cell production until week 20, when hematopoiesis takes place in bone marrow, the origin of synthesis of blood for the remainder of the human life span.

Under certain pathological conditions, the bone marrow ceases to be a hospitable site for blood cell production; hematopoiesis may then return to the liver and to other organs, a condition called *myeloid metaplasia*. These changes in the location of hematopoiesis reflect where the soil is fertile for growth, replication, and differentiation of the hematopoietic pluripotent stem cell. These cells have the capacity both to differentiate into all types of blood cells—the erythrocytes, granulocytes, lymphocytes, and platelets—and to renew themselves. The rate of renewal and differentiation of stem cells must keep pace with the death rate of peripheral blood cells under various states of demand in order to maintain the peripheral blood cell concentration at a level compatible with the proper functioning of the organism.

STEM CELL PHYSIOLOGY

The hematopoietic stem cell is present in normal bone marrow in very small concentrations. The ratio of stem cells to nucleated bone marrow cells is about 1:2000. The stem cell has only recently been isolated in pure form. Both the physiologist and the clinician usually evaluate the stem cell by its offspring, the differentiated blood cells. Several types of stem cells can be defined experimentally by this approach (Fig. 28-1).

The Pluripotent Stem Cell

In mice subjected to amounts of ionizing radiation—about 9 Gray*—sufficient to destroy all hematopoiesis, and then given intravenous infusions of bone marrow from untreated mice, colonies of blood cells appear in the spleen. These discrete colonies contain erythrocytes, phagocytes, lymphocytes, and megakaryocytes, indicating that the donor infusion must have contained hematopoietic progenitor cells capable of differentiating into all blood cell types. Such pluripotent stem cells are capable of replicating themselves as required to respond to peripheral demands for differentiation into cells committed to the production of erythroid, phagocytic, and platelet lines. Physiologists refer to these cells as colony-forming units, stem cell, or simply CFU-S.

---

* One Gray is the radiation dose yielding 10^{10} ionizations per gram of tissue.

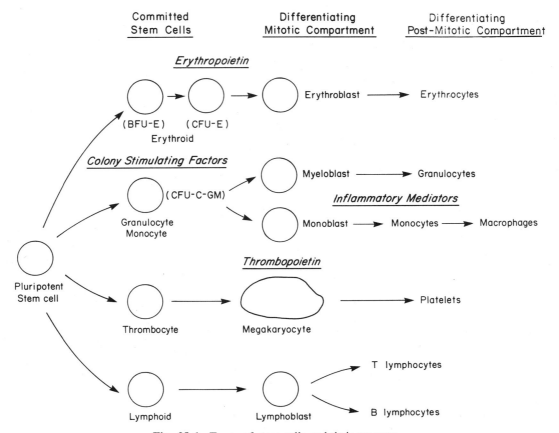

Fig. 28-1. Types of stem cells and their progeny.

Committed Stem Cells

The cultivation of bone marrow or peripheral blood in an appropriate medium can lead to the formation of colonies of cells differentiating into either phagocytic, erythroid, or megakaryocytic cells. These culture techniques are therefore believed to select for the expression of committed stem cells, designated CFU-C. The cultivation of bone marrow or peripheral blood in semisolid medium leads to the growth of discrete colonies containing cells having the morphology of phagocytes, polymorphonuclear leukocytes, and macrophages. This procedure is said to recruit colony-forming units for granulocytes and macrophages, abbreviated CFU-GM. Growth of peripheral

blood or bone marrow in plasma clots to which is added a source of erythropoietin leads to the outgrowth of different types of colonies containing erythroid cells. Large clusters of immature erythroid cells are defined as primitive burst-forming units, erythroid (BFU-E), named for the resemblance of these colonies to sunbursts. Smaller colonies are designated mature burst-forming units, erythroid; small cell colonies containing erythroid cells are believed to be the expression of relatively more mature erythroid stem cells, called colony-forming unit, erythroid (CFU-E). Appropriate cultivation techniques can also lead to the selection of stem cells committed to growth into megakaryocytes, colony-forming units, megakaryocytic (CFU-M). Current research is directed toward defining different stages of maturation of the committed stem cells, with the focus on the difference in the numbers and colonial morphology of the cells appearing under different cultural conditions.

The relevance of these culture systems to hematopoiesis in humans and in experimental animals is evident from the fact that the presence, absence, or number of colony-forming units obtainable from the bone marrow or peripheral blood often changes in parallel with alterations in the production of blood cells in the intact organism. Moreover, humoral factors can be shown to stimulate growth of particular blood cells, both in animals and the culture systems. For example, erythropoietin will enhance red cell production in mice and is also required for the expression of CFU-E in plasma clot cultures. Endotoxin, a lipopolysaccharide cell wall constituent of gram-negative bacteria, is a potent stimulus to granulocytopoiesis in animals and humans; it also induces macrophages and other cells to produce the colony-stimulating factors described in Chapter 1 (Table 1-1). Recently, the activity of hematopoietic hormones has been directly demonstrated in humans by the infusion of recombinant erythropoietin and colony-stimulating factors with subsequent enhancement of erythropoiesis and myelopoiesis, respectively.

Stem cells can be harvested from peripheral blood as well as from bone marrow. This fact suggests that the stem cells may sense the environmental demands for differentiation and replication by coursing through the blood and peripheral organs, as well as waiting in the bone marrow for humoral signals to provide this information. This circulation of stem cells might also explain how leukemic cells and other malignant stem cells are almost invariably found throughout the bone marrow at the outset of clinical disease. Furthermore, it explains how infusions of bone marrow stem cells into the peripheral blood can lead to engraftment of the bone marrow during the procedure of bone marrow transplantation (Ch. 32).

STEM CELL DISORDERS

Diseases affecting the pluripotent stem cell fall into four main categories (Table 28-1): (1) reversible or permanent stem cell failure; (2) qualitative abnormalities of stem cells; (3) uncontrolled proliferation of stem cells, and (4) malignant transformation of the stem cells.

The diseases in which stem cell proliferation leads to elevations in one or more peripheral blood cell types have historically been termed *myeloproliferative disorders*, simply meaning "proliferation of marrow." The diseases described in this section overlap with each other, as well as with some of the acute leukemias, especially the acute nonlymphocytic leukemias (see Ch. 19).

Many acquired stem cell diseases are disorders exhibiting abnormal stem cell clones. These clones may be manifested as increased, decreased, or qualitatively altered production of peripheral blood cells and in almost all cases involve the entire bone marrow. Yet at some time the clone must have arisen from one area of the bone marrow, another factor in support of the idea that stem cells leave the bone marrow and return to it in other locations.

Table 28-1. Stem Cell Disorders

Initial Disorder	Evolutionary Disorder
Bone marrow failure	
Aplastic anemia	Acute nonlymphocytic leukemia
Bone marrow dysplasia	
Paroxysmal nocturnal hemoglobinuria	Aplastic anemia or acute nonlymphocytic leukemia
Myelodysplasia	
Cyclic neutropenia	
Chronic idiopathic neutropenia	
Bone marrow hyperplasia	
Polycythemia vera	Myelofibrosis or acute nonlymphocytic leukemia
Myeloid metaplasia	Myelofibrosis
Bone marrow neoplasia	
Chronic granulocytic leukemia	Blast crisis
Essential thrombocythemia	Acute nonlymphocytic leukemia
Erythroleukemia	

Failure of the Pluripotent Stem Cell; Aplastic Anemia (Pancytopenia)

A large number of disease processes can interfere temporarily or permanently with the viability of the pluripotent stem cell. The end result is a single dismal clinical syndrome somewhat incompletely designated aplastic anemia, because the patient has leukopenia and thrombocytopenia as well as anemia, that is, pancytopenia.

The consequences of pancytopenia are depressingly straightforward: weakness, pallor, infection, and bleeding. The erythrocyte morphology is usually normal, and the anemia is therefore classifiable as normocytic and normochromic; but often, for unexplained reasons, the mean corpuscular volume may be abnormally high. Usually, the reticulocyte count is low, especially in the face of the anemia, indicating a failure of an erythroid response to the low circulating hemoglobin concentration. All the leukocyte forms are reduced in concentration, but especially the phagocytes, the polymorphonuclear leukocytes, and mono-

cytes, leaving the differential white blood cell count a monotonous picture of typical and a few atypical lymphocytes. Even the total lymphocyte count will be reduced, and the lymphocytes remaining presumably are long-lived memory cells. Few platelets will be seen on the blood smear, and the actual count confirms the presence of thrombocytopenia.

The known causes of aplastic anemia are physical, chemical, and biological agents capable of attacking the pluripotent stem cell in the bone marrow. These various insults presumably damage the genetic material of the pluripotent stem cell with sufficient vigor to cause cell death.

Physical Agents

Ionizing radiation directed against the entire bone marrow above a dose of 7 Gray will destroy all bone marrow stem cells and induce permanent pancytopenia. External radiation must be of the γ-ray or x-ray type capable of penetrating the body and gaining access to bone marrow cells. Lower doses of ionizing radiation are progressively less damaging, but reduce the reserve capacity of the bone marrow to respond to demands imposed by bleeding or infection. Radiation is most destructive to rapidly dividing cells, the mitotic compartment described in Chapter 1. It is evident from the rates of maturation of erythrocytes and granulocytes that basophilic normoblasts, myeloblasts, promyelocytes, and myelocytes turn over rapidly and are therefore susceptible to irradiation damage and other genetic insults. However, the fact that the bone marrow can recover from sublethal damage indicates that a portion of the stem cells are in a dormant or nondividing state at the time of exposure and are recruited into differentiation and replication after bone marrow aplasia. Indeed, one can show that the total number of CFU-GM in culture falls in the bone marrow of patients receiving cytotoxic chemotherapy or radiation toxic to the bone marrow.

Causes of Bone Marrow Failure

Physical agents
    Ionizing radiation

Chemical agents
    Organic solvents (benzene)
    Medications (chloramphenicol)

Biological agents
    Abnormal amino acid metabolism
      (ketotic hyperglycinemias)
    Metastic cancer and leukemia
    Granulomatous infections
    Congenital disorders (Fanconi's anemia)

Chemical Agents

Chemicals and drugs are frequently suspect in the causation of bone marrow failure, although only a few agents can be implicated definitively. Since the early 1900s, a frequent association of industrial exposures to benzene and benzene derivatives has made these organic solvents the prime culprits responsible for bone marrow damage and even leukemia. The mechanism of this effect is unknown. The extensive use of these chemicals for multiple uses in modern society creates the problem that an exposure to such chemical agents cannot always be identified. Certain medications are implicated as stem cell toxins. The most clear-cut examples are drugs used in cancer chemotherapy that are designed to kill tumor stem cells.

Acute damage to the bone marrow stem cells by toxins or drugs may be manifested primarily be neutropenia. The basis of this fact is the short life span of the neutrophil. About 7 days after the differentiation of stem cells is impaired, the bone marrow reserve of mature neutrophils will be depleted. Within 6 to 12 hours, the last blood neutrophil will leave the circulation; the profound neutropenia that results is commonly called *agranulocytosis*. The longer life span of reticulocytes and erythrocytes (120 days) and of platelets (7 days) buffers the impairment of production of these cells, and the resumption of stem cell activity will replenish erythrocytes and platelets faster than neutrophils, the generation time of erythrocytes and platelets being 4 days and 5 days, respectively, in contrast to 7 days for neutrophils. Drugs frequently associated with acute agranulocytosis are listed below.

Chloramphenicol, an antibiotic with a broad antibacterial spectrum, causes two types of bone marrow failure. The first is a dose- and time-dependent phenomenon in which the drug induces bone marrow suppression that is reversible after administration of the medication is discontinued. Most, if not all, patients receiving chloramphenicol are subject to this

---

Medications Associated with Acute Agranulocytosis

Psychoactive drugs
  Phenothiazines

Antithyroid drugs
  Thiourea compounds

Antibiotics
  Semisynthetic penicillins
  Sulfonamides

---

effect, which is manifested initially by a decrease in the reticulocyte count and a concomitant rise in serum iron, a result of cessation of erythropoiesis. Examination of the bone marrow at this time indicates vacuolation of the normoblasts. Subsequently, the white blood count, mainly the polymorphonuclear leukocyte count, falls, ultimately followed by a drop in the platelet count. This common and reversible toxicity of chloramphenicol on the bone marrow is overshadowed by the devastating permanent destructive effect of chloramphenicol on the bone marrow of the occasional patient.

Ethanol is also toxic to the bone marrow, although its direct effects on hematopoiesis are usually only apparent in the setting of heavy alcoholism, with or without concomitant vitamin (folic acid) deficiency. In the absence of folate deficiency, the anemia, leukopenia, and thrombocytopenia of alcohol are self-limited and rapidly reversible. Chronic alcoholism, however, can precipitate serious pancytopenia and complications thereof when associated with hepatic cirrhosis. Spur cell anemia and, more commonly, congestive splenomegaly can contribute to anemia. Hypersplenism together with alcoholic bone marrow suppression may aggravate thrombocytopenia, which together with coagulation factor deficiency resulting from the failing liver predisposes to bleeding.

The development of aplastic anemia in patients receiving a large variety of drugs commonly used in clinical medicine has raised the suspicion that these medications have a causal role, although proof thereof is hard to document. Nevertheless, a first step in the evaluation of a patient with pancytopenia should be to determine whether there has been an exposure to solvents or drugs and, whenever possible, to discontinue the exposure.

Biological Agents

Biological agents are also capable of causing the clinical picture of aplastic anemia. In disseminated tuberculosis, a granulomatous inflammatory infiltrate can replace the bone marrow. Neoplasms such as metastatic cancer, acute leukemia, multiple myeloma, and the lymphomas are capable of producing similar effects. Neutropenia, thrombocytopenia, or pancytopenia are concomitants of certain rare inborn errors of amino acid metabolism associated with accumulation of ketone bodies and glycine in the blood and urine. These disorders, grouped under the designation of *ketotic hyperglycinemias*, are methylmalonic acidemia, propionic acidemia, and isovaleric acidemia. It is presumed that one of the organic acids that accumulates in these disorders is toxic to the bone marrow stem cells. A genetic disorder predisposes to the development of aplastic anemia. Patients with Fanconi's anemia are found to have breaks in their chromosomes as well as various skeletal abnormalities. At about 5 to 7 years of age, progressive bone marrow failure occurs. The pluripotent stem cells in these patients are either programmed to fail after a finite life span or are abnormally susceptible to factors in the environment.

In most cases of aplastic anemia, none of the aforementioned causes can be identified, and the aplastic anemia is said to be of unknown cause, that is, idiopathic, Idiosyncratic reactions to unidentified toxins are difficult to rule out. A possible role of viral infections is suggested by the occasional finding of aplastic anemia after a case of viral hepatitis. A parvovirus has been associated with the transient aplasia occurring in patients with hemolytic disorders (aplastic crisis) but not with aplastic anemia.

Because many diseases including blood disorders are attributable to autoimmunity, it is appealing to speculate that autoimmunity against hematopoietic stem cells accounts for aplastic anemia. Except for some of the entities described in Chapter 29, this mechanism seems to be applicable in only a minority of cases where patients suffering from aplastic anemia have a response or even remission induced by immunosuppressive therapy (see below).

The success of bone marrow transplantation in reconstituting normal stem cell function in many patients with idiopathic aplastic anemia (Ch. 32) is evidence that whatever it was that destroyed the bone marrow is no longer present; otherwise, it would destroy the engrafted stem cells. The success of engraftment with bone marrow from identical twins, a setting in which no immunosuppression is required to prevent rejection of the donated bone marrow graft by the recipient's immune system, argues further against an important role of autoimmunity in the pathogenesis of many cases of idiopathic aplastic anemia.

The failure of hematopoiesis is not demonstrably attributable to lack of the erythropoietic or other hormones that stimulate blood cell synthesis, because the levels of these factors that can be measured are markedly elevated in patients with aplastic anemia.

Diagnosis and Management of Aplastic Anemia

Pancytopenia is an indication for examination of the bone marrow by both aspiration and biopsy. The biopsy is essential because infiltration of the bone marrow with granulomas or cancer cells can produce fibrosis, which in turn can result in an inability to aspirate marrow cells. Because bone marrow aplasia yields the same dry aspirate encountered in these other diseases, a diagnosis of aplastic anemia might be made in error, whereas a bone marrow biopsy would indicate the presence of tuberculosis, cancer, or fibrosis. The approach to the management of these various diseases differs considerably, hence a correct diagnosis is essential.

The biopsy specimen in aplastic anemia shows bone spicules; fat; marrow stromal cells, including fibroblasts, mast cells, and macrophages; some lymphocytes; and either a reduction or absence of normal hematopoietic cells, that is, cells of the erythroid, granulocytic, or megakaryocytic lineages. Occasionally, a bone marrow biopsy specimen of a patient with pancytopenia will have only slightly reduced normal or even increased numbers of hematopoietic cells. This finding may simply mean that the sample obtained is not representative of the total bone marrow mass. Alternatively, the observation of normal or increased hematopoietic cells in the face of pancytopenia can be a reflection of ineffective hematopoiesis. This finding is characteristic of a preleukemic syndrome. There is no completely reliable method for evaluating the hematopoietic activity of the total bone marrow. Ferrokinetic studies yield a characteristic picture in bone marrow failure. After injection of radioactive iron, the uptake of the iron into the bone marrow from the plasma is delayed or nonexistent. This pattern contrasts with that in ineffective erythropoiesis, in which the iron rapidly enters the bone marrow but, as in aplastic anemia, fails to appear in peripheral red blood cells.

Treatment of Stem Cell Failure

The first management principle is supportive care of the patient with pancytopenia; if, however, a remediable cause of the bone marrow failure is detectable, treatment should be begun as soon as possible. The approach to supportive treatment is essentially identical to that outlined for the patient with acute leukemia. Anemia is treated with transfusions of packed erythrocytes and thrombocytopenia with platelet transfusions. Infection must be diagnosed early with appropriate cultures of body fluids and excreta and must be treated vigorously with appropriate antibiotics.

Supportive care can maintain a reasonable existence for long periods of time in some patients with pancytopenia. However, for the profoundly thrombocytopenic patient, transfusions of platelets are needed at least weekly, and the supportive care becomes both expensive and tedious. Long-term transfusions with erythrocytes can lead to iron overload and the organ damage characteristic of hemochromatosis. Eventually, the development of antibodies against transfused erythrocytes and platelets limits the effectiveness of transfusion support. Moreover, the state of the art of phagocyte transfusion is not up to that of erythrocyte and platelet transfusions (see Ch. 30). Therefore, the patient with severe bone marrow depression is at high risk for overwhelming sepsis with low-grade pathogens.

It is possible to minimize infections in the pancytopenic patient by literally sterilizing the patient and his/her environment. The patient's skin is bathed with antiseptic solutions. Food is autoclaved, and the patient ingests nonabsorbable broad-spectrum antibiotics to remove microorganisms from the gastrointestinal tract. The patient is placed in a meticulously cleaned room the air intake of which is filtered to clear out microorganisms. These heroic measures can be effective, but their expense, effort, and negative psychological impact limit their utility.

Idiopathic aplastic anemia is probably the final common dénouement of different pathological processes. The relative rarity of idiopathic aplastic anemia—fewer than 1500 cases in the United States per year—makes it difficult to establish prognostic and therapeutic guidelines. Left untreated, most patients with profound pancytopenia and very empty marrows as shown by aspirate and biopsy are condemned to a permanent state of aplasia. However, some patients, especially those with some evidence of residual bone marrow activity, may show transient or even long-standing improvement in their hematopoiesis with time. The use of androgens may induce such improvement in a few cases.

Androgenic hormones have a mild stimulatory effect on hematopoiesis, especially on erythropoiesis, in normal physiological conditions. The higher red blood cell mass of males compared with that of females is the most obvious manifestation of the androgenic effect. Androgens appear to act primarily by increasing the production of erythropoietin in the kidney. Because most patients with aplastic anemia have high levels of circulating erythropoietin, androgens cannot be expected to be helpful in aplastic anemia unless they stimulate hematopoiesis directly. That such is the case is suggested by the occasional striking responses of patients with aplastic anemia to androgens. Reticulocyte counts and erythrocyte concentrations rise initially, followed by an increase in granulocytes and lastly, if at all, by the platelets.

Of the various androgen preparations available, the natural androgen, testosterone, has the disadvantage that it is not absorbed from the gastrointestinal tract and therefore must be given by injection, a disagreeable and potentially dangerous route in a patient with low platelet counts. Synthetic androgens that can be given by mouth have the disadvantage of having a propensity to cause damage to the liver. The side effects of androgens, especially virilization in females, make their continued administration less than desirable. After discontinuation of the androgens, the blood counts may remain at near-normal levels or may decline.

Unfortunately, only a few patients with severe aplastic anemia respond to androgen therapy. In a sense, this is not surprising, because a hormone has to have a target to work on, and the target in this case, the stem cells, is often depleted in this disease.

The treatment of choice for patients with severe aplastic anemia is now bone marrow transplantation, the repletion of stem cells by infusion of bone marrow from a histocompatible donor, usually a sibling (Ch. 32).

Therefore, an early step in the evaluation of a patient with aplastic anemia is to establish whether suitable bone marrow donors are available and to begin histocompatibility testing procedures as soon as possible. The urgency is based on the premise that (1) infection can set in at any time and either kill the patient or compromise the success of transplantation, and (2) the more transfusions the patient receives for support, the greater the risk of sensitization against antigenic determinants on the cells of the potential bone marrow donor. For the patient who lacks a potential bone marrow donor, it is reasonable to arrange for a program of supportive care and a trial of immunosuppressive therapy. In particular, commercially available antithymocyte globulin has produced therapeutic responses in about half of treated patients, and these patients have had longer survivals than patients given supportive care alone.

Bone Marrow Dysplasia

Cyclic Neutropenia

Cyclic neutropenia is a genetically inherited disease in which the activity of the pluripotent stem cell oscillates with a regular periodicity to create cyclic hematopoiesis. The principal expression of this intermittent hematopoiesis is a cyclic fluctuation in the peripheral blood neutrophil and monocyte counts, although subtle variations in reticulocyte, erythrocyte, and platelet counts can be detected. The reciprocal variations between neutrophil and monocyte counts reflect the shorter bone marrow maturation time of the monocyte compared with that of the neutrophil. The reason for the waxing and waning of the stem cell differentiation is unknown. Patients with cyclic neutropenia may become symptomatic when the granulocyte count is at its nadir. Such patients develop mouth ulcers and fevers at this time and, rarely, life-threatening infections. Cyclic neutropenia also exists in a strain of gray collie dogs. The disease can be cured by bone marrow transplantation from normal dogs, indicating that the disease process resides in the stem cell.

Congenital Neutropenia

Neutropenia in the newborn can arise from severe infection, from the presence of maternal isoantibodies against neutrophils, or as a genetically inherited trait. Inherited neutropenia, a rare condition, may be transmitted as a dominant recessive trait. The manifestations of inherited neutropenia are variable. For example, in some families affected members show depressed monocyte, lymphocyte, and neutrophil counts, whereas in other families affected members show elevated monocyte, lymphocyte, or eosinophil counts. The tendency of the affected person to acquire bacterial infections is inversely related to the average neutrophil count (see Ch. 18). For patients who manage to survive beyond early childhood with congenital neutropenia. the infection rate may decrease as other defenses become better developed. It is likely that many cases of congenital neutropenia are the result of an inborn defect in the stem cell. However, an interesting observation is that bone marrow from some of these neutropenic patients yields many mature neutrophils in tissue culture, suggesting some environmental insults in the patient's bone marrow.

Paroxysmal Nocturnal-Hemoglobinuria

Paroxysmal nocturnal hemoglobinuria is an acquired disorder, presumed to be clonal, of the pluripotent stem cell. The disease has a variety of clinical manifestations. The abnormal pluripotent stem cell clone coexists to a variable degree with the normal stem cells and yields progeny having altered surface membranes. These subtle and as yet uncharacterized alterations in membrane structures on the external surfaces of erythrocytes, phagocytes, and platelets cause the membranes under certain circumstances to appear foreign to the components of the alternative pathway of complement activation. The sequential attachment of alternative complement pathway proteins, C3, followed by the late-acting complement components to the membrane of the erythrocyte leads to its lysis.

Although the fundamental defect in the paroxysmal nocturnal hemoglobinuria cell membrane is unknown, it has recently become evident that a number of phenomena related to these cells can be explained by a common abnormality, the failure to synthesize or retain a class of membrane proteins normally bound to the lipid bilayer by a phosphatidylinositol-peptidoglycan linkage. One such protein is the enzyme acetylcholinesterase, long known to be deficient on paroxysmal nocturnal hemoglobinuria cells. Others are surface receptors including the class III Fc receptor that is normally present on polymorphonuclear leukocytes and macrophages (but not monocytes) (Ch. 18) and one of the lymphocyte adhesion molecules known as LFA1 and lately shown to be missing from or decreased in paroxysmal nocturnal hemoglobinuria neutrophils and lymphocytes, respectively. More pertinent to the functional abnormalities of the disorder is the fact that decay-accelerating factor (DAF), an entity that inhibits the propagation of complement action by participating in the inactivation of C3 on the cell surface, is one of these sugar-lipid-linked proteins. Its deficiency on paroxysmal nocturnal hemoglobinuria cells can explain at least in part the complement sensitivity of those cells.

The significance of the hemolysis in a given patient depends on the size of the abnormal stem cell clone and on the circumstances alluded to above. If the abnormal clone is small, a small number of complement-sensitive erythrocytes may turn over rapidly; the only clinical evidence of the disease will be a small increase in the reticulocyte count and possibly evidence of hemosiderin in the urine. At the other extreme, the patient may have massive intravascular hemolysis and chronic brisk hemolysis can lead to iron deficiency from iron loss as hemosiderin into the urine.

In the test tube, the binding of complement components to erythrocytes is promoted by increasing the hydrogen ion concentration or by decreasing the ionic strength of the medium. The latter is accomplished by diluting the blood with a sucrose solution adjusted for a physiological osmotic strength. Paroxysmal nocturnal hemoglobinuria, but not normal erythrocytes, bind complement components in this medium of low ionic strength; after centrifugation of the erythrocytes, the supernatant fluid over the normal erythrocytes is colorless, whereas that over the paroxysmal nocturnal hemobglobinuria cells is red. This procedure is the sucrose hemolysis test (or sugar water test), which is used to diagnose paroxysmal nocturnal hemoglobinuria.

The factors that determine the degree of complement fixation and hemolysis in the patient with paroxysmal nocturnal hemoglobinuria are unclear. The nocturnal exacerbation of hemolysis sometimes observed in which hemoglobulin appears in the urine at night—hence the name of the disease—has been ascribed to lowering of the blood pH by alveolar hypoventilation during sleep. Whether true or not, hemolysis in paroxysmal nocturnal hemoglobinuria can be quite variable in severity and can occur at any time.

Another clinical problem of paroxysmal nocturnal hemoglobinuria is arterial and venous thrombosis and the attendant infarction of organs, the circulation of which becomes compromised. Paroxysmal nocturnal hemoglobinuria is one cause of a hypercoagulable state possibly because platelets and granulocytes fix complement and aggregate. Platelets and granulocytes are more resistant to complement-mediated lysis than are erythrocytes, hence neutropenia and thrombocytopenia in paroxysmal nocturnal hemoglobinuria cannot be ascribed to direct complement-mediated destruction. However, the membrane perturbations inflicted by complement deposition on these cells render them "sticky," leading to their inappropriate aggregation in the vasculature.

Because hypoplasia of the bone marrow and pancytopenia are manifestations of paroxysmal nocturnal hemoglobinuria, this disease is one cause of the clinical spectrum of aplastic anemia. Although paroxysmal nocturnal hemoglobinuria is a rare disease, a sufficient number of cases have evolved after variable periods of time into acute myelogenous or myelomonocytic leukemia to merit consideration of paroxysmal nocturnal hemoglobinuria as a preneoplastic disorder.

The treatment of paroxysmal nocturnal hemoglobinuria in its hemolytic phase is the same as that of any chronic hemolytic anemia of comparable severity. The treatment of paroxysmal nocturnal hemoglobinuria-associated bone marrow hypoplasia is similar to that of bone marrow failures in general.

Myelodysplastic Syndromes

This group of interrelated stem cell diseases presents a spectrum ranging from chronic anemia unresponsive to iron, vitamins, or other measures without other blood cell abnormalities to a blatantly "preleukemic" state with anemia, rising percentage of blasts in the bone marrow, thrombocytopenia, and bizzare myeloid and erythroid maturation. The cause and pathogenesis of the refractory anemias are unknown, but all evidence points to their being manifestations of acquired genetic changes in the pluripotent stem cell that programs a wide variety of phenotypic abnormalities in blood cell maturation, morphology, and function. The refractory anemias may be chronic and stable or may evolve to either pancytopenia or leukemia.

The anemias are refractory in that most do not respond to treatment of the patient with iron, folic acid, vitamin B_{12}, or pyridoxine, agents that would be expected to be effective against deficiency disorders involving these compounds and that present with similar erythroid morphology. The erythrocytes are frequently macrocytic. Ringed sideroblasts may be prominent in the bone marrow along with varying degrees of megaloblastic maturation. The anemias are of variable severity, and some patients require frequent red cell transfusions. Numerous deficiencies of enzyme activities involved in heme synthetic pathways have been observed in the bone marrow cells of such patients.

Thrombocytopenia, a neutrophilic leukocytosis, and monocytosis sometimes may be present. Abnormalities of neutrophilic polymorphonuclear leukocyte maturation reminiscent of the myelodysplastic changes seen in the maturation pattern in acute granulocytic leukemia are frequently encountered. These aberrations include giant pink or azure granules coexisting in the same granulocytic cells, the Pelger-Huet anomaly of the nuclei of neutrophils, or marked nuclear hypersegmentation of the neutrophils.

That myelodysplasia has a neoplastic aspect is strengthened by the fact that these disorders are one of the complications of treatment of cancer and leukemia with mutagenizing therapy. Furthermore, the bone marrow cells from a majority of patients with myelodysplasia have discernable chromosomal abnormalities, particularly hypoploidy and loss of specific chromosomal segments. The most common finding is monosomy or partial loss of the long arm of chromosome 7 ($7q^-$). Alterations of chromosomes 3 and 5 are also frequent findings.

The classification of the myelodysplastic syndromes (Table 28-2) depends on the morphology and course of the refractory anemias. The propensity of the disorder to progress to frank leukemia is related to the number of affected cell lines and the degree of immaturity and dysplasia of the bone marrow. The presence of chromosomal abnormalities, especially complex changes, is associated with increased risk of leukemic progression.

Abnormal Proliferation of Stem Cells

Polycythemia Vera

General Features

Polycythemia vera is the name historically given to a chronic myeloproliferative disorder in which the production of erythrocytes, phagocytes, and platelets is increased and in which the accumulation of erythrocytes is the dominant feature. The erythrocyte mass may increase to very high levels. In patients who have two glucose 6-phosphate-dehydrogenase (G6PD) isoenzymes in addition to polycythemia vera, the erythrocytes contain a single G6PD isoenzyme. This feature indicates that polycythemia vera is a disorder of a pluripotent clone stem cell that acquires a selective advantage through a reduction in control over

Table 28-2. French-American-British (FAB) Classification of the Myelodysplastic Syndromes

Classification	Characteristics
Refractory anemia (RA)	Anemia unresponsive to iron. 15% progress to acute nonlymphocytic leukemia (ANLL)
Refractory anemia with ringed sideroblasts	> 15% of marrow erythroblasts are ringed sideroblasts. 15% progress to ANLL
Refractory anemia with excess blasts (RAEB)	5–20% of nucleated marrow cells are blasts. Dysplastic features are prominent, and thrombocytopenia is common. 30% progress to ANLL
Chronic myelomonocytic leukemia (CMML)	Refractory anemia, thrombocytopenia, monocytosis, 5–20% bone marrow blasts, 40% progression to ANLL
RAEB "in transformation"	20–30% bone marrow blasts, anemia, thrombocytopenia, invariable progression to ANLL

its proliferation. Erythropoietin levels are low in the urine of patients with polycythemia vera, further illustrating that the blood proliferation that occurs in this disease is autonomous. The neutrophil and platelet counts are often elevated but to levels less than 25,000/μl and 800,000/μl; respectively. Leukocyte alkaline phosphatase activity is usually elevated. The basophil count is frequently increased and may be responsible for elevations in blood and urinary histamine in patients with polycythemia vera. The peripheral blood morphology is usually normal.

The main clinical manifestation of the increased hematopoiesis of polycythemia vera is ascribable to the effects of the elevated red blood cell concentration on blood flow. The relationship between blood flow and erythrocyte concentration is complex and depends on cardiac output, blood vessel size, and the hematocrit. A relatively small hematocrit elevation above the normal range can cause blood flow in an organ to fall by one-third to one-half. Therefore, symptoms of polycythemia vera are often those of deficient cerebral blood flow, such as headaches, dizziness, and abnormalities of vision. Engorgement of skin blood vessels can cause a ruddy color and, for reasons that are unclear, patients with polycythemia vera suffer from itching of the skin after a warm bath. Some patients with polycythemia vera have abnormally activated platelets that aggregate spontaneously or after minimal stimulation. This platelet hyperactivity, in some instances combined with elevated platelet counts, can contribute to vascular insufficiency by promoting coagulation in engorged capillaries with slow blood flow. Paradoxically, the hyperactive platelets may not function properly in hemostasis, and a bleeding tendency can result as well. The increased cell turnover in polycythemia vera can lead to hyperuricemia

Diagnosis and Management

First, erythrocytosis must be diagnosed by showing that the patient actually has an elevated red cell mass. An elevated hematocrit, the usual presenting finding, only suggests the presence of erythrocytosis; it does not establish it. The distinction between an elevated hematocrit and erythrocytosis is important; in fact, the combination of a modest elevation in the hematocrit and a normal red cell mass is common. Known as Gaisböck's syndrome or stress erythrocytosis, this combination is typically seen in hard-driving middle-aged men who tend to be smokers, overweight, and hypertensive. The red cell mass in these patients is generally on the high side of normal, whereas plasma volumes are in the low-normal range, leading to a high hematocrit without an increase in red cell mass. Stress erythrocytosis is important to diagnose, because patients with this condition may be at risk for heart attacks and other vascular occlusive disease.

The red cell mass can be measured by labeling a known quantity of the patient's red cells with ^{51}Cr, reinjecting them, and after sufficient time for complete mixing, determining by what factor the tagged cells were diluted by the patient's own circulating red cells.

The second task is to differentiate polycythemia vera from the various causes of secondary polycythemia (described in Ch. 12), which are physiological responses to tissue hypoxemia. These diseases can be diagnosed by measurements of arterial oxygen saturation or the hemoglobin oxygen dissociation curve. Certain clinical features are helpful in pointing to a diagnosis of polycythemia vera. Patients with polycythemia vera tend to be middle-aged or elderly men with elevations in the granulocyte and platelet counts as well as the hematocrit, absence of pulmonary disease, and moderate splenic enlargement. The serum uric acid level is often elevated in conditions of accelerated myelopoiesis. Uric acid is a breakdown product of purine metabolism. The bone marrow examination shows an excessive number of normal red cell precursors.

The goal in the treatment of polycythemia is to reduce the red cell mass. This reduction can be easily achieved in many patients by means of monthly phlebotomies. Unfortunately, bleeding promotes platelet production and, when the abnormal platelets of polycythemia increase in number, the bleeding and thrombotic manifestations of the disease become more of a problem. Therefore, treatment is often directed at the abnormal stem cell. Radioactive phosphorus, ^{32}P-phosphoric acid, injected into the circulation is incorporated into the DNA of the bone marrow stem cells. The β-radiation emitted by the radionuclide kills some of these cells. The treatment is sufficient to reduce the proliferation of polycythemia vera bone marrow for prolonged periods of time. The relative permanence of the treatment together with the control of platelet production are somewhat offset by the carcinogenic risk of ionizing radiation. However, the carcinogenic potential of radioactive phosphorus is lower than that accompanying the administration of alkylating agents to suppress the proliferation of the bone marrow.

Polycythemia vera can be managed successfully by means of the treatments mentioned for long periods of time. The disease may evolve slowly over a period of years into a burnt-out phase wherein the bone marrow proliferation returns to normal. Thereafter, the bone marrow may even begin to develop fibrosis, and pancytopenia may ensue.

Idiopathic Myelofibrosis

Although focal fibrosis of the bone marrow can be an accompaniment of inflammatory disease and of metastatic cancer, a distinct disease entity is idiopathic myelofibrosis. In this disorder, a progressive fibrosis of the bone marrow is accompanied to a variable degree by evidence of increased proliferation of granulocytes and by the development of myeloid metaplasia, that is, foci of hematopoiesis in the liver and spleen. This extramedullary hematopoiesis differs from the extraosseous blood cell development associated with severe hemolytic anemias, in which the bone marrow expands by direct extension into neighboring tissues. In idiopathic myelofibrosis with myeloid metaplasia, the bone marrow develops in the organs of hematopoiesis of fetal life: the liver and spleen. It is not known why myeloid metapla-

sia occurs in response to idiopathic myelofibrosis and why it is unusual in other diseases that infiltrate the bone marrow, such as lymphomas and solid tumors. Idiopathic myelofibrosis is sometimes the sequel of long-standing polycythemia vera.

Studies of G6PD isoenzymes in idiopathic myelofibrosis have indicated that the granulocyte proliferation reflects the expansion of a single clone of stem cells, whereas the fibroblasts populating the bone marrow are not of a single clonal origin. From this work it is concluded that the bone marrow fibrosis represents a reaction to some stimulus elaborated by the clonal disorder. To some extent, the accumulation of granulocytes in the blood is itself a reaction to the fibrosis. The peripheral blood picture is usually initially that of a leukoerythroblastic reaction with immature granulocytes and erythrocytes in the peripheral blood. The erythrocyte morphology is abnormal, featuring misshapen red cells, especially teardrop forms.

The cause of idiopathic myelofibrosis is unknown. The clonality of the disorder implies an acquired genetic disease resembling cancer or leukemia. In addition, chromosomal abnormalities are frequent in idiopathic myelofibrosis, particularly deletions of the long arm of chromosome 13 (13q⁻) and t[1;13] translocations. One hypothesis relates the frequent presence of morphologically abnormal and dysfunctional platelets in idiopathic myelofibrosis (see Ch. 14) to the fibrotic process. Platelets contain a growth factor called platelet-derived growth factor (PDGF), which is mitogenic for a variety of cells including fibroblasts. Interestingly, one of the two polypeptides comprising PDGF is highly homologous to an oncogene product of the acute transforming primate retrovirus, the simian sarcoma virus *c-sis*. It is proposed that elaboration of PDGF or PDGF-related peptides by the aberrant megakaryocytes in idiopathic myelofibrosis stimulates fibroblastic proliferation, resulting in a net increase in collagen deposition in the bone marrow.

The clinical manifestations of idiopathic myelofibrosis are initially the effects of splenomegaly, which can become massive. The enlarged spleen can impair digestion and appetite by compressing the stomach and can create an unpleasant feeling of heaviness in the left upper quadrant. The enlarged spleen can also sequester and destroy peripheral blood cells. The enlarged spleen may become infarcted, resulting in acute left upper quadrant pain radiating into the left shoulder. A friction rub may be audible in the left upper quadrant when the patient respires in such cases. The spleen can even rupture after minimum trauma in this area, causing an acute abdomen and possible death from hemorrhage.

Later in the course of idiopathic myelofibrosis, bone marrow failure and pancytopenia become dominant, as the myeloid metaplasia cannot compensate for the loss of bone marrow function incurred by the myelofibrosis. The liver may fail from compromised parenchymal function caused by progressive myeloid metaplasia within the organ. The patient eventually dies of liver failure, hemorrhage, or infection. The usual treatment for idiopathic myelofibrosis is palliative, involving support for the progressive pancytopenia, packed erythrocyte transfusions for the anemia, and platelet infusions for thrombocytopenia. Splenectomy can alleviate the symptoms of massive splenomegaly and occasionally lead to an improvement in peripheral blood counts when splenic sequestration of cells dominates splenic hematopoiesis.

The rate of progression of idiopathic myelofibrosis is variable. In some cases the course may be relatively slow and stable. Patients who present without large spleens, severe anemia, or thrombocytopenia may have a median survival of 10 years. Others with these findings, however, may succumb with a year or two.

Intensive cytotoxic treatment followed by allogeneic bone marrow transplantation (Ch. 32) has led to the cure of a few patients with idiopathic myelofibrosis. This outcome is not only of importance for the patients eligible for such therapy but also because it demonstrates that the primary disorder resides in the hematopoietic stem cell, not the fibrous stroma that proliferates. Also remarkable is the fact that the normal transplanted hematopoietic cells engrafted in the fibrotic bone marrow space and that the fibrosis resolved following transplantation.

Neoplasms of the Stem Cells

Chronic Granulocytic Leukemia

Chronic granulocytic leukemia, also called chronic myelogenous leukemia, is a disease characterized by a proliferation of a malignant clone of pluripotent stem cells usually expressed as an exuberant production of granulocytes, especially neutrophils and basophils. This aspect of chronic granulocytic leukemia, called the *chronic phase*, may persist, causing relatively little morbidity to many patients for a variable duration averaging 2 to 3 years. After this time, the malignant nature of the process becomes more striking. The proliferating cells become predominantly immature blasts that manifest the malignant propensity to invade organs, and the disease comes to behave like an acute leukemia. The acute leukemic phase of chronic granulocytic leukemia is designated chronic granulocytic leukemia in blastic crisis. The incidence of chronic granulocytic leukemia is highest in middle-aged persons, affects males more than females, but may occur in childhood.

In the chronic phase of chronic granulocytic leukemia, the peripheral blood contains granulocytes, usually 15,000/μl and often up to 100,000/μl; the granulocytes are of all stages of maturation. The increased granulocyte mass is also evident in the bone marrow and spleen, and the latter can often be massively enlarged. The crowding effect of the proliferative process in the bone marrow can produce a leukoerythroblastic picture such that misshapen erythrocytes and teardrop forms appear in the peripheral blood. Chronic granulocytic leukemia in the chronic phase is easily distinguished from other myeloproliferative disorders and leukemoid reactions, which may also express leukoerythroblastic pictures in the peripheral

Fig. 28-2. Origin of the Philadelphia chromosome.

blood, as well as splenomegaly by the presence of two phenomena unique to chronic granulocytic leukemia.

The first is a chromosomal aberration wherein a translocation of genetic material takes place between the long arms of the 22nd and 9th chromosomes. This translocation is most evident from the short-legged appearance of chromosome 22 in karyotypic analyses (Fig. 28-2). This chromosome is called the *Philadelphia chromosome* (abbreviated Ph_1) after the city in which it was first observed. The presence of the Philadelphia chromosome is not only diagnostic of chronic granulocytic leukemia, but has also provided the evidence, in addition to G6PD isoenzyme typing of erythrocytes and leukocytes, for the clonal origin of chronic granulocytic leukemia. Furthermore, the abnormal chromosome can be found in dividing cells of lymphocytic as well as granulocytic lineage, indicating that chronic granulocytic leukemia is a disorder of the pluripotent stem cell.

The second feature of chronic granulocytic leukemia, which is only slightly less specific for the disease than the Philadelphia chromosome, is a low level of activity of the enzyme *alkaline phosphatase* in the mature-appearing polymorphonuclear leukocytes. Only occasionally is a low alkaline phosphatase score found in other disorders, including some cases of the myeloproliferative diseases and paroxysmal hemoglobinuria.

Molecular Pathogenesis

Chronic granulocytic leukemia was the first example of a consistent genetic abnormality associated with neoplastic disease. The key event in the balanced translocation between chromosomes 9 and 22 is the placement of an oncogene usually on chromosome 9 to chromosome 22. The oncogene is *c-abl*, which is related to the transforming gene *v-abl* of the Abelson virus, a retrovirus that produces a lymphoid neoplasm in mice. The *abl* oncogene is a representative of the class described in Chapter 19 that has tyrosine kinase activity believed to be involved in the stimulation of cell division. The region on chromosome 22 where *c-abl* lands is called the *bcr cluster gene*. What then happens is that a fusion product of *bcr* and *c-abl* is produced constitutively that has tyrosine kinase activity that is greater than that of the normal *c-abl* gene product. On the other hand, *abl* is not the whole story in the neoplastic behavior of chronic granulocytic leukemia. The *bcr/abl* fusion gene product does not by itself transform fibroblasts in transfection assays, and other oncogenes, which include *myc* and *ras*, can be expressed in chronic granulocytic leukemia cells. Moreover, once chronic granulocytic leukemia goes into blast crisis, the *bcr/abl* gene may be deleted without alteration in the progress of the disease.

Clinical Features

The initial effects of chronic granulocytic leukemia on the patient are manifestations of the enlarged granulocyte mass. The enlarged spleen may cause a feeling of discomfort in the left upper quadrant or even impair the patient's appetite and digestion by compressing the stomach. When the granulocytic proliferation becomes extensive, the patient begins to suffer from loss of appetite and weight loss. Anemia and thrombocytopenia may result from crowding of the bone marrow by the granulocytic proliferation. Occasionally, a plethora of granulocytes in the peripheral blood can cause obstruction of the blood circulation with signs and symptoms of cerebral hypoxia or organ infarction. Nevertheless, in many patients with chronic granulocytic leukemia in the chronic phase, the disease may present relatively few problems.

The onset of blast crisis is heralded by progressive immaturity of the peripheral blood granulocytes, by increases in the basophil count in the peripheral blood, and by the appearance of chromosomal abnormalities in addition to the Philadelphia chromosome. Treatment of the chronic phase does not influence the time of onset of blast crisis in chronic granulocytic leukemia.

The blasts in blast crisis chronic granulocytic leukemia may resemble myeloblasts or lymphoblasts, a variability reflecting the pluripotent stem cell origin of the leukemic process. When the lymphoblastic morphology is evident, an event seen in one-third of cases, the blasts contain the enzyme terminal deoxyribonucleotide transferase, a marker of lymphoblasts in acute lymphoblastic leukemia and also may express clonal immunoglobulin gene rearrangements characteristic of B-cell maturation.

Treatment

The goal of therapy of the chronic phase of chronic granulocytic leukemia has traditionally been to keep the granulocyte count from rising above 25,000/μl. This has been relatively easily accomplished by means of small doses of alkylating agents or with hydroxyurea (see Ch. 31). Following these treatments, the white blood cell count falls, the hematocrit may rise, and the spleen may decrease in size. A recent addition to the therapeutic armamentarium has been the recombinant lymphokines, α and γ interferon. Although the responses to these agents are less reliable than to chemotherapeutic agents, they are potentially less toxic. Either low dose alkylating agents or interferons represent suppressive and not curative treatment. The Philadelphia chromosome persists in the setting of normal blood counts, indicating the lingering specter of the malignant clone.

Stable-phase chronic granulocytic leukemia invariably progresses to the blast phase, and the blasts have proved extremely resistant to chemotherapy. Vincristine and prednisone, drugs useful in the treatment of acute lymphoblastic leukemia, can yield responses when the blastic phase of chronic granulocytic leukemia is lymphoid in appearance and markers, but the responses are transient. To avoid an inevitably fatal outcome, therefore, it is necessary to replace the malignant stem cell with allogenic bone marrow transplantation. This is theoretically the treatment of choice for patients with suitable marrow donors (Ch. 32). Seventy to 90 percent of patients thus transplanted have had prolonged leukemia-free survival. Preferably this approach would be taken long before the emergence of blasts resistant to cytotoxic agents used to ablate the host bone marrow before transplantation. Unfortunately, bone marrow transplantation is not uniformly successful and risk-free, and its failures and risks must be balanced against the median survival of relatively asymptomatic patients with chronic granulocytic leukemia.

These uncertainties have encouraged investigators to stratify patients in the chronic phase according to features that may predict the duration of this phase. In general, patients with relatively low white blood counts, low percentages of blasts, small spleens, lack of anemia and thrombocytopenia, and relatively few chromosomal abnormalities can expect longer survival. Researchers are determining whether it is possible to prolong the chronic phase of chronic granulocytic leukemia in patients not eligible for bone marrow transplantation by administration of combinations of chemotherapeutic agents. Another approach is to freeze bone marrow from the chronic-phase patient and then perform an autologous bone marrow transplant when the patient enters blast crisis in an effort to restore the chronic phase (see Ch. 32). An even "higher technology" variation on this theme is to treat the bone marrow with drugs that might kill the malignant blast cells. Interestingly, cultivation of blast crisis bone marrow resulted in the dropout of malignant blast cells followed by outgrowth of normal hematopoietic cells, raising the theoretical possibility of returning marrow cultured in vitro to a leukemic patient treated to ablate endogenous bone marrow stem cells. Recently, it was found that the antitumor antibiotic mithramycin can induce differentiation of chronic granulocytic leukemia blasts and concomitantly diminish expression of *c-abl* and *c-myc*. Treatment of some patients in blast crisis with mithramycin and hydroxyurea returned patients from blast crisis to the chronic phase, although continuous treatment was required. The utility of these now experimental modalities is unclear.

SUGGESTED READINGS

Bartram, C.R., Janssen, J.W.G., Becher, R., et al. (1986). Persistence of chronic myelocytic leukemia despite deletion of rearranged *bcr*/c-*abl* sequences in blast crisis. J. Exp. Med. *164*:1389.

Bennett, J.M., Catovsky, D., Daniel, M.T., et al. (1982) Proposals for the classification of the myelodysplastic syndromes. Br. J. Haematol. *51*: 189.

Berk, P.D. (1986) Therapeutic recommendations in polycythemia vera based on Polycythemia Vera Study Group protocols. Semin. Hematol. *23*:132.

Champlin, R.E., & Golde, D.W. (1985) Chronic myelogenous leukemia: Recent advances. Blood *65*:1039.

Clark, S.C., Kamen, R. (1987) The human hematopoietic colony stimulating factors. Science *236*: 1229.

Goldman, J.M., Apperley, J.F., Jones, L., et al. (1986) Bone marrow transplantation for patients with chronic myeloid leukemia. N. Engl. J. Med. *314*:202.

Koller, C.A., Campbell, V.W., Polansky, D.A., et al. (1985) In vivo differentiation of blast-phase

chronic granulocytic leukemia. Expression of c-*myc* and c-*abl* protooncogenes. J. Clin. Invest. *76*:365.

Koller, C.A., & Miller, D.M. (1986) Preliminary observations on the therapy of the myeloid blast phase of chronic granulocytic leukemia with plicamycin and hydroxyurea. N. Engl. J. Med. *315*:1433.

Liu, E., Hjelle, B., Bishop, R.M. (1988) Transforming genes in chronic myelogenous leukemia. Proc. Natl. Acad. Sci. USA *85*:1952.

Low, M.G., Ferguson, M.A.J., Futerman, A.H., & Silman, I. (1986) Covalently attached phosphatidylinositol as a hydrophobic anchor for membrane proteins. Trends Biochem. Sci. *11*:212.

Marsh, J.C.W., Hows, J.M., Bryett, K.A., et al. (1987) Survival after antilymphocyte globulin therapy for aplastic anemia depends on disease severity. Blood *70*:1046.

Sokal, J.E., Baccarani, M., Russo, D., & Tura, S. (1988) Staging and prognosis in chronic myelogenous leukemia. Semin. Hematol. *25*:49.

Spangrude, G.J., Heimfeld, S. & Weissman, I.L. (1988) Purification and characterization of mouse hematopoietic stem cells. Science *241*:58–62.

Talpaz, M., Kantarjian, H.M., Kurzrock, R., Gutterman, J. (1988) Therapy of chronic myelogenous leukemia: Chemotherapy and interferons. Semin. Hematol. *25*:62.

Thomas, E.D., & Storb, R. (1984) Acquired severe aplastic anemia: Progress and perplexity. Blood *64*:325.

Ward, H.P., & Block, M.H. (1971) The natural history of agnogenic myeloid metaplasia (AMM) and a critical evaluation of its relationship with the myeloproliferative syndrome. Medicine *50*: 357.

Whang-Peng, J., Young, R.C., Lee, E.C., et al. (1988) Cytogenetic studies in patients with secondary leukemia/dysmyelopoietic syndrome after different treatment modalities. Blood *71*:403.

Immune Destruction of Blood Cells

GENERAL PRINCIPLES

The destructive potential of the immune system is ordinarily directed against foreign microorganisms. When blood cells from one person are purposefully or accidentally infused into another genetically unrelated person, components on the cell surface, antigens, may be recognized as foreign and fall prey to the immune mechanisms. Such immune reactions generated by humans against other humans are called *isoimmune* reactions; the antibodies produced by humans against the blood cells of other humans are called *isoantibodies*. Isoantibodies limit the survival of transfused blood cells, and the destruction of transfused blood cells can produce systemic symptoms, called a *transfusion reaction*. Isoantibodies may also arise from the sensitization of a mother by the blood cells of her fetus. Isoantibodies of the IgG class cross the placenta and can destroy the blood cells of the fetus.

The immune system can occasionally become perverse and active against itself. This general pathological process is called *autoimmunity* (Ch. 21). Autoimmunity, or autoaggression as it was first called, can be viewed as a loss of the tolerance ordinarily possessed by the immune system for self-antigens. Blood cells are susceptible to autoimmune destruction, and the immunological reactions may be active against stem cells, erythroid cells, plate-lets, lymphoid cells, phagocytes, or combinations of blood cells.

All the effector mechanisms of the immune system—antibody and complement-mediated cell lysis, antibody and complement-mediated opsonization, and lymphoid cell-mediated cell destruction—may be operative in the attack on normal blood cells. Antibodies directed against self-antigens are called *autoantibodies*. Autoimmune blood cell destruction is said to be primary if it occurs in the absence of other diseases known to affect the immune system. Otherwise, the autoimmune disorder is designated secondary. Clearly there must be some reason for the onset of autoimmunity in the primary setting, but the predisposing causation is simply not obvious. Frequently the onset of antibody-mediated blood cell destruction follows a viral infection, especially in children. In this setting, the autoimmune reaction may be the result of immune complexes composed of virus antigens and antibodies against these antigens. The autoimmune disorder of this type frequently remits permanently after a period of months. In older patients, in whom the onset of autoimmune blood cell destruction is less frequently preceded by an obvious infection, the disease tends to be chronic, although variable, in severity.

Disorders predisposing to secondary autoimmune blood cell destruction include the congenital and acquired immunodeficiency states, collagen-vascular diseases such as systemic lupus erythematosus, and malignant lymphoid neoplasms, especially of the B-cell variety. Mediations, some of which are used frequently in medical practice, are capable of inciting immune-mediated blood cell destruction by a variety of mechanisms.

MECHANISMS OF IMMUNE-MEDIATED BLOOD CELL DESTRUCTION

Agglutination

IgM antibodies activate complement and agglutinate cells. It is possible that agglutinated blood cells become trapped in capillaries of organs rich in mononuclear phagocytes such as the liver, lungs, and particularly the spleen, where their exposure to the phagocytes and lymphoid cells that can destroy them is maximized. Agglutination is probably not a major mechanism of blood cell destruction but is a useful phenomenon for identifying the presence of IgM antibodies directed against certain blood cells.

Complement-Mediated Cytolysis

IgM and IgG antibodies can activate complement components, leading to the deposition of complement components C1–C9, the production of membrane lesions, and loss of cytoplasmic components (Ch. 17).

Opsonization

Opsonization of blood cells leading to recognition by phagocytes is the principal and most prevalent mechanism in operation in immune-mediated blood cell destruction. The Fab region of IgG molecules binds to surface antigens of blood cells, leaving the Fc regions exposed to interact with receptors on phagocytes and lymphoid cells. The phagocytes can bind and either partially or totally engulf the antibody-coated blood cells. Total phagocytosis clears the opsonized cells from the circulation. Partial phagocytosis removes membrane from the blood cells, reducing their volume as well as their capacity to cope with osmotic stresses.

IgG or IgM antibodies against blood cell surface antigens can bind to these antigens and activate complement, leading to the deposition of C3b, the opsonic fragment of C3 on the blood cell surface. This deposition sets the cell up for total or partial engulfment by phagocytes as well. It will be recalled that C3b is attacked by an enzyme complex, the C3b inactivator, and β-1H. The balance between the rates of deposition of C3b on the cell and of the rate of C3b inactivation determines, among other factors, whether the cells are susceptible to attack by phagocytes.

The phagocytes primarily involved in the destruction of blood cells are the fixed phagocytes; these macrophages of the mononuclear phagocyte system are located in the organs of clearance, where they come into intimate contact with the opsonized blood cells. The removal of blood cells by phagocytes is most efficient in the spleen, because of its sluggish flow and sievelike structure. Therefore, lightly opsonized blood cells may be destroyed primarily in the spleen, although more heavily coated cells can be removed by the Kupffer cells of the liver. Cytotoxic lymphocytes can also recognize antibody-coated target cells and lyse them.

Role of Temperature in Immune-Mediated Blood Cell Destruction

Antibody reactions against blood cell reactions are sensitive to the ambient temperature. IgG antibody molecules against blood cell antigens almost always bind to the blood cells at 37°C, normal body temperature; they have been historically designated *warm-reacting antibodies*. IgM antibody molecules directed against blood cells often bind to the antigens better at lower temperatures; they have been historically termed *cold-reactive antibodies*. Because IgM antibodies agglutinate cells, cold-reactive antibodies have also been termed *cold agglutinins*. The thermal amplitude of the antibody reaction can be determined by incubating blood cells with a variety of dilutions of antibody-containing serum at different temperatures and observing the maximal dilution or titer of serum that agglutinates the cells.

Cold-reactive IgM antibodies can arise during infections. Viral infections associated with such antibodies include infectious mononucleosis caused by the Epstein-Barr virus, bacterial infections including syphilis (EBV), and infections caused by *Mycoplasma*. Occasionally, antibody-secreting lymphoid neoplasms produce monoclonal IgM antibodies in large quantities that react with blood cells at low temperatures. The practical importance of the thermal amplitude of cold-reactive antibodies is that blood cell destruction may be initiated or exacerbated by exposure of the patient to cold temperatures.

The presence of antibody molecules or complement components on the surface of blood cells is a necessary condition, but it is not sufficient to cause immune-mediated blood cell destruction. Destruction of blood cells by immunoproteins requires either that the entire complement sequence leads to membrane lysis or that the Fc region of the immunoglobulin molecule, with or without participation of the third component of complement, causes the blood cell to be recognized as foreign by phagocytes or lymphocytes. Therefore, these molecules must be oriented on the blood cell surface so as to engender such recognition. When the Fab domains of IgG antibody molecules bind to blood-cell surface antigens, the Fc portions of the antibody molecules are oriented appropriately to interact with phagocyte Fc receptors or with C1 for complement activation. On the other hand, it will be recalled that B lymphocytes contain surface immunoglobulin. This immunoglobulin is presumably oriented with its Fc region buried within the plasma membrane, and therefore it will not elicit either complement fixation or recognition by phagocytes. However, the surface immunoglobulin can be detected by another antibody molecule specific for immunoglobulin. In a similar fashion, IgG antibodies bound to Fc receptors on cells also have their Fc regions masked. Therefore, only antibodies with the Fab domains apposed to blood cell surface antigens would be expected to have Fc portions free to interact with complement or phagocytic receptors. Even correctly oriented immunoglobulin molecules on blood cell membranes may fail to result in destruction of the blood cells.

Depending on the class of antibody, the propensity for destruction varies. For example, IgM usually has no direct opsonic effect but requires complement deposition for destruction of the target. The effect of complement fixation will depend on the relative rates of complement addition and inactivation. If inactivation of C3b exceeds its deposition, C3 fragments remain on the membrane of the target cell, but the fragments are incapable of fixing later complement components or of expressing opsonic activity. Finally, aggregated immunoglobulins are much more effective than dispersed immunoglobulins in eliciting complement fixation or recognition by phagocytes. Therefore, the antigen density and mobility on the blood cell surface that will influence the aggregation state of the surface molecules can determine whether or not destruction occurs. This factor explains in part why certain red blood cell antigens are more important in the transfusion setting than others.

GENERAL PRINCIPLES OF TREATMENT OF IMMUNE-MEDIATED BLOOD CELL DESTRUCTION

Some cases of secondary immune blood cell destruction caused by medications, neoplasms, or collagen-vascular disorders can be successfully managed by treating the underlying condition. In other cases, treatment involves the use of immunosuppressive therapy designed to reduce the concentration of immunoproteins directed against the target blood cells or to interfere with the destructive mechanisms aimed at the coated cells. There are a number of problems with such therapy, however. Initial treatment is usually the administration of corticosteroids, which impair the clearance of opsonized blood cells by mononuclear phagocytes. Even if corticosteroids are effective, their continued use is hazardous because of their potent side effects, which include excessive weight gain, causation of a diabetic state in susceptible patients, and osteoporosis.

Splenectomy is another treatment for autoimmune blood destruction. Many cases treated with splenectomy respond well to a markedly reduced dose of corticosteroids, thereby minimizing or eliminating harmful side effects. In other cases the drug can even be discontinued after surgical removal of the spleen. However, the absence of this most efficient clearance organ may permit the bone marrow production of blood cells to outstrip the rate of production. In this situation, instead of being cured of the autoimmune process, the patient is in a compensated state wherein the concentration of affected blood cells is maintained by a greater rate of production than normal. This elevation in blood cell turnover with its increased demand on bone marrow productivity raises the patient's requirement for folic acid and can lead to a folic acid deficiency; such patients should receive supplemental folic acid therapy. When splenectomy and corticosteroids fail to control immunological destruction, more potent immunosuppressive drugs and other radical therapies are enlisted (Ch. 31).

The therapies include antineoplastic agents. The ones used most frequently in addition to corticosteroids are the vinca alkaloid vincristine and the alkylating agent cyclophosphamide. For reasons that are unclear, danazol, an androgenic compound with minimal virilizing activity, can diminish autoimmune blood cell destruction in some cases. Other treatments aim at saturating the clearance capacity of the mononuclear phagocyte system. In one, gamma globulin is administered intravenously in amounts sufficient to increase significantly the total plasma IgG concentration. This maneuver has been shown in some cases to decrease by mass action the binding of specific antibody-coated blood cells to macrophages and thereby to diminish the clearance of the coated cells. The amounts of pooled gamma globulin required make this treatment very expensive. A variation of this approach is to infuse Rh-positive erythrocytes (see below) coated with anti-Rh antibodies. Although the injected red cells are gradually hemolyzed in the patient, the interaction between the iatrogenically coated cells and the mononuclear phagocyte system diverts the latter from binding and clearing the patient's own cells. In the future, monoclonal antibodies of peptides that inhibit macrophage Fc receptor binding of sensitized platelets may be useful.

SPECIFIC DISEASES OF IMMUNE-MEDIATED BLOOD CELL DESTRUCTION

Immune-Mediated Stem Cell Destruction

In a small number of cases of bone marrow failure, the pancytopenia appears to be the result of cell-mediated or antibody-mediated autoimmunity against pluripotent stem cells. The recovery of a few patients with aplastic anemia after immunosuppressive therapy is consistent with this hypothesis (Ch. 28). Serum or lymphoid cells from some patients with bone marrow failure has prevented the outgrowth of erythroid or granulocyte-macrophage colonies in cultures of normal bone marrow, suggesting the presence of immunological factors capable of inhibiting hematopoiesis. The antigens on the stem cells that might be targets of immune-mediated stem cell destruction are unknown.

Immune-Mediated Red Blood Cell Destruction

Pure Red Cell Aplasia

Anemia, an absence of reticulocytes, and normal concentrations of platelets and leukocytes in the peripheral blood characterize pure red cell aplasia. This disorder displays an absence or marked diminution of red blood cell precursors in the bone marrow, yet normal numbers of megakaryocytes and granulocyte precursors. Pure red cell aplasia occurs mainly in adults and is frequently associated with neoplasms of the thymus. It is possible to document the presence of circulating complement-fixing antibodies against erythroid cells by permitting bone marrow erythroid cells to incorporate radioactive iron, mixing the bone marrow with a patient's immunoglobulin and complement, and assessing release of the radioactive iron caused by complement-mediated cell lysis. Pure red cell aplasia may respond to treatment with immunosuppressive medication and, when associated with thymoma, to removal of the thymic tumor.

Immune Hemolysis

Red Blood Cell Antigens Involved in Immune Hemolysis

The red blood cell membrane surface has more than 300 components capable of producing antibodies when injected into animals. Such antigens are designated *blood groups*. A catalog of a patient's red blood cell antigens defines the individual blood type. Only a small number of these antigens are important in immune-mediated red blood cell destruction.

The most important blood groups from the standpoint of immune-mediated red cell destruction are in the *ABO system*. The antigens of this system are polysaccharides attached to red blood cell membrane lipids and proteins; each particular antigen is defined by the sugar residing at the end of the carbohydrate chain. Genes that program these antigens reside on the long arm of the ninth chromosome and encode for glycosyltransferase enzymes, which attach the terminal sugars to the oligosaccharide chains. In the case of type A, a specific enzyme puts *N*-acetyl-D-galactosamine on the chain; the type B transferase adds D-galactose (Fig. 29-1). The person who has neither the genes for A or B transferases builds red cell surface glycolipids and glycoproteins containing a terminal fucose residue. This structure is the foundation on which the sugars of the A and B antigens reside in persons possessing the requisite genes. A person lacking these genes is said to have red blood cell type O. The expression of the A and B blood group genes is codominant, so that persons with the genotype AA or AO both have A antigens on their red blood cells. Similarly, persons with the genotype BB or BO express the B antigen, and those with the genotype AB possess both A and B red blood cell antigens. Person who have neither A nor B genes have type O red blood cells.

The A and B red blood cell antigens are extremely effective in eliciting antibodies; the antigens are so richly endowed on the red blood cell surface that the destructive capacity of such antibodies is great. Furthermore, carbohydrate sequences identical to those found on the red blood cell antigens are widespread in nature, existing on the surface of enteric bacteria and on a variety of plant seeds and pollen. Thus, most people have antibodies in their plasma against either the A or B blood group antigens, whichever is not expressed on their own red blood cells. For example, a person who is red blood cell type A has B antibodies, a person who is red blood cell type A has anti-B antibodies, and a person who is red blood cell type O has both A and B antibodies. Only the person whose red blood type is AB lacks serum antibodies against these antigens (Fig. 29-2). For this reason, persons with red blood cell types A, B, or O will not tolerate

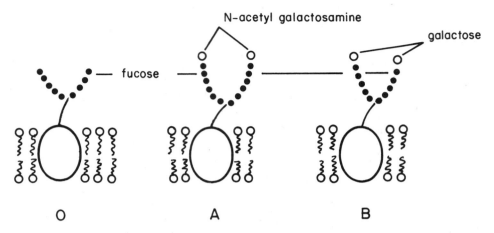

Fig. 29-1. Structure of major blood groups.

red blood cell transfusions that are not matched for these antigens. Type AB persons can theoretically accept red blood cells from persons of any type in this system, although unmatched transfusions are rarely given in practice.

About two-thirds of the population synthesize the A and B carbohydrate sequences on various body secretions. The body fluids of these secretors contain the A and B substances as well as their red blood cells.

The next most important red blood cell antigen system is called the *Rhesus (Rh) system*. Although well-defined genetically, the cell-surface structures that elicit the antibodies are much less well characterized than is the case for the ABO antigens. As best as can be deter-

mined, the immune system recognizes determinants on proteins in close approximation to lipids in the membranes of their blood cells. The genes coding for this expression, located in the first chromosome, program a set of antigens designated C, D, E; the absence of expression of a set of these antigens is termed by convention c, d, e. The inheritance of the antigens occurs in sets, such as CDe, cde, and eDE.

The D antigen is the most active of the Rh antigens in inciting antibodies. A single infusion of erythrocytes containing the D determinant into a patient who does not have this antigen (i.e., whose red cells are defined as Rh-negative) is associated with a 50 percent

Plasma Antibody	Anti B	Anti A	None	Anti A & B
Cell Antigens	A	B	AB	O
Genotype	AA or AO	BB or BO	AB	OO

Fig. 29-2. Blood group antigen and antibody profiles.

probability that red blood cells in a subsequent infusion of this type will be destroyed.

A variety of other antigens are occasionally of importance for immune-mediated red blood cell destruction. The structural definition of many of these antigens is unknown. Of the various red cell antigens, the Lewis system differs from others in that it is not produced by developing red blood cells during maturation; rather, it is taken up as glycolipid molecules from the plasma. The Ii system is of interest because the i antigen is expressed on fetal red blood cells. During the first year of life, its expression is reduced and is replaced by the I antigen. Autoantibodies against I or i antigens arise in certain infectious diseases and in malignant lymphoid neoplasms. The Duffy blood group is named for the patient in whom antibodies to it were first discovered. It is relatively commonly found on the red cells of whites but is rare in blacks. A possible basis for this difference in distribution is the finding that the Duffy antigen is the receptor to which the malaria parasite *Plasmodium vivax* binds in order to enter the red cell.

Isoimmune hemolysis in adults nearly always arises from the transfusion of imperfectly matched red blood cells. Antibodies against the A and B antigens fix complement, thereby leading to massive intravascular hemolysis and the most serious transfusion reactions. Such reactions may be associated with hypotension caused by the release of vasoactive complement fragments, as well as manifestations of serious hemolysis, hemoglobinuria, hemoglobinemia, and renal failure (Ch. 8). The principal effect of isoantibodies directed against other erythrocyte antigens is to compromise the survival of the transfused red cells.

Isoimmune red blood cell destruction can usually be avoided by carefully matched donors with recipients of blood transfusions. However, such matching may be difficult when the potential recipient has an unusual blood type or requires long-term transfusion support. The latter class of patients is likely to begin to produce antibodies against antigens that are ordinarily of minor importance.

Neonatal Isoimmune Hemolysis

Fetal erythrocytes that carry paternal cell-surface antigens not found on the maternal erythrocytes can leak across the placenta to enter the maternal circulation; the mother is thus sensitized, causing her to produce antibodies to the paternal and fetal antigens. IgG antibodies directed against these antigens can then cross the placenta in the other direction and begin to destroy the fetal erythrocytes. All fetal erythrocyte antigens have the potential to elicit isoantibodies, but the Rh system, particularly the D antigen, is most important in this regard. The Rh antigens are highly antigenic, because antibodies against them are very destructive to erythrocytes and because, unlike some other antigens, they are not found on other body tissues that could soak up the isoantibodies and divert them from the attack on erythrocytes.

The severity of hemolysis in the fetus is variable, but tends to become worse as sensitization occurs with successive pregnancies. The peripheral blood of the fetus and neonate with isoimmune hemolytic anemia shows reticulocytosis, spherocytes, and nucleated erythrocytes, explaining the name historically given this disease: *erythroblastosis fetalis*. In severe cases, the liver and spleen are enlarged and contain foci of extramedullary hematopoiesis. If the hemolysis is sufficiently serious to cause fetal hypoxia and death, the dead fetus is edematous and is said to have died of hydrops fetalis.

Presumably, the principal mode of erythrocyte destruction in this setting is IgG-mediated opsonization and clearance by the mononuclear phagocyte system. Partial destruction and symmetrical membrane removal from the erythrocytes by the phagocytes are responsible for the spherocytosis that ensues. Excessive erythrocyte destruction leads to hyperbilirubinemia. In contrast to the adult, who can tolerate large quantities of unconjugated bilirubin, in the fetus and the neonate the brain, especially the basal ganglia, is damaged when the plasma bilirubin level exceeds 20 g/L for any period of time. In fatal cases, the basal ganglia are stained a brownish yellow color called *kernicterus*. Neonatal isoimmune hemolysis with kernicterus was previously a common cause of mental retardation in those infants who survived.

A mandatory element of present-day prenatal care is to check the Rh type of the maternal red blood cells. If the mother's red blood cells are negative for the presence of the RhD antigen, she is at risk for Rh isosensitization by the fetus. It is then necessary to test the mother for the development of anti-RhD antibodies during the pregnancy, although it is unusual for the anti-RhD titer to rise in a first pregnancy.

In previous years, a rapidly rising maternal anti-RhD titer required amniocentesis, the removal of amniotic fluid by means of a needle inserted through the abdomen and measurement of bilirubin in the fluid. A sufficiently high amniotic fluid bilirubin level might require the infusion of Rh-negative erythrocytes by a needle into the amniotic cavity. These cells would find their way into the fetal circulation and replace hemolyzed Rh-positive fetal cells. Clearly, this was risky and invasive treatment. For infants born with erythroblastosis fetalis, a bilirubin rising to levels associated with the danger of kernicterus required the exchange of the fetal erythrocytes with RhD-negative cells by means of catheters inserted into the umbilical vessels.

Since the mid-1960s, it has been standard practice to administer an intramuscular injection of anti-Rh IgG to all Rh-negative women giving birth to Rh-positive infants. Anti-Rh IgG is prepared by injecting normal male volunteers with Rh-antigen-bearing erythrocytes. This passive immunization with anti-Rh antibodies prevents the maternal immune system from mounting an active response against any Rh-bearing erythrocytes that enter the maternal circulation. The routine immunization of mothers at risk with anti-Rh IgG has virtually eliminated isoimmune neonatal hemolytic anemia in the United States.

The erythrocyte antigens of the ABO system can also react with maternal antibodies directed against them. For example, a fetus with type B erythrocyte antigens can sensitize a mother with type A erythrocyte antigens. However, these antibodies are less problematic than anti-Rh antibodies in this setting because (1) the antibodies are usually of the IgM class, which do not cross the placenta; and (2) the carbohydrate components of the A and B antigens are present in secretions of most persons. These secretory molecules soak up IgG antibodies crossing the placenta directed against A or B sequences, thereby lowering the impact against erythrocytes. Nevertheless, mild to moderate neonatal hemolysis is occasionally ascribable to isoimmune reactions involving A and B antigens.

Autoimmune Hemolytic Anemia

In autoimmune hemolytic anemia, the development of autoantibodies against the erythrocyte surface leads to increased erythrocyte clearance and shortened erythrocyte survival. Sometimes the antibodies are directed against the Rh antigens on the erythrocyte, but usually they attack undefined surface constituents present on all erythrocytes. All cells are coated with the autoantibodies, irrespective of cell age. Therefore, the hemolysis is persistent and the disappearance curve of cells labeled with a marker such as radioactive chromium is exponential in nature. The shortened erythrocyte survival causes anemia and pallor. The hemolysis results in hyperbilirubinemia and attendant jaundice. The anemia and resulting hypoxia stimulate increased erythrocyte production, expressed as increased erythroid cells in the bone marrow and a rise in the peripheral blood reticulocyte count. The destructive effect of the autoantibodies in conjunction with the mononuclear phagocytes is to remove membrane in a symmetrical fashion from the red cells, thereby resulting in the production of spherocytes. Prolonged autoimmune hemolysis is associated with the hypertrophy of macrophages in the spleen that, along with the sequestration of antibody-coated erythrocytes in the spleen, leads to splenomegaly.

Serological Procedures in Autoimmune Hemolysis

Because erythrocytes lack Fc receptors and do not synthesize immunoglobulin, antibodies on the surface of erythrocytes are nearly always oriented with their Fab regions bound to the erythrocyte-surface antigens. This positioning leaves the Fc region of the molecules available to interact with complement components or with Fc receptors on mononuclear phagocytes in the spleen or elsewhere. Therefore, the detection of IgG antibodies on the erythrocytes usually indicates that hemolysis is taking place. The presence of complement alone on erythrocytes indicates usually that IgM binding to the erythrocytes resulted in the fixation of the third component of complement.

Customarily, laboratories test for the presence of IgG or C3 on erythrocytes using specific antibodies against these proteins. The erythrocytes are washed free of serum and suspended at 37°C in an isotonic salt solution to which rabbit antihuman IgG or anti-C3 is added. If the erythrocytes are coated with IgG or C3 molecules, the respective antibodies complex with them. Because the added antibodies are divalent, they have two binding sites for the antigens. They can therefore bridge the molecules coating adjacent erythrocytes and stick the red cells together. A positive reaction is therefore recognized by agglutination of the erythrocytes.

The antiglobulin agglutination test is named for its originator, R.A.F. Coombs. The aggregation of a patient's erythrocytes by anti-IgG or anti-C3 is called a positive *direct Coomb's test*. If the patient's serum is reacted with normal erythrocytes and agglutination is observed after the cells are washed and incubated with the anti-IgG or anti-C3, the result is a positive *indirect Coomb's test*. For an indirect test to be positive, free antierythrocyte an-

tibodies must have been present in the patient's serum. This situation is observed in about two-thirds of cases of autoimmune hemolytic anemia.

Most cases of autoimmune hemolytic anemia are caused by IgG warm-reactive antibodies. Some of these cases follow viral infections, whereas others occur in the setting of systemic lupus erythematosus (SLE), immunodeficiency disorders, or B-cell neoplasms.

IgM cold-reactive autoantibodies are usually encountered in two settings. In patients with EBV or *Mycoplasma* infections, IgM antibodies are directed against the erythrocyte's I antigen. In this setting of infection, the antibodies may be present without overt hemolysis, or the hemolysis may be mild to moderate. The antibodies disappear once the infection is controlled. On the other hand, other patients, many of whom have, or subsequently develop, B-cell neoplasms, acquire high concentrations of IgM cold-reactive antibodies often directed against the i antigen. Hemolysis in this setting may be relatively severe and exacerbated if the patient becomes chilled. Cold-reactive antibodies are detected by reducing the temperature of a blood sample below 37°C to room temperature or less. Because IgM antibodies can agglutinate the targets with which they react, clumping of the erythrocytes at the lowered temperature reveals the presence of the autoantibodies. Blood containing cold-reactive red cell autoantibodies may show overt erythrocyte agglutination when refrigerated and is said to have *cold agglutinins*. In a rare disorder called *paroxysmal cold hemoglobinuria*, IgM cold-reactive antibodies are directed against the erythrocyte surface antigen designated P_1. Chilling of the patient is associated with severe hemolysis. Paroxysmal cold hemoglobinuria is observed as a complication of syphilis and other infectious diseases.

The treatment of autoimmune hemolytic anemia entails interference with the pathological removal of antibody-sensitized erythrocytes by inhibiting the clearance function of the mononuclear phagocytes. Corticosteroids are effective in this regard and will control the disorder in two-thirds of cases. The remaining patients require more aggressive treatment, such as splenectomy. If splenectomy proves ineffective, immunosuppressive medications may also be needed. The increased erythroid cell turnover may deplete the patient's stores of folic acid, and it is wise to give the patient folic acid supplements. As for treatment of immune-mediated blood cell destruction in general, there are a number of problems with the use of high-dose corticosteroids and splenectomy.

Drug-Induced Immune Hemolysis

A variety of medications result in conditions that produce positive direct Coomb's tests and occasionally overimmune hemolysis. Such drugs are known to act by at least three mechanisms.

In the first mechanism, a medication or its metabolites react with antibody against itself, and the medication–antibody combination binds to the erythrocyte surface. The complex sensitizes the erythrocyte to immunologic destruction, usually by initiating the participation of complement. The erythrocyte has been called an innocent bystander in this reaction. The antibodies are often of the IgM class. Quinidine and quinine are examples of drugs that act in this fashion.

In the second mechanism, the medication or its metabolites bind first to the erythrocyte. The antimedication antibody, usually IgG, reacts with the cell-bound medication and sensitizes the cell for clearance. Penicillin is a drug that has this effect.

The third mechanism is a case wherein the medication or its metabolites somehow cause the patient to generate antibodies directed against erythrocyte antigens. The drug is required to generate and maintain the antibody, but it need not be present in order for the antibodies, usually of the IgG class, to bind to erythrocytes and sensitize them for immune destruction. How the medication causes the immune system to look at erythrocytes as nonself in such circumstances is unclear. Erythro-

cyte autoantibodies arising in the setting of treatment with alpha methyldopa, used as an antihypertension drug, is the prototype of such reactions.

Medication-associated antibodies reacting with erythrocytes need not lead invariably to hemolysis. When erythrocyte destruction is a problem, the clinical manifestations are identical to those described for autoimmune hemolytic anemia. Treatment, which is invariably effective, is to withdraw the offending medication.

Immune-Mediated White Blood Cell Destruction

The understanding of the principle that the dominant mechanism by which iso- or autoantibodies destroy blood cells is that the Fab domain of the antibody molecule binds to an antigen on the target cell surface and that the Fc region of the antigen-bound antibody then initiates a variety of effects arose primarily from laboratory studies employing red blood cells as targets of antibodies and in the clinical setting of antibody-mediated erythrocyte hemolytic disorders. Besides the ready availability of cells to study and the susceptibility of erythrocytes to complement-mediated lysis, the red cell was a suitable subject because it lacks Fc receptors. Therefore, antibodies do not ordinarily bind to erythrocytes, and the mere presence of antibody molecules on the red cell surface, detectable by the Coombs' test, is strongly suggestive of a potentially destructive state. This is not the case with white blood cells that have membrane Fc receptors. White blood cells, therefore, ordinarily have immunoglobulins bound to their surfaces, and a Coomb's type of assay would always report these antibodies. The detection of pathogenetically relevant immunoproteins on the white cell surface has thus depended on tests designed to bring out functions such as opsonic expression of Fc domains of cell-bound immunoglobulins or else on the ability to mea-

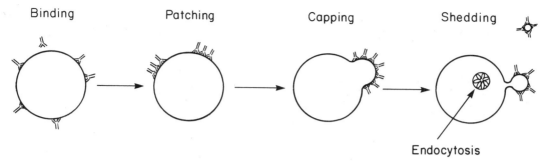

Fig. 29-3. Modulation of cell-bound antibodies by leukocytes.

sure amounts of immunoglobulin above background quantities.

The complexity of the interaction between immunoproteins and erythrocytes is further compounded in the case of living white blood cells, which can process or modulate cell-surface antibodies in ways that erythrocytes cannot. As shown in Figure 29-3, white blood cells reacted with antibodies against their cell surface antigens can aggregate the antigen–antibody complexes into *patches*. The patches coalesce to form a protuberance, or *cap*, at one pole of the cell. The cell may then either internalize the antigen–antibody complexes by endocytosis or release them into the extracellular space, a process called *shedding*. Hence, white blood cells may be capable of cleaning antibodies from their surfaces, and thereby escape immunological destruction.

A few patients with lymphopenia or subnormal immune function have been shown to possess circulating antilymphocyte antibodies. Some of these patients had systemic lupus erythematosus.

Antibodies against antigens on polymorphonuclear leukocytes have been detected in the serum of neonates with neutropenia and in the serum of their mothers. The antibodies disappear from the infants bloodstream after about 4 weeks of age, the time it takes for the infant to clear IgG, and the neutrophil counts rise at that time. This disorder, *neonatal isoimmune neutropenia*, is the equivalent of erythroblastosis fetalis. Some infants with neonatal isoimmune neutropenia acquire bacterial infections because of the reduction in phagocytic activity.

Autoantibodies against polymorphonuclear leukocytes can cause neutropenia. *Autoimmune neutropenia* has variable manifestations, depending on the severity of the condition. The destructive effect of antibodies may be directed against both peripheral blood granulocytes and granulocyte precursors in the bone marrow when neutropenia is profound. A wide variety of medications can cause neutropenia by means of antibodies. Some medications frequently associated with immune-mediated leukopenia are semisynthetic penicillins, sulfonamides, and thiourea antithyroid drugs.

Immune-Mediated Platelet Destruction

Destruction of Transfused Platelets

Antibodies directed against a platelet surface antigen (PLA_1), an epitope of platelet membrane glycoprotein IIb/IIIa, are very destructive to the platelets. However, the PLA_1 antigen is present on platelets of more than 98 percent of persons. Therefore, antibodies against PLA_1 antigens only rarely are a problem in platelet transfusion therapy. However, persons who lack the PLA_1 antigen on their platelets and also receive transfusions of PLA_1-bearing platelets may develop a condition called *post-transfusion purpura*. The platelets contained in whole blood transfusions are sufficient to elicit this disorder. At some time following the transfusion, the patient generates anti-PLA_1 antibodies. These antibodies are believed to bind PLA$_1$ antigen released from the transfused platelets, and the antigen–antibody complex then binds to the patient's own PLA$_1$- negative platelet. The binding of these complexes causes the destruction of the patient's platelets. The disorder is self-limited and remits completely.

PLA$_1$-positive infants of PLA$_1$-negative mothers can sensitize the mother, and the resulting anti-PLA$_1$ antibodies cause thrombocytopenia and hemorrhage in the first weeks of life. Infants with *neonatal isoimmune thrombocytopenia* can be treated with transfusions of PLA$_1$-negative maternal platelets until the anti-PLA$_1$ antibodies disappear after 4 to 6 weeks of age.

Thrombocytopenia caused by bone marrow failure is a common problem in hematology. It is treated with supportive care with platelet transfusions. However, platelet surfaces have histocompatibility (HLA) antigens (Ch. 32), and anti-HLA antibodies arise in many patients and become a limiting factor in the effectiveness of platelet support therapy. The time of detection of anti-HLA antibodies against infused platelets correlates with the onset of refractoriness to the hemostatic effectiveness of the transfusions; the platelet count in the recipient no longer rises in response to such transfusions from the donor to whose platelet antigens the recipient is sensitized. Judicious HLA antigen matching of donors with recipients can prevent such isosensitization and eventually find platelets that will survive in a sensitized recipient. Unfortunately, HLA matching is a somewhat laborious and expensive procedure.

Autoimmune Thrombocytopenia

IgG autoantibodies against platelets can sensitize the platelets for destruction. The structure of the antigens involved is unknown, and these antigens are present on the platelets of most persons. Platelet autoantibodies may be primary or secondary and, in the latter case, arise in the setting of SLE, immunodeficiency disorders, or B-lymphocyte neoplasms. Auto-immune thrombocytopenia may be the first sign of HIV infection and is found in about 10% of patients with AIDS. In children, acute autoimmune thrombocytopenia often follows a viral infection and remits spontaneously, whereas in adults the onset is usually more insidious and not clearly related to another illness and takes a chronic and intermittent course.

The antibodies causing neonatal isoimmune- or post-transfusion purpura or directed against HLA antigens are detectable by complement-mediated platelet lysis. In contrast, the autoantibodies responsible for autoimmune thrombocytopenia do not induce complement-mediated lysis and have been difficult to measure. Platelets resemble white blood cells in bearing Fc receptors that bind immunoglobulins. In addition, states of increased platelet turnover are often associated with large platelets that have more membrane and hence more Fc receptors than normal platelets. The detection, therefore, of greater than normal background immunoglobulin on the surface of platelets does not necessarily mean that the antibodies have something to do with the high turnover state.

Autoimmune platelet destruction results in thrombocytopenia and manifestations of hemorrhage in the patient. Unless severe acute or chronic bleeding has occurred, the erythrocyte and white blood cell counts are normal. A bone marrow aspirate characteristically reveals plentiful megakaryocytes. It is uncommon for the spleen to be enlarged. The serum contains antiplatelet antibodies of the IgG class, and the few circulating platelets can be shown to be coated with antiplatelet IgG, C3, or both. IgG antiplatelet antibodies cross the placenta, and therefore newborns of mothers with autoimmune thrombocytopenia are at risk for thrombocytopenia and hemorrhage in the neonatal period.

Patients with autoimmune thrombocytopenia are customarily treated with corticosteroids to reduce the clearance of sensitized platelets. If thrombocytopenia persists despite corticosteroid therapy or if prolonged corticosteroid therapy is required to maintain the platelet count, splenectomy is usually performed. Most patients respond to splenectomy, but occasionally more potent immunosuppressive therapy, danazol or intravenous gammaglobulin or antibody-coated erythrocyte infusion, are required. Because of the rapid clearance of platelets in autoimmune thrombocytopenia, platelet transfusions are of little benefit in this disease. If a patient bleeds massively and is going to have an emergency splenectomy, transfusion of enormous numbers of platelets may be necessary to control hemorrhage before and during splenectomy.

Medication-Associated Immune Platelet Destruction

Medications can induce immune-mediated platelet destruction. Penicillin, quinidine, and quinine elicit antibodies that cause reactions resembling the hemolytic disorders produced by these drugs. Antibodies against the anticoagulant heparin may produce thrombocytopenia, possibly because the heparin–antibody complexes bind to the platelets and activate them. In some cases, switching from bovine to porcine heparin alleviates the thrombocytopenia. Although the incidence of this complication of heparin is unusual, the large-scale use of the anticoagulant in clinical medicine makes the problem familiar to most physicians.

SUGGESTED READINGS

Bell, C.A., Ed. (1981) Seminar on Immune-Mediated Cell Destruction. American Association of Blood Banks, Washington, D.C.

Clarkson, S.B., Bussel, J.B., Kimberly, R.P., et al. (1986) Treatment of refractory immune thrombocytopenic purpura with an anti-Fcγ-receptor antibody. N. Engl. J. Med. *314*:1236.

Fehr, J., Hoffman, V., & Kappeler, U. (1982) Transient reversal of thrombocytopenia in idiopathic thrombocytopenic purpura by high-dose intravenous gamma globulin. N. Engl. J. Med. *306*:1254.

Karpatkin, S. (1980) Autoimmune thrombocytopenic purpura. Blood *56*:329.

Karpatkin, S. (1988) Immunologic thrombocytopenic purpura in HIV-seropositive homosexuals, narcotic addicts and hemophiliacs. Semin. Hematol. *25*:219.

Logue, G.L., & Schimm, D.S. (1980) Autoimmune granulocytopenia. Annu. Rev. Med. *31*:191.

Marcus, D.M., Ed. (1981) Blood group immunochemistry and genetics. Semin. Hematol. *18*:1.

Petz, L.D., & Garratty, G. (1980) Acquired Immune Hemolytic Anemias. Churchill Livingstone, New York.

Salama, A., Kieffel, V., & Mueller-Eckhardt, C. (1986) Effect of IgG anti-Rh(D) in adult patients with chronic autoimmune thrombocytopenia. Am. J. Hematol. *22*:241.

Schreiber, A.D., Chien, P., Tomaski, A., & Cines, D.B. (1987) Effect of danazol in immune thrombocytopenic purpura. N. Engl. J. Med. *316*:503.

Sheridan, D., Carter, C., & Kelton, J.G. (1986) A diagnostic test for heparin-induced thrombocytopenia. Blood *67*:27.

Swisher, S., Ed. (1976) Autoimmune hemolytic disorders. Semin. Hematol. *13*:247.

Blood Transfusion Therapy

A significant accomplishment of modern biomedical technology has been the development of blood transfusion therapy. The initial successes of blood transfusion therapy were in the realm of whole blood transfusions and directed at red blood cell and plasma replacement. In recent years the trend has progressively evolved toward transfusion of blood components. There have been several reasons for this tendency. First, frequently only one component of blood is required by a patient, for example, red blood cells, plasma, individual plasma proteins, or platelets. Second, many components, especially plasma, can be stored indefinitely, whereas whole blood cannot be kept for very long time intervals. Third, each component of a whole blood transfusion has the capacity to exert toxic effects. By restricting the transfusion to fewer components, the total toxicity of the transfusion can be minimized. The technology for selective transfusion of erythrocytes, plasma, and to a lesser extent platelets, has evolved to a high degree. Transfusion of blood phagocytes, principally neutrophils, is possible but lags behind in its technology.

PROCUREMENT OF WHOLE BLOOD AND PLASMA

The usual procedure for obtaining whole blood is to bleed (phlebotomize) a 450-ml unit of blood from a blood donor. This amount of blood loss is inconsequential to a healthy adult weighing more than 50 kg. The technique is to insert a needle into a suitable vein in the donor's antecubital fossa. To the needle is attached a length of plastic tubing that inserts into a plastic phlebotomy bag containing 40 ml of an anticoagulant solution. The bag is held below the level of the needle. The venous pressure of the donor, enhanced by a tourniquet on the upper arm, is sufficient to maintain flow of blood until 450 ml of blood is in the bag. At that point, blood flow stops because of the increase in pressure in the filled bag. In addition, the bag may be suspended on a balance beam at the opposite end of a counterweight; when filled, the bag tips the beam, signaling to the phlebotomy technician that the bag is filled.

Before a phlebotomy, simple selection and screening measures establish that the donor is sufficiently healthy. These measures include an inquiry as to the donor's state of health and as to whether there is a history of diseases that can be transmitted by blood transfusion. The donor must have a normal body temperature and blood pressure, both of which are examined before donation. Certainly the donor must not be anemic. A simple test for anemia is to obtain a drop of blood by means of a finger prick and to allow it to fall into a copper sulfate solution of defined density. If the red blood cell hemoglobin concentration is below about 13 g/100 ml, the drop of red blood will not sink into the blue copper sulfate solution.

If the red blood cell mass is above this level, the drop sinks to the bottom. A healthy blood donor can be bled of a unit of blood every 6 weeks.

With modern equipment, the entire phlebotomy and subsequent fractionation of whole blood can be done without ever exposing the blood to the air. At the end of the phlebotomy, the tubing leading to the phlebotomy bag is clamped and tied, the needle is cut off distal to the knot, and the bag is then available for transfusion or storage.

The complications of phlebotomy are minimal. The major problem is fainting of inexperienced donors. In many blood banks donors lie supine in special chairs that can be adjusted to lower the donor's head during phlebotomy, a measure that relieves the symptoms of a fainting reaction. Verbal reassurance is also very helpful in this situation.

WHOLE BLOOD AND WHOLE BLOOD FRACTIONS AND THEIR USES

Whole Blood

Whole blood contains all the cells and plasma proteins of the blood. Platelets, phagocytes, and many plasma proteins rapidly become inactivated during storage, so that for practical purposes, whole blood can be considered to consist of erythrocytes and plasma. Fresh whole blood may be indicated for patients suffering from massive hemorrhage. In this circumstance, all blood components are being rapidly lost. Even in this situation, not all components need to be replaced to an equivalent extent. In other words, the principal danger to the hemorrhaging patient is loss of blood volume and oxygen-carrying capacity. However, in the circumstance of massive hemorrhage, platelets and clotting factors may be lost to the degree that the hemorrhagic problem is compounded by impaired hemostasis. Therefore, in this circumstance about one of every eight units of transfused blood should be fresh.

Theoretically, whole blood is indicated when a patient needs both erythrocytes for anemia and plasma protein for replacement of intravenous volume. In point of fact, it is recommended in such cases that erythrocytes and plasma be given as separate components, because the plasma for purposes of colloid replacement can be stored indefinitely. It is therefore less wasteful to keep plasma than whole blood, because the erythrocytes and plasma would have to be discarded once the whole blood passed the expiration date during storage. Viewed in this way, there are very few indications for the administration of whole blood.

Separation of Packed Erythrocytes and Plasma

The whole blood in its plastic bag is spun in a centrifuge that drives the erythrocytes to the bottom. The transfusion bag has several outlets to which plastic tubing can be attached for fractionation. By rolling up the bottom of the packet, the supernatant plasma can be expressed into the exit tubing, which is attached to a transfer pack. This tubing is then clamped, sealed, tied, and cut, as was done after phlebotomy, when the transfer is completed. The plasma is available for transfusion and storage as are the packed erythrocytes. This procedure can also be used in plasmapheresis to remove abnormal plasma from patients with paraproteinemias. During plasmapheresis, the plasma can be discarded and the packed erythrocytes returned to the patient. Conversely, when patients with polycythemia are subjected to therapeutic phlebotomy, the erythrocytes are discarded and the plasma may be returned to the patient. Packed erythrocytes are the treatment of choice for most chronic anemias requiring blood transfusions. Whole plasma is given to patients requiring intravascular volume, especially if depleted of plasma proteins. Fresh plasma or plasma frozen immediately after separation and stored at $-20°C$ (fresh frozen plasma) is needed for certain coagulation disorders (see Ch. 13).

Plasma Fractionation

The chemical separation of plasma proteins was initiated during the 1940s. The classic methods involve addition of salts or solvents to the whole plasma, the addition of which causes the major component proteins, albumin and the immunoglobulins, to precipitate differentially. The precipitates are removed from the liquid by centrifugation and redissolved in water. Albumin can be used to provide this plasma component in patients with liver disease who are unable to synthesize it or in patients with protein-losing disorders. Immunoglobulin is used in the treatment of antibody deficiency diseases.

During the 1960s, procedures for precipitating coagulation factor VIII along with fibrinogen by subjecting plasma to low temperatures revolutionized the treatment of classic hemophilia. In recent years, the isolation of plasma proteins has become increasingly sophisticated and has provided complexes of coagulation factors in varying states of activation. The great advantage of many plasma fractions is their longevity during storage. Many of the fractions can be kept almost indefinitely in a dried state and reconstituted with sterile water or salt solution. The principal problem with such fractions is that they are rather expensive to prepare.

Storage of Whole Blood and Packed Erythrocytes

The problem of erythrocyte preservation is related to factors determining erythrocyte survival. It is necessary to maintain the red blood cell's redox potential, energy charge, and ultimately its membrane integrity. Through trial and error, conditions have evolved for the optimal storage of erythrocytes. The anticoagulant solutions contain glucose as a substrate for glycolysis and citric acid as anticoagulant to chelate the calcium. In addition to preventing fibrin formation during phlebotomy, the low calcium concentration prevents the slow leak of calcium into red cells associated with stiffening of the membrane skeleton. The citrate anticoagulant is buffered with sodium citrate and citric acid or, more commonly, sodium phosphate to maintain the blood pH at about 6. The inclusion of adenine in the preservative mixtures helps maintain the ATP level of the stored red cells. In such solutions, the cells remain viable for about 21 days at 4°C. The incubation at low temperature slows the glycolytic rate of the cells to a level that sustains viability but that does not lead to a depletion of glucose or an accumulation of waste lactic acid to a toxic level. Under these conditions, the erythrocyte membrane remains able to retain cytoplasmic constituents and to maintain the gradients of sodium and potassium at nearly normal levels, that is, 100 mEq/L of potassium inside and 100 mEq/L of sodium outside. Glucose fuels the reduction of the redox potential to prevent oxidation of glutathione, hemoglobin, and membrane components. If one considers that about 11 million units of blood are transfused per year in the United States, the importance of improving storage conditions can be appreciated. A 1 percent lengthening of the preservation of blood is equivalent to providing 100,000 units that would otherwise have to be procured.

Some changes do take place in erythrocytes during storage. In particular, the high glucose and phosphate concentration in the medium raises the 2,3-diphosphoglycerate concentration of the erythrocytes. The cells also lose some potassium ions and accumulate sodium ions from the medium. The pH of the suspending solution continues to fall because of accumulation of lactic acid. Nevertheless, these storage lesions are reversed when the erythrocytes are infused into the recipient's circulation. The 2,3-diphosphoglycerate falls, and the potassium:sodium ratio rises. The reversibility of the lesions persists until 20 days of storage. Beyond that time, the cells begin to leak increasing quantities of hemoglobin and the number of irreversibly damaged cells becomes intolerably high.

PROCEDURES INVOLVED IN RED BLOOD CELL TRANSFUSION

Cross-Matching

When a whole blood or packed or red blood cell transfusion is contemplated for a patient, the first priority is to obtain a small sample of blood from the patient. The sample is allowed to clot in a glass tube and is taken to the blood bank, where the serum is separated from the clot by centrifugation. Both the serum and the erythrocytes in the clot are used for the process of *cross-matching*, which is the determination of the blood product most suitable immunologically for the recipient.

The cells are checked for agglutination by serum from type B and type A persons, sera containing anti-A and anti-B IgM antibodies, respectively. Anti-A serum agglutinates erythrocytes containing A antigens, whereas anti-B serum agglutinates erythrocytes containing B antigens. Both will agglutinate erythrocytes from a person with the AB phenotype, as the erythrocytes have both A and B antigens. Neither antiserum reacts with erythrocytes of a person with a type O, whose erythrocytes have neither A nor B antigens. To be doubly sure of the ABO cross-match, as this procedure is called, the ability of the patient's serum to agglutinate known type A and B cells is checked. The result should be symmetrical with the test on the patient's cells. If the cells were found to be type A, the serum should agglutinate only type B cells. If type B cells were found, the serum should agglutinate type A cells. If the cells were type O, the serum should agglutinate both type A and B erythrocytes. If the cells were type AB, the serum should not agglutinate any cells. The cross-match for ABO of compatibility is particularly important, be-cause immunological reactions involving this system elicit complement-mediated intravascular hemolysis and inflict serious toxicity on the recipient.

Cross-matching for Rh compatibility is performed by reacting the potential recipient's cells with anti-D antisera in a medium containing a high albumin content, which allows these antibodies, usually of the IgG class, to cause agglutination. The tendency of the IgG antibodies to aggregate after being bound to erythrocytes is enhanced in this protein rich medium. At this point in the cross-match it is possible to identify the recipient's major blood group and Rh status, for example, A Rh-positive, B Rh-negative, O Rh-positive, AB Rh-positive, and, in theory, to select a suitable unit of whole blood or packed erythrocytes for infusion. However, if feasible, a further cross-match procedure is often carried out that determines whether the recipient has antibodies against other erythrocyte antigens. This matching is done by means of an indirect antiglobulin or Coomb's test. One approach is to mix the recipient's serum with erythrocytes from the donor.

After the first incubation, the cells are washed free of the recipient's serum by centrifugation and are then suspended in a solution of rabbit anti-human IgG antibody. If the recipient's serum contains any IgG antibodies that react against one or more of the antigens on the donor's red cells, the anti-IgG will now cause those cells to agglutinate. A positive reaction in the pool test then requires that the procedure be repeated against a panel of cells of defined antigenic composition in order to identify the antigen(s) involved. Thereafter, erythrocytes containing this antigen can be avoided in transfusions.

Erythrocytes matched for ABO and Rh blood groups, or even in extreme circumstances, unmatched type O Rh-negative erythrocytes alone, can be used in emergencies. However, it is advantageous whenever possible to take the cross-match one step further, especially when patients have had previous transfusions. Furthermore, the procedure must be repeated when a patient requires additional transfusions.

The Infusion of Packed Erythrocytes or Whole Blood

Blood taken right out of the blood bank is cold, has relatively low pH, and has high citrate, lactate, and potassium contents. If the blood is given rapidly and in large amounts, these properties can be toxic. Of special concern are the ability of citrate to sequester calcium and the effect of the potassium ion on suppressing neuromuscular function. If possible, the blood should be warmed (not burned) infused as slowly as possible; some recommend that calcium infusions be given when massive transfusions are delivered. The recipient's serum potassium concentration should be monitored if massive transfusion therapy is in progress, especially if there is a question as to the patient's renal function.

Frozen Erythrocytes

The 21-day storage limit for the whole blood and packed red blood cells is adequate for most transfusions. However, certain circumstances make longer storage desirable. First, if anemic patients requiring repeated transfusions have an unusual red blood cell antigen profile, they will eventually develop antibodies against most erythrocytes in the general population. It may not be possible to phlebotomize persons with compatible blood types as frequently as the recipient needs the cells. However, if a supply of an unusual type of erythrocytes can be collected over a long time and stockpiled in a frozen state, the problem may be solved. Second, frozen blood can be transported to remote locations and stored wherever freezer facilities are available.

The major problem in frozen storage, cryopreservation, is to avoid damage to cell constituents, especially membranes, by ice crystals that form during freezing. This problem is approached by means of colligative compounds that can both lower the freezing point of water as well as penetrate the cell's membrane to prevent intracellular as well as extracellular freezing. Cryoprotective agents of this type include glycerol and dimethylsulfoxide. In addition to the use of cryoprotective agents, the temperature must be lowered slowly to prevent ice formation and abrupt phase transitions in cellular components. Therefore, freezing of blood cells requires technology for addition of cryopreservative agents, controlled freezing, frozen storage (usually at $-20°C$ or lower), controlled thawing, and finally, removal of the cryopreservative. Removal of the cryopreservative is accomplished by extensive washing of the cells. Therefore, an additional advantage of frozen blood is the fact that it is extensively washed free of plasma, a process that reduces its risk of transmitting diseases.

After freezing and thawing, about 10 to 15 percent of erythrocytes are lysed. An additional 10 to 15 percent have a short survival after infusion. The rest have a survival nearly equivalent to that of conventionally stored erythrocytes. However, the thawed cells deteriorate rapidly on further storage and must therefore be transfused within 24 hours after thawing. Moreover, a point worth noting is that the frozen and thawed erythrocytes have almost entirely lost their potassium content to the extracellular fluid. The cell will normalize this ionic imbalance after infusion into the circulation by pumping sodium ions out and potassium ions in. Because the initial infusion medium is very rich in potassium, a transient increase in serum potassium can occur in the recipient. On the other hand, if enough frozen and thawed erythrocytes are infused into a recipient, the cells act as potassium traps and can actually pump enough potassium out of the plasma into themselves to cause a transient hypokalemia.

Despite the advantages of frozen erythrocytes, the expense and logistical problems caused by the complex technical procedures involved and the additional requirements for freezer space limit the practicality of freezing as a routine method for erythrocyte processing and preservation at the present time.

PLATELET TRANSFUSIONS

Procurement of Platelets

The size and shape of platelets are sufficiently different from those of erythrocytes to allow them to be relatively easily separated from the whole blood. The simplest procedure for this separation, called *plateletpheresis*, is to remove a unit of whole blood, to centrifuge it gently at about 500 times gravity, and to express the platelet-rich plasma into a transfer pack and return the packed red cells to the donor. In the usual centrifugation procedure described for preparation of plasma, the blood is spun more rapidly at 1000 times gravity, causing the platelets to collect in the buffy coat. A unit of platelet-rich plasma contains on the order of 10^{11} platelets.

Despite the ease of this procedure, the usual thrombocytopenic patient requires more than 10^{11} platelets. A rule of thumb is that an infusion of a unit of platelets, that is, the platelets derived from a unit of whole blood, will increase the platelet count of a 70-kg person by 10,000 platelets per microliter of blood. To increase the yield of platelets from a donor, it is possible to process up to 1200 ml of plasma from a single donor per week. A more sophisticated approach is to remove blood from one antecubital vein of a donor by means of a pump and to drive the blood into a centrifuge. The blood, depleted of platelet-rich plasma, is pumped back into the antecubital vein in the donor's other arm. The centrifuge device separates platelet-rich plasma from the erythrocytes in the whole blood. The blood flow from the patient into the machine and back may be continuous or intermittent, depending on the technology used. The more platelets that can be obtained from a single donor, the lower the

risk of sensitization of the recipient against different HLA antigens on the infused platelets.

Platelet cross-matching for immunological reasons is not routine because of its expense, but in some instances it is indicated and required when prolonged platelet support is necessary.

Storage of Platelets

Platelets can be maintained in a viable state in platelet-rich plasma for about 2 days at either room temperature or in the cold (4°C). Interestingly, platelets stored in the cold have a shorter average survival time in a recipient's circulation than do platelets stored at room temperature. However, the basis of the longer survival seems to be that the platelets stored at room temperature are less active in hemostasis than are the cold-storage platelets. Therefore it has been argued that the cold-storage platelets should be used when immediate hemostasis is required and room temperature storage platelets should be employed for more prolonged hemostasis.

Procedures for freezing of platelet-rich plasma are being developed. Although frozen platelets have been shown to function for hemostasis, they are not yet widely employed.

Phagocyte (Neutrophil) Transfusions

The turnover rate of blood phagocytes, predominantly neutrophils, is on the order of 10^{10} per day under normal circumstances and up to 10 times that value in states of bacterial infection. If we consider that a 450-ml unit of whole blood contains about 2×10^9 neutrophils, it is obvious that five or preferably more units of whole blood need to be processed and gleaned of neutrophils if the turnover in a recipient is to be approximated. Several technical procedures have been developed to try to accomplish this feat. The major procedures currently under investigation involve extracorporeal centrifugation of multiple units of blood in a manner described for platelet-pheresis. Blood is centrifuged in a cylindrical container to yield erythrocytes and plasma. However, instead of removing platelet-rich plasma, the devices skim off a neutrophil-enriched buffy coat at the plasma–erythrocyte interface. Unfortunately, this leukopheresis procedure can routinely generate on the order of only 10^{10} neutrophils from an acceptable volume of whole blood. To increase this amount two to three times, a viscous polymer, hydroxyethyl starch, that coats erythrocytes causing them to separate more efficiently from neutrophils is added during the procedure. In addition, donors are often given corticosteroids before leukopheresis to increase their concentration of circulating neutrophils.

The technological feat of obtaining phagocytes in large numbers has unfortunately not in and of itself solved the problem of phagocyte support for patients with phagocyte deficiency who are susceptible to bacterial and fungal infection. First, even the impressive numbers of neutrophils acquired are at the theoretical lower limit of maintaining the required neutrophil turnover. Second, it is not clear that the neutrophils obtained are either totally functional or, on the other hand, completely nontoxic. There is some evidence that damaged neutrophils aggregate and collect in the lungs, where they have the potential to injure pulmonary capillary endothelium and produce edema and inflammation. The resulting reaction may destroy lung substance and block the pulmonary microcirculation, both effects resulting in hypoxemia. In addition, neutrophils have a very short survival in the living organism and deteriorate even more rapidly during conditions of storage that have been tried. Another problem is that there is relatively definitive information concerning the antigens of neutrophils, a deficiency that limits the practicality of cross-matching. Finally, the technology associated with neutrophil transfusion is not only expensive but potentially hazardous to the healthy blood donor. This hazard results from the need to treat the donor with hydroxyethyl

starch, corticosteroids, and anticoagulants. For all these reasons, phagocyte transfusion must be considered of limited utility at the present time

COMPLICATIONS OF BLOOD TRANSFUSION THERAPY

Immunological Reactions

As described in Chapter 29, the infusion of ABO-incompatible erythrocytes leads to various hemolytic reactions mediated by the natural IgM isoantibodies directed against A and B antigens and the interaction of these antibodies with the complement system. These types of reactions lead not only to immediate intravascular destruction of the infused cells, but to circulatory instability and possibly serious renal damage as well. Transfusions of Rh-incompatible blood cause generally less serious and delayed hemolytic reactions. In addition, such a transfusion in women of childbearing age sensitizes the Rh-negative mother against an Rh-positive fetus and sets that fetus up for erythroblastosis fetalis. Immunological reactions against other erythrocyte antigens cause variable degrees of delayed hemolysis of the transfused blood.

The major consequence of immunological reactions against infused platelets and white blood cells appears to be the short survival of those cells and limitation of their usefulness. However, antibodies against white cells may also damage them and cause them to produce pulmonary and other tissue damage as discussed above.

Occasionally immunological reactions occur against plasma components. Genetically determined plasma IgA deficiency is fairly common. IgA-deficient persons receiving whole plasma may produce anti-IgA antibodies. When blood or plasma containing IgA is subsequently infused into the IgA-deficient recipient, various types of immunological reactions such as urticaria, anaphylactic shock, or serum sickness may occur. One uncommon immunological consequence of transfusion is the passive transfer of IgE antibodies from an allergic donor to a recipient. Exposure of the previously nonallergic recipient to the antigen to which the donor was allergic results in an allergic reaction in the recipient.

Cardiovascular Overload

If through miscalculation or some other reason more blood product is given to the intravascular space than the cardiovascular system can tolerate, pulmonary edema can occur. This complication may arise following a blood transfusion into an anemic person who either because of severe anemia or underlying cardiac disease is in borderline cardiac failure. This complication can sometimes be avoided by giving blood transfusions slowly to patients with underlying cardiovascular disease. The volume of blood coagulation factor infusions can be minimized by employing concentrated coagulation factor fractions presently available. However, some of these preparations contain high concentrations of fibrinogen, and relatively small increments in plasma fibrinogen can cause large increases in blood viscosity.

Infectious Complications Associated with Transfusion Therapy

With modern technology the overt contamination of blood products with microbes as a result of procurement and storage techniques is unusual. The major infectious complication of blood transfusion therapy is the spread of diseases that are latent in the donor. In theory, any infection in which the offending organism circulates in the blood can be transmitted by blood transfusion therapy. The infections caused by the hepatitis B virus, the (presumed viral) agent causing non-A, non-B hepatitis, the AIDS virus (HIV-1), and to a lesser extent the cytomegalovirus, are the major offenders.

The fraction of adults having infectious hep-

atitis or AIDS viruses in the bloodstream is high among populations living under conditions of poor sanitation and among drug addicts who make a practice of sharing the needles with which they indulge their habits. For these reasons, the probability that a unit of blood will be infected with hepatitis virus is heavily dependent on the population from which it was obtained. In general, blood banks that use blood products from volunteer donors tend to have a lower infection transmission rate than do blood banks that pay their donors. A reason for this difference is the fact that blood is one commodity that drug addicts can sell to finance their habits.

With the great advances that have come in understanding of the structure and pathogenicity of the hepatitis B and AIDS viruses in recent years, it has become increasingly possible to use immunological methods to detect the presence of hepatitis B or HIV infection in blood. In patients who are carriers of hepatitis B, virus particles or parts thereof are present in sufficiently high concentrations in blood that sensitive immunochemical tests can efficiently detect them. To improve the discrimination of hepatitis testing and to screen for persons with non-A, non-B hepatitis, an assay for the certain liver enzymes is also performed on the presumption that elevated levels of these enzymes in the blood represent possible hepatic infection. Recent success in cloning the virus responsible for non-A, non-B hepatitis promises a direct test for this pathogen. In the case of AIDS, the virus exists at such low levels in blood that it makes little sense to try to detect it. The current approach to HIV testing, therefore, uses the serological assays for anti-HIV antibodies described in Chapter 21. Although these tests are very reliable, there persists a "window of vulnerability" of possibly several months in which a person recently exposed to HIV has yet to generate antiviral antibodies.

Fractionation of blood into components can serve to some extent to reduce the risk of infection. The hepatitis virus is remarkably hardy and survives the normal vicissitudes of blood storage including freezing and thawing.

However, the prolonged storage attendant in the processing of blood for plasma, plasma albumin, and immunoglobulins causes the virus to become nonviable with time or to be removed during the fractionation process. Unfortunately, most coagulation protein fractions are so enriched for the hepatitis virus that these fractions are associated with a high risk of infection. A safe and effective hepatitis B vaccine is now available, however, and whenever possible, patients requiring blood protein concentrates should be vaccinated before their first factor infusions.

Other methods available to reduce the risk of infection from blood protein fractions include application of organic solvents, steam pasteurization, and additional purification by means of monoclonal antibodies. The techniques vary in expense and are currently undergoing evaluation. Blood proteins manufactured by recombinant genetic technology are likely to be safe. The major problem now is to make their preparation less expensive.

In the United States today, even with precautions in effect, the risk of infection increases cumulatively with each unit of whole blood infused. The absolute risk in a given situation varies with the locale and the sources of blood. It can be appreciated that after therapy of massive hemorrhage or open heart surgery, the risk of infection is relatively high. A hopeful prospect for such patients is the use of autotransfusion. The patient anticipating modest blood loss during elective surgery can donate blood on several occasions before surgery and take iron tablets to stimulate new red cell production. For massive hemorrhage, surgeons are now using devices to remove debris from blood leaking into body cavities during trauma and surgery and reinfusing this blood into the patient's circulation.

SUGGESTED READINGS

Aach, R.D., Szmuness, W., Mosley, J.W., et al. (1981) Serum alanine aminotransferase of donors in relation to the risk of non-A, non-B hepatitis in recipients. N. Engl. J. Med. *304*:989.

Bove, J.R. (1987) Transfusion-associated hepatitis and AIDS. What is the risk? N. Engl. J. Med. *317*:242.

Chaplin, H., Jr. (1984) Frozen red cells revisited. N. Engl. J. Med. *311*:1696.

Garratty, G., Ed. (1986) Red Cell Antigens and Antibodies. American Association of Blood Banks, Arlington, VA.

Masouredis, S.P. (1982) Pretransfusion tests and compatibility: Questions of safety and efficacy. Blood *59*:873.

Snyder, E.L., Ed. (1983) Blood Transfusion Therapy: A Physician's Handbook. American Association of Blood Banks, Arlington, VA.

Toy, T.C.Y., Strauss, R.G., Stehling, L.C., et al. (1987) Predeposited autologous blood for elective surgery. A national multicenter study. N. Engl. J. Med. *316*:517.

Zuck, T.F. (1988) Transfusion-transmitted AIDS reassessed. N. Engl. J. Med. *318*:511.

31

Principles of Therapy for the Hematologic Malignancies

Treatment of hematologic malignancies is directed toward the destruction of malignant stem cells. The goal is to achieve selectivity, that is, the maximal destruction of tumor stem cells with minimal damage to healthy stem cells. Some biological principles are useful in thinking about the development and application of such therapy.

HOW CAN MALIGNANT CELLS BE KILLED?

Surgery is effective against many localized epithelial and connective tissue tumors but is rarely applicable to hematological malignancies, because the tumor cells are usually disseminated at the time of diagnosis. Surgery is primarily used for obtaining tissue for histological analysis.

The killing of dispersed malignant cells requires some agent that can seek them out and then attack their mechanisms for living or their capacity to replicate. Some properties of cells affect their susceptibility to such therapeutic attacks, and these properties vary at different stages in their life cycle. The *cell cycle* is summarized in Figure 31-1 and Table 31-1. Therefore, the susceptibility of cells to killing by different methods varies with the type of cell

and the stage of its life cycle. Most treatments act best on rapidly dividing cells, because the metabolic demands of these cells and a maximal number of structural rearrangements may be occurring. Treating dividing cells is analogous to throwing a wrench into a moving (as opposed to a stationary) machine. The susceptibility to killing by various agents also depends on the ability of the cells to permit the entry of the toxic agents and on whether the cell can destroy the toxins. It is fortunate that some malignant stem cells are, for various reasons, more susceptible to damage than are normal stem cells. This selectivity can arise from a number of factors:

1. A higher number of the tumor stem cells are in cycle and/or are cycling more rapidly than are normal cells. Agents that are especially toxic to cycling cells then kill more tumor cells than normal cells.

2. The tumor stem cell has a unique, unusually active, or missing metabolic pathway that renders it more susceptible to a toxin than normal cells.

3. The tumor stem cell is less able to protect itself or recover from toxic damage than the normal cell.

An observation made for tumors in experimental animals is that many toxic agents kill a

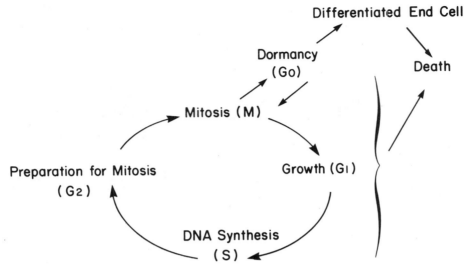

Fig. 31-1. Cell cycle.

fixed *fraction* of tumor cells rather than a fixed number of cells and the size of the fraction killed is proportional to the dose of treatment. The major importance of such fractional killing and its dose-dependence is that the treatment by a single agent given once will only be curative when the treatment dose is high and/or the tumor burden is small. For example, even if a treatment kills a high fraction, say 99 percent, of tumor cells, and 10 billion cells were originally present, 100 million cells will still survive the treatment. This phenomenon partly explains why combinations of treatment are more effective than single agents, because each can reduce the tumor cell burden by a fraction until a sufficiently low level of cells is reached below which their survival is no longer possible. Another reason favoring the use of treatment combinations is improved selectivity. A combination of agents acting against tumor stem cells by different mechanisms may be less toxic to normal cells than a higher dose of a single agent. For all of these reasons, it is customary to treat neoplasms beyond the time when obvious tumors have disappeared; such therapy of inapparent disease is called *adjuvant treatment*. When all is said and done, the "best" combination and timing of treatments for a given time and a given disease are usually arrived at by a mixture of theoretical ideas and of trial and error. As new therapies become available, the "best" treatments change.

Table 31-1. The Cell Cycle

Phase of Cell Cycle	Metabolic and Structural Events
All	Maintenance of energy charge for metabolic reactions (ATP synthesis)
	Maintenance of redox potential (to keep components reduced)
	Maintenance of membrane integrity and ion gradients
G1, G2	Synthesis of structural molecules (RNA, protein, lipids, sugars)
S	DNA synthesis
M	Construction and disassembly of chromosomes and mitotic spindle
	Dissolution and restructuring of nuclei
	Formation of cleavage furrow
	Movements for cell separation (cytokinesis)

WHY ARE TUMOR STEM CELLS RESISTANT TO TREATMENT?

First, tumor stem cells sometimes have a growth rate equal to or less than that of normal stem cells. In such cases, treatments active against rapidly growing cells have no selective effect. Second, tumor stem cells can generate protective mechanisms that repel assaults against them. The genetic makeup of tumor stem cells tends to be unstable, and antitumor treatment itself can select for tumor stem cells resistant to the treatment. For example, enzymes can be induced that inactivate the effects of the treatment. This resistance can evolve along several lines. One that has been elucidated in recent years is the induction by tumor cells of a gene that encodes a transport system that efficiently pumps a remarkably diverse spectrum of structurally unrelated cytotoxic drugs out of the cell. This gene has been cloned and sequenced and is referred to as the multidrug resistance or *mdr* gene. Alternatively, the cells may increase the content of enzymes that detoxify the drugs or bypass the blocks in key metabolic pathways caused by certain agents. These and other mechanisms explain why cytotoxic drugs may be effective for a while, yet become ineffectual later in time. The use of treatment combinations may block this trend toward resistance. By attacking cells at multiple vulnerable points, it is hoped that the ability of a few cells to survive and develop resistance can possibly be prevented.

THERAPIES USED AGAINST HEMATOLOGICAL MALIGNANCIES

Ionizing Radiation

Use of Ionizing Radiation in Hematological Malignancies

Ionizing radiation is used for the cure or palliation of hematological tumors. Its curative potential is mainly in localized Hodgkin's disease (stages I–III) and in a few cases of localized non-Hodgkins lymphomas of the large-cell type. Short of cure, ionizing radiation has extensive value in the palliative treatment of lymphoma, leukemia, and multiple myeloma. Tumor masses often melt away in response to radiation. Effects of tumor infiltrates on tissues and organs such as pain, neurological dysfunction, and compression of intestinal, urinary, or airway pipelines, can be rapidly and dramatically reversed. A recent application of radiation therapy in hematology has been its use in bone marrow transplantation (Ch. 32). In the treatment of congenital disease affecting blood cells, ionizing radiation directed at the entire bone marrow, essentially total-body irradiation, destroys the genetically abnormal bone marrow stem cells in preparation for engraftment with histocompatible normal cells. In addition, this type of therapy is under evaluation for the treatment of nonlymphocytic and stem cell leukemias. *Total-body irradiation* is used in this setting in an effort to destroy all leukemic stem cells. Thereafter, normal bone marrow is given.

Types of Ionizing Radiation

x-Rays and γ-rays are of the electromagnetic wave spectrum and are also considered high-energy photons. x-Rays are emitted when rapidly moving electrons are suddenly decelerated in a vacuum. The energy of x-rays is defined by the voltage used to produce them. Thus, kilovoltage x-rays, used primarily in former years, emerge from devices generating 200 to 400 kv. Modern machines use several million, up to 25 million, volts to produce megavoltage x-rays. Still higher-energy x-rays, up to 40 million volts, can be generated by a device called a *betatron*. γ-Rays arise from changes of energy states during the decay of certain radionuclide elements. A frequently used source of γ-rays is cobalt 60 (^{60}Co). A mass of ^{60}Co used for radiation therapy may be housed in a shielded container; it undergoes about 10^{16} disintegrations per minute. The *cu-*

rie is the unit of radioactive decay expressed in disintegrations per minute, 1 curie being equal to 2.2×10^{12} disintegrations per minute. Therefore, a clinical ^{60}Co source has several thousand curies. The ^{60}Co emits γ-rays with energies of 1.33 and 1.7 million electron volts.

Electrons are generated with high velocities from a linear accelerator or a betatron. The emitted electrons can have energies from 6 to 18 million electron volts or higher.

Heavy particles, such as protons, neutrons, π mesons, and α-particles can be produced with a cyclotron. Because of their large masses, these particles can be very destructive to cells; the rate of transmission of energy from the radiation to the cell components per unit distance, the linear energy transfer (LET), is highest for these particles. The LET for the particles is highest when they have slowed to a particular speed, and this state of high-energy transfer is called the *Bragg peak*. Therefore, by adjusting the geometry of the incident beam, it is possible to limit heavy particle damage to a very discrete area.

The therapeutic or toxic dosage of radiation is ultimately determined by the energy transfer from radiation to tissue and is quantified as the amount of energy absorbed per unit mass of tissue. The current standard usage to indicate this sum is the *Gray* (abbreviated Gy), which is equivalent to one joule of energy absorbed per kilogram of tissue. The Gray is equivalent to 100 rad, rad being the units of dosage used in the past and still frequently encountered. The rad is similar to the roentgen (abbreviated R), which is the amount of radiation able to ionize air.

Mechanisms of Action of Ionizing Radiation

Various types of ionizing radiation damage vital cell components. The mechanism of destruction may be either direct or indirect. Direct damage occurs when the radiation ionizes and thereby breaks bonds in nucleic acids and proteins. Such direct damage is predominant in the action of heavy particles. A significant amount of the cytotoxic effect is indirect in that the radiation ionizes water molecules and oxygen dissolved in the water to yield free radicals that secondarily oxidize and destroy cell components. This indirect damage explains why the capacity of ionizing radiation to kill cells is in part proportional to the oxygen tension of the cell and why the center of large, bulky, and poorly vascularized tumors is relatively resistant to radiation damage. This effect has also encouraged therapists to devise ways to increase the oxygen tension of tumors with hyperbaric oxygen or other techniques and to experiment with chemicals, radiation sensitizers that mimic the effect of oxygen on radiation damage. Metronidazole, a drug originally used to treat infections caused by the protozoan *Trichomonas vaginalis*, is a radiation sensitizer.

The relationship between radiation dose and a cytotoxic effect in experimental cell systems can be shown to fit a curve in which the number of cells surviving falls exponentially as the dose of radiation increases, a finding consistent with a random hit mechanism (Fig. 31-2). The exponential curve is straightened out by plotting the radiation dose against the logarithm of surviving cells. It should be noted that there is a threshold radiation dose below which no killing occurs. Below this dose, the damage is insufficient and/or repair processes are adequate to prevent cell killing. The position of the threshold and the steepness of the slope of the curve depend on the type of radiation involved and on the characteristics and environment of the cells. In general, cells that (1) are dividing rapidly, (2) have a long mitotic phase, and (3) are relatively undifferentiated are most easily damaged by ionizing radiation. Tumor stem cells of hematological malignancies often have these properties, making them highly radioresponsive.

Fractionation

One aspect of selectivity in radiation therapy is the finding that malignant cells are less effective than normal cells in recruiting new cell growth and repairing radiation damage. Therefore, the delivery of a tumoricidal dose of radi-

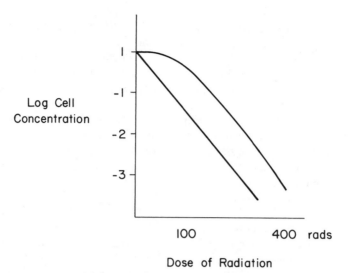

Fig. 31-2. The relationship between radiation dose and cytotoxic effect in experimental cell systems.

ation therapy in fractions rather than all at once can kill a tumor, but with less damage to normal tissue. Furthermore, as a tumor shrinks, its oxygenation may improve, enhancing the indirect damaging effect of later radiation fractions.

General Principles of Treatment with Radiation

The technology of radiation therapy is very sophisticated and currently permits the therapist to select methods that deliver maximal destructive energies to a tumor with minimal damage to other cells. For example, the high-voltage x-rays and γ-rays and heavy particles available can penetrate the body without damaging the skin and superficial tissues. On the other hand, kilovoltage x-rays and electron beams can be used for superficial tumors, such as mycosis fungoides or symptomatic leukemic infiltrates. The radiation therapist works with a physicist and a technologist to establish the geometry and extent of the dosage applied to the patient. In the process, heavy metal templates may be designed and built for each patient to limit the beams to where they are intended by shielding normal tissues. Modern devices can

minimize the complications of irradiation to both patient and medical personnel.

Complications of Radiation Therapy

Complications of radiation therapy are the result of cell necrosis and genetic damage. The tissues most susceptible to these effects are those containing cells in rapid turnover, such as the skin, hematopoietic tissue, and the gastrointestinal tract. Therefore, the acceptable dosage of radiation therapy varies inversely with the amount of susceptible tissues exposed: A high dose is acceptable over a small area, but a relatively low dose may be lethal over the entire body. Nevertheless, sufficiently high doses of radiation can damage fibroblasts of connective tissue, bone, and even muscle and nerve cells. Therefore, high amounts of radiation therapy must be carefully directed to minimize the exposure of normal tissues, and only rarely can local doses exceed 50 Gy. In the radiation therapy of lymphoid organs, for the treatment of Hodgkin's disease, for example, the usual dose is 45 Gy given in fractions over 6 weeks.

Despite careful precautions, radiation therapy can lead to certain complications. Irradiation of large areas of the body often causes fatigue and nausea. Irradiation of the pelvis, spine, and long bones can produce transient bone marrow failure, and a total body dose of 4.5 Gy yields permanent bone marrow aplasia. Radiation of the abdomen, by damaging intestinal stem cells, can cause abdominal cramps, watery diarrhea, and gastrointestinal hemorrhage. In children, radiation of growing cartilage and bony epiphyses may result in growth retardation. Pulmonary damage, cardiac fibrosis, premature coronary atherosclerosis leading to acute myocardial infarction, and interstitial nephritis have all been described as late consequences of radiation therapy.

Ionizing radiation is potentially carcinogenic. The development of nonlymphocytic leukemia and of solid tumors (carcinomas and sarcomas) in tissues exposed to radiation is an infrequent but definite complication of this therapy. The mechanism of carcinogenesis is unknown but probably has something to do with damage to the stem cell's genetic material. Cells in tissues exposed to ionizing radiation express various manifestations of such damage, including chromosomal breaks and chromosomal rearrangements. The damage is not sufficient to kill the cell but causes mutations that in some cases lead to malignant behavior.

Chemotherapy

Chemotherapy is defined as the treatment of tumor stem cells by means of medications and hormones. Chemotherapy has the advantages of penetrating many areas and of lodging an active attack against disseminated tumors. Nevertheless, chemotherapy cannot easily infiltrate large, bulky, and poorly vascular tumors, and many drugs do not penetrate the blood–brain barrier. For the treatment of acute lymphatic leukemia, it is necessary to give radiation therapy to the cranium or to inject drugs into the cerebrospinal fluid, or both, in addition to oral and intravenous chemotherapy in order to eradicate malignant cells in the central nervous system.

It is customary to use combinations of drugs having different mechanisms of action. For some diseases, drug therapy is continued after the induction of a remission, with the goal of eradicating, or at least repressing, clinically latent but nonetheless finite numbers of tumor stem cells. This rationale supports the use of maintenance therapy in the acute leukemias and adjuvant therapy after the surgical resection or localized radiation therapy of tumors.

Development of Chemotherapeutic Agents

Occasionally chemotherapeutic agents are developed by an inductive process, that is, they are synthesized or engineered to inhibit a particular metabolic reaction of tumor cells. More often than not, however, drugs enter the clinical arena by a screening process in which they are found to kill tumors in animals. The usual approach is to try various agents against animal tumors, using an approach that lends itself to rapid, reproducible evaluation. These tumors are usually virulent, that is, small numbers inoculated into the animal will grow rapidly and kill the organism within a short time. One example is a lymphoid neoplasm of mice, called L1210 leukemia. In such a system, the ability of a drug to cure for increased survival time of the inoculated animals is taken as an index of its effectiveness. Although many effective chemotherapeutic agents are active in these animal models, it is disconcerting that some drugs very active against human cancers occasionally are unimpressive in the animal screening tests.

When new compounds are judged worthy of clinical trial, they are initially given in research institutions to consenting patients with malignant neoplasms, in order to determine the toxicity of the drug. Because the tumors in these patients are usually far advanced, determination of efficacy is not a major goal in such phase I trials. Once the toxicity of the drugs is determined, the drugs are compared in phase II trials against other drugs in patients with a variety of tumors, preferably in a carefully controlled manner. In further phase III trials, dose and schedule adjustments and combinations with other treatments are compared for relative efficacy. Because of the inherent variability in the growth rates and responsiveness of tumors of similar histology, large numbers of patients are needed to evaluate in such studies. Furthermore, because so many factors can influence the natural history of tumors, concurrent controlled trials in which patients are randomly allocated to groups receiving the two treatments being compared are optimal for determining the effectiveness of various treatments.

Mechanism of Action of Various Chemotherapeutic Agents

Alkylating Agents

Many drugs used in chemotherapy are alkylating agents (Table 31–2). These are bifunctional or multifunctional compounds with reactive electron-negative groups appropriately spaced to form adducts with macromolecules. Their ultimate toxicity may be mechanical insofar as the alkylating agents cross-link side groups of nucleic acids and proteins, thereby impairing their biological functions, such as transcription, translation, replication, and enzymatic activity.

The differences between these drugs in clin-ical terms largely rest in their routes of administration, rates and onset of action, and mechanisms of elimination, which, in some instances, influence their toxicity. For example, cyclophosphamide itself is not an alkylating agent, but it is converted by the liver microsomal system into phosphoramide mustard, an alkylating compound. Also, unlike other alkylating agents, the alkylating agents derived from cyclophosphamide are excreted in the urine. Contact of these compounds with the bladder can cause a hemorrhagic cystitis and possibly bladder cancer. In contrast to other alkylating agents, cyclophosphamide is relatively selective in its bone marrow toxicity and does not suppress megakaryocyte turnover to the degree obtained with other aklylating agents.

The general toxicity of alkylating agents for normal cells involves inhibition of growth of relatively rapidly dividing stem cells in the bone marrow, skin (especially the hair follicles), and the gastrointestinal tract. Not surprisingly, their principal side effects are pancytopenia, hair loss, and ulceration of mucous membranes. Some alkylating agents have particular side effects.

More by convention than anything else, different alkylating agents are used to treat different diseases. When rapid tumor destruction is neither necessary nor possible, as for example in multiple myeloma, the convenience of oral administration of medication is a factor in the selection of melphalan as the treatment of

Table 31-2. Alkylating Agents

Alkylating Agent	Route of Administration	Usual Use	Unique Toxicity
Mechlorethamine	IV	Hodgkin's disease	
Chlorambucil	Oral	Chronic lymphatic leukemia	
Cyclophosphamide	Oral or IV	Non-Hodgkin's lymphomas, solid tumors	Hemorrhage cystitis
Melphalan	Oral	Multiple myeloma	
Nitrosoureas	Oral or IV	Lymphomas, solid tumors	Renal damage
Busulfan	Oral	Chronic granulocytic leukemia	Pulmonary fibrosis
Procarbazine	Oral	Lymphomas	
Cisplatin	IV	Solid tumors, lymphomas	Auditory nerve damage

choice. Once a malignancy becomes resistant to the action of a particular alkylating agent, others prove ineffective as well, suggesting that the final biochemical cytotoxic effect is the same for all such agents.

Antimetabolites

Chemicals that inhibit specific enzymes required for the survival of tumor stem cells are antimetabolites (Table 31-3). The relevant metabolic pathways are dedicated to the synthesis of RNA and DNA, and the compounds used are generally analogues of normal substrates of these pathways. The toxic complications of antimetabolites are generally very similar to those of alkylating agents.

Folic acid is a methyl group donor for the conversion of deoxyuridine-5'-phosphate (dUMP) to thymidine-5'-phosphate (dTMP), a precursor of thymidine triphosphate (TTP) and the thymine base of DNA. The chemotherapeutic antimetabolite methotrexate is a folic acid analogue that binds competitively to the enzyme tetrahydrofolate reductase. Inhibition of this enzyme prevents the conversion of folic acid to tetrahydrafolic acid, the active form of the vitamin. One feature of methotrexate treatment is that it is possible within a few hours after administration of the drug to give formyl tetrahydrofolate, also known as folinic acid or citrovorum factor. This compound is distal to the metabolic block and can reverse the toxic effects of the methotrexate. Rescue with citrovorum factor has been used after administration of very large doses of methotrexate. This strategy, which uses grams of intravenous methotrexate (the usual dose being measured in milligrams), followed by orally administered folinic acid, is effective against some neoplasms. Most methotrexate given in this way is excreted by the kidneys and, because of the high concentrations involved, can precipitate in the nephrons, especially at acid pH, causing renal damage. Therefore, renal function must be normal before attempting such treatment, and vigorous hydration and alkalinization of the urine with sodium bicarbonate should be attempted.

Purine and pyrimidine bases containing sulfhydryl groups or other substituents can be incorporated into and lead to the formation of abnormal DNA or RNA, which are ineffective for cell survival. Cytosine arabinoside, 6-mercaptopurine, and 6-thioguanine are examples of this class of antimetabolites and are used in the treatment of acute leukemia. 5-Fluorouracil is an agent used in the treatment of solid tumors, and azathioprine is an antimetabolite used for immunosuppression in the treatment of autoimmune disorders and for organ transplantation.

The efficacy of purine antagonists depends on the uptake and phosphorylation of the analogues. Resistance to these agents may in part

Table 31-3. Antimetabolites

Antimetabolites	Route of Administration	Mechanism of Action	Usual Use	Usual Toxicity
Methotrexate	Oral or IV	Inhibition of tetrahydrofolate reductase	Lymphatic leukemias, solid tumors	Hepatic cirrhosis (rare)
6-Mercaptopurine	Oral or IV	Inhibition of DNA synthesis	Acute leukemias	Hepatic
6-Thioguanine	Oral or IV	Inhibition of DNA synthesis	Acute leukemias	Hepatic
6-Azacytidine	Oral or IV	Inhibition of DNA synthesis	Acute nonlymphocytic leukemias	Hepatic
Azathioprine	Oral	Converted to GMP in vivo	Immunosuppression	Hepatic
5-Fluorouracil	IV	Inhibition of thymidilate synthase	Solid tumors	
Cytosine arabinoside	Continuous IV infusion	DNA polymerase	Acute nonlymphocytic leukemias	

derive from the induction in tumor stem cells of phosphatases, which dephosphorylate the base analogues, thereby preventing their incorporation into DNA. Cytosine arabinoside is rapidly deaminated and must therefore be infused rapidly or continuously. Another interaction of importance is the inactivation of 6-mercaptopurine by the enzyme xanthine oxidase. Allopurinol, a xanthine oxidase inhibitor, is often given to patients with neoplasms to prevent urate overproduction resulting from cell lysis and release of purines. Allopurinol can therefore delay inactivation of 6-mercaptopurine, causing a normal dose to become toxic. Methotrexate is a competitive inhibitor of tetrahydrofolate reductase; therefore, a mechanism of resistance of tumor stem cells is the production of greater amounts of the enzyme. Indeed, in cultured cells resistant to methotrexate, it is possible to document the presence of reduplicated DNA segments coding for the tetrahydrofolic acid reductase enzyme.

Antibiotics

Compounds with antitumor actions originally extracted from living organisms are classified as antibiotics. These compounds act as cell toxins by diverse methods.

Vinca Alkaloids. The vinca alkaloids are compounds isolated from the periwinkle plant. The active principles are vincristine and vinblastine. The known biochemical actions of these agents are that they bind with very high affinity to the cell protein tubulin and inhibit the assembly of this protein into microtubules, one of the cell's important fiber systems that in particular forms the mitotic spindle. Because these compounds bind to the ends of preformed microtubules, substoichiometric quantities can profoundly affect the balance between assembled and unpolymerized tubulin in cells.

The toxicity of the two vinca alkaloids used in practice differs. Vinblastine is primarily suppressive to the bone marrow, whereas vincristine produces a dose-dependent neuropathy. This neuropathy is both sensory and motor and may be manifested initially by paresthesias in the toes, followed by loss of deep tendon reflexes in the ankles and then difficulty with gait. Automatic neuropathy may occur, leading to constipation and even ileus. The neuropathy is reversed after cessation of treatment, although the remission of symptoms may be slow.

Anthracycline Compounds. These antibiotics are brightly colored multiple-ring chemicals with conjugated sugars. They have two known effects: (1) they bind directly to cellular DNA; and (2) they appear to generate toxic oxygen metabolites, and may thereby damage cells by a process analogous to the microbicidal effect of activated phagocytes or the indirect effects of radiation therapy.

The anthracyclines are toxic to rapidly growing cells, especially the bone marrow and hair follicles. Anthracyclines, like nitrogen mustard, are very toxic to subcutaneous tissues and cause extensive necrosis if extravasation occurs during an intravenous infusion. The most troublesome toxicity unique to anthracyclines is damage to the heart. The mechanism for this relatively specific toxicity has not been established. This toxicity is expressed as heart failure, which occurs when a critical cumulative dose is exceeded. Although the critical dose can be approximated below which cardiac failure is rare, the threshold for a given patient is impossible to predict. Furthermore, there is no simple test that currently permits the physician to predict that congestive heart failure is impending in a given patient. Therefore, the dose of anthracyclines must be restricted to the population threshold for most patients and reduced further or avoided for patients with preexisting cardiac disease. Because anthracyclines are very effective broad-spectrum chemotherapeutic agents, this cardiac damage is frustrating.

Bleomycin. A mixture of sulfur-containing polypeptides, bleomycin has been shown to sever DNA strands. Its principal advantage is its lack of bone marrow toxicity; it has been used for the treatment of lymphomas. It causes allergic reactions and skin and pulmonary toxicity.

Hormones Used in the Treatment of Hematological Diseases

Corticosteroids

Natural and synthetic glucocorticoids are used in the treatment of leukemias, Hodgkin's disease, and non-Hodgkin's lymphomas. They are also frequently used in hematology for immunosuppression of autoimmune disorders. Glucocorticoids have many actions on many organ systems. Their ability to kill lymphoid cells appears to be associated with their binding to cytoplasmic receptors, which then go into the nucleus. Beyond this, their mode of action is unknown. The limiting factor in corticosteroid therapy is the myriad of side effects (Table 31-4) associated with Cushing's syndrome, the name granted to the endogenous overproduction of glucocorticoids.

Androgens

In addition to the use of androgens in the treatment of bone marrow failure, androgens are occasionally useful in the palliative treatment of breast cancer.

Enzymes

Theoretically, a selective nutritional requirement of tumor stem cells could be exploited by depriving the system of that nutrient. Acute lymphoid leukemia cells, unlike normal cells, have a requirement for the amino acid asparagine. Because infusion of the bacterial enzyme asparaginase can effectively starve acute lymphatic leukemia cells, it is used in the treatment of human acute lymphatic leukemia. Such enzyme preparations, if contaminated with other bacterial substances, can lead to allergic reactions and other toxic effects, including acute pancreatitis and disorders of the coagulation system.

Toxicity of Chemotherapeutic Drugs

Side effects of chemotherapy are listed in Tables 31-2 through 31-4. Certain common toxic manifestations of chemotherapy deserve elaboration.

Bone Marrow Failure

The willingness to accept bone marrow failure during chemotherapy is a relative matter. In an attempt to induce a complete remission

Table 31-4. Side Effects of Chemotherapy

Hormone	Use in Hematology	Side Effects
Glucocorticosteroids	Therapy of lymphoid neoplasms Immunosuppression Therapy of hypercalcemia Therapy of malignant disease	Fluid retention Hypokalemia Osteoporosis Myopathy Aseptic necrosis of the femoral head Protein catabolism Hirsutism Dental atrophy and purpura Mental alterations Neutrophilia caused by inhibition of phagocyte function Suppression of lymphoid function
Androgens	Therapy of breast cancer Therapy of bone marrow failure	Fluid retention Virilization Liver toxicity Erythrocytosis

in the acute leukemias, total bone marrow failure is a planned integral part of the treatment, and the risk of bleeding and infection and the supportive measures directed against these risks are usually acceptable. In contrast, for other hematological malignancies, such profound bone marrow suppression is not warranted; the physician monitors the numbers of peripheral red blood cells, platelets, and granulocytes to ascertain whether an occasional patient is having an extraordinarily profound bone marrow effect from the treatment. This effect may occur in patients receiving chemotherapy who have previously received radiation therapy to large areas of the bone marrow. It may be necessary in such cases to reduce dosages of drugs.

An aspect of hematology that is presently quite interesting and exciting is the possibility that hematopoietic hormones such as GM-CSF, G-CSF, and M-CSF (Ch. 1) may shorten the duration of chemotherapy-induced bone marrow failure by increasing the rate of repopulation of normal blood cell progenitors. Early research indicates that this is the case, and the theoretical concern that these growth factors might stimulate neoplastic cell proliferation has not yet been borne out.

Carcinogenesis

Certain chemotherapeutic agents have the property of inflicting sublethal damage on normal stem cells, eventually causing evolution to a malignant state. Acute nonlymphocytic leukemia is the most frequent neoplasm to arise after chemotherapy. Alkylating agents are especially active in this regard, and risk of chemotherapy increases if ionizing radiation was included in the treatment. The increasing effectiveness of chemotherapy in the treatment of certain cancers has allowed more patients to live long enough to manifest the carcinogenic complication of their earlier therapy. Recognition of this complication of chemotherapy has led therapists to try to establish the minimal treatment required to eradicate malignant disease and minimize the carcinogenic risk.

Metabolic Effects of Tumor Killing

When chemotherapy or radiation therapy work effectively against a large mass of tumor cells, the body may be exposed to the debris released by the dead and dying cancer cells. One troublesome component is uric acid, which accumulates as a result of breakdown of tumor cell nucleic acids. Uric acid can deposit in the joints and other tissues, producing gout or causing renal stones and even urinary outflow obstruction. Treatment of this complication includes liberal administration of fluids in order to maintain urine flow and dilute the uric acid concentration. Maintenance of an alkaline urinary pH level by means of sodium bicarbonate can also minimize precipitation of the uric acid. However, uric acid accumulation can be prevented by priming patients with allopurinol before instituting chemotherapy. Allopurinol functions as an inhibitor of xanthine oxidase— the enzyme responsible for converting purines to uric acid (at the steps where hypoxanthine is changed to xanthine, and subsequently to uric acid).

In the occasional case of excessive tumor lysis, cellular destruction can lead to hyperkalemia, hyperphosphatemia, and hypocalcemia.

Nausea and Vomiting

Both chemotherapy and radiation therapy can cause nausea and vomiting. The cause of this disagreeable side effect is multifactorial. Direct damage to the gastrointestinal mucosa can play a role. Perturbation of certain areas of the brain stem—one being called the chemoreceptor trigger zone—and of the vestibular system may be involved. Finally, a conditioning effect takes place once patients come to dread the nausea and vomiting of treatment: They may actually begin to retch at the thought of an appointment with the physician. Unfortunately, there are no foolproof answers to these problems. Antihistamines, phenothiazines, anticholinergic antiemetics, corticosteroids, and butyrophemones are useful in some patients.

Sedation with barbiturates and minor tranquilizers such as lorazepam may reduce the agony and the memory of nausea and vomiting, especially in the case of drugs showing a high incidence of this complaint. The alkylating agents, especially nitrogen mustard, nitrosoureas, cisplatin, and procarbazine, are particularly problematic in this regard. Care must be taken not to oversedate; otherwise the patient runs the risk of aspirating gastric contents into the lungs while vomiting. Some patients, particularly young people, may obtain relief from nausea and vomiting if given tetrahydrocannabinol, the active principle of the marijuana plant. Older persons tend to find the cerebral effects of this drug unpleasant. Psychiatric assistance and hypnosis can be useful in dealing with the conditioning aspects of nausea and vomiting.

Malnutrition

Patients with cancer are very concerned with nutrition, having been conditioned about the wasting caused by the disease. Alimentation can be disturbed by the nausea and vomiting associated with therapy, problems with chewing and swallowing resulting from cases in which radiotherapy has been delivered to the head and neck, and from anxiety. In addition, there is considerable speculation as to the nutritional aspects of cancer. A very vocal and persuasive group has promoted the idea that nutritional imbalances and deficiencies are of great importance in the causation and spread of malignancies. Although these theories currently have debatable scientific merit, patients with neoplasms are often aware of these ideas and are concerned about them. Therefore, the physician should be sympathetic to the patient's nutritional concerns. A nutritionist is a valuable ally in the treatment team and can advise the physician and the patient about types of feeding useful for a given patient. In some cases the use of total parenteral nutrition, the infusion of needed calories and vitamins by the intravenous route, may be appropriate.

Immunotherapy

It would be helpful if the immune system could deal with tumor stem cells as well as it handles microorganisms. Immune destruction of tumor cells would have the advantage over most current anticancer treatments of not requiring that the target cells be especially active or in cycle.

Unfortunately, human cancer cells appear to be too much a version of self to be perceived as foreign and disposed of by immunological defenses. This ability of tumors to avoid detection by the immune system exists despite the fact that many tumor cells do have unique surface antigens. In an effort to make use of these antigens, attempts were made to stimulate the immune system in a general way by administering relatively nontoxic microbial products such as the bacillus Calmette-Guerin (BCG). It was hoped that the "angry" immune system consisting of lymphocytes and macrophages activated by the microbial materials would now eliminate tumor cells. This nonspecific immunotherapy seemed beneficial in a few cases, but on the whole was not very successful.

Monoclonal antibodies have the theoretical advantage of very great specificity for unique tumor antigens. The antibodies could then target tumor cells for killing by the body's immunological effector mechanisms. Alternatively, these antibodies can be tagged with chemotherapeutic agents or toxins. This approach takes advantage of a limitation of "straight" antibody therapy—the problem of antigenic modulation (see Ch. 29). Tumor cells, like lymphocytes and phagocytes, can internalize surface antigens reacted with antibodies, thereby removing from their surfaces the signals needed for immunological destruction. However, if the surface-bound antibodies contain toxins, these entities could be brought into the cell like Trojan horses. Unfortunately, the theoretically appealing elements of monoclonal antibodies as antitumor agents have only rarely been realized at the practical level.

Other "Biological" Therapies

Reference has been made in other chapters to the responsiveness of certain neoplasms to "natural" products of the body. These include hairy cell leukemia, which can remit during therapy with α-interferon; chronic granulocytic leukemia, which can be controlled by either α- or γ-interferons; and a very few cases of non-Hodgkin's lymphoma, which have responded to γ-interferon. The mechanisms by which these antiviral agents affect neoplasms are unknown. The interferons can be shown to inhibit the growth of cells in tissue culture, and such antiproliferative effects may be one of their antineoplastic actions. On the other hand, they also activate mononuclear phagocytes, and it may be that they enhance other aspects of host responses to the tumor.

Another "biological response modifier" under study is interleukin 2. This lymphokine (Ch. 1), among other effects, activates natural killer cells to increased cytotoxicity against a variety of tumors in tissue culture and has caused some striking regressions of solid tumors, notably renal cell cancers and melanomas. Unfortunately, interleukin 2 is very toxic, causing, among other effects, impressive capillary permeability leading to serious body fluid shifts, such that intensive nursing care has been required to care for patients receiving this agent.

OVERVIEW

The treatment of the hematological malignancies—the leukemias and lymphomas, and, when specialists act as medical oncologists, the solid tumors—is in a continuing state of evolution. Improved therapeutic strategies are best sought in well-designed controlled therapy trials in which large numbers of patients are enrolled. Although only a few large medical centers will have enough patients to test hypotheses regarding treatment, cooperative treatment groups have been organized to include participation of physicians with relatively small practices in such studies. Participating physicians must be willing to take the time required to obtain laboratory data and record results of therapy. They must also be sufficiently motivated to convince a patient to enter the protocol, pointing out that the patient's individual interests, as well as posterity, are well served and dispelling the notion that the patient is merely a guinea pig. Patients and physicians alike are understandably desirous of the "best" treatment, but both must be made to understand that it takes therapeutic trials to establish the "best" therapy as fact rather than opinion.

Few therapies can be considered routine. The treatment plan against lymphomas, solid tumors, and occasionally the leukemias may require surgery to make the diagnosis, and, in the case of solid tumors, as treatment. Radiation therapy will often be required in the treatment plan. Nursing and social service personnel are part of the team as well. This interdisciplinary approach requires intensive cross-consultation among members of the therapeutic unit to arrive at an integrative treatment that is best for a given patient. In this consortium of expertise, however, someone must act as the primary physician to guide the discussion and keep very close track of the patient and his or her family. In the case of hematological malignancies, the hematologist or hematologist–oncologist will often have this role, although an internist or other generalist may take it on with assistance from specialists.

The treatment of a localized or of a slowly evolving malignancy may be relatively straightforward and create little morbidity. But the therapy of many hematological malignancies constitutes an extreme physical, emotional, and economic strain on the patient and the patient's family. The physician must mobilize all necessary resources to deal with the problems that arise. The physician has to use all measures of support to anticipate and deal with the physical complications of the diseases and treatment. The primary physician must also be prepared to manage patiently the patient's anxieties and those of the patient's family. The patient must be encouraged occasionally to bear up when appropriate and forge ahead with the sometimes grueling and disagreeable aspects of therapy. Sometimes assistance from social service personnel may be helpful in dealing with economic problems and in minimizing the disruptive effects of the disease on the family. For example, with help from visiting nursing services, it may be possible to avoid repeated visits to the medical center. Honestly appraised, the practice of hematology is no more depressing than that of many other specialties of internal medicine. Nevertheless, experience has shown that it is helpful for members of the treatment team to discuss their feelings about some of the very ill patients and about the terminal illnesses of patients with each other and with interested psychiatrists.

Patients with malignancy especially fear pain. There is no excuse in nearly all cases for this fear to become a reality. Pain often arises from the infiltration and disruption of normal tissues by malignant cells and from penetration of nerve roots. Both processes can be amplified by anxiety. Pain medication should not be withheld or limited out of fear of addiction. Medication should usually be given by a regular schedule to control pain rather than "as needed," because the patient may be too frightened, concerned about addiction, or inca-

pable of making the appropriate requests. The effectiveness of opiates and other pain medications can be enhanced by the appropriate use of tranquilizing drugs.

Despite spectacular advances in the management of hematological malignancies and the increasing proportion of "cures," many patients will die as a result of their disease. The goal of the physician should be to make the patient's remaining life as useful and comfortable as possible. Although a discussion of terminal care is beyond the scope of this text, common sense dictates that intelligent and supportive palliative treatment should be as challenging and rewarding to the physician as curative treatment.

SUGGESTED READINGS

Berger, N.A. (1986) Cancer chemotherapy: New strategies for success. J. Clin. Invest. *78*:1131.

Casarett, A.P. (1968) Radiation Biology. Prentice-Hall, Englewood Cliffs, NJ.

Coldman, A.J., Goldie, J.H. (1987) Impact of dose-intense chemotherapy on the development of permanent drug resistance. Semin. Oncol. *14* (Suppl):29.

Croop, J.M., Gros, P. & Housman, D.E. (1988) Genetics of multidrug resistance. J. Clin. Invest. *81*:1303.

Legha, S.S. (1988) Tamoxifen in the treatment of breast cancer. Ann. Intern. Med. *109*:219.

Bone Marrow Transplantation

The replacement of failed, abnormally functioning, or malignant bone marrow with normal marrow is a relatively recent achievement. Its accomplishment and increasing utility grew out of the following developments. First, except for autologous marrow transplantation (i.e., the procedure of saving a patient's own marrow stem cells in a frozen state and infusing them back to the donor at a later time), it was necessary to overcome the problems of graft rejection and graft-versus-host disease. Second, it was necessary to gain sufficient experience with the procedure to learn what factors affect the outcome. This information, together with careful documentation of the natural history of diseases in which marrow grafting was contemplated, have begun to inform us as to when and for whom marrow transplantation is indicated. Although growing in successes and scope, bone marrow transplantation requires a considerable investment in hospital personnel, space, support resources, and laboratory expertise. It is therefore currently a high-technology activity of hematology.

IMMUNOLOGY OF BONE MARROW TRANSPLANTATION

Histocompatibility

The factors determining the probability of engraftment of bone marrow from another person, known as *allotransplantation*, are more or less the same as those that influence the acceptance of kidney or other solid organ allografts. The principal factors are the ability to avoid or suppress the expression of a cell-mediated immune response against the graft, or by the graft against the host. In these immune responses, the structures recognized as nonself by the immune system, primarily T lymphocytes, are histocompatibility antigens on the surfaces of the cells of engrafted organs. These antigens, first identified on the surfaces of lymphocytes, are designated human lymphocyte antigens, or HLA.

HLA are in large part defined in the laboratory by their reactivity with specific antibodies against them. The antibodies are found in the serum of persons who have been exposed to foreign tissues: women who have had numerous pregnancies, persons who have had many blood transfusions, and others who have rejected tissue grafts. The reactivity of the antibodies with lymphocytes is documented by their capacity to bind to target lymphocytes and fix the entire complement cascade to the lymphocyte membrane, thereby causing it to leak. This leakage can be detected by measuring the release of intracellular constituents labeled with radioactive chromium or by observing for the seepage of certain dyes into the cell from the extracellular medium. The result of years of cooperative effort involving many laboratories that accumulated antisera and reacted them with lymphocytes of several generations of multiple families has generated a descriptive panel of HLA antibodies that define corresponding antigens. This information has been supplemented with data on the genetic distribution of various cellular enzymes and plasma proteins known to be coded by particular genes. On the basis of this collection of data, it is evident that HLA are encoded by DNA on the short arm of the sixth chromosome. The positions of different HLA variants on this chromosome have been mapped (Fig. 32-1).

The HLA system has been divided into four major groups: HLA-A, HLA-B, HLA-C, and HLA-D. Groups A–C, also known as class I histocompatibility antigens, are defined by the complement-fixing reactions described above. These HLAs are expressed on the surfaces of T and B lymphocytes. These structures are composed of two polypeptide chains: a large one that spans the membrane bilayer from the cytoplasmic to the extracellular surface, and a small one that is totally external to the cell. This smaller polypeptide is also called β_2 microglobulin because it was recognized first

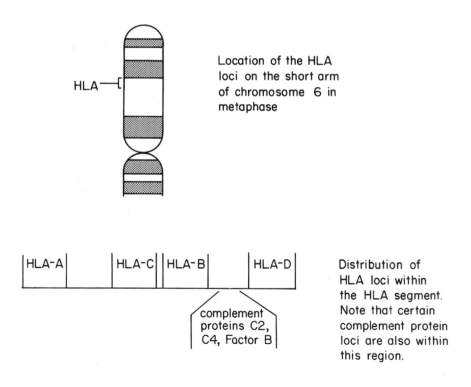

Location of the HLA loci on the short arm of chromosome 6 in metaphase

Distribution of HLA loci within the HLA segment. Note that certain complement protein loci are also within this region.

Fig. 32-1. Chromosome 6 map showing loci relevant for histocompatibility.

as a circulating plasma protein, presumably shed from cell surfaces. A particular HLA phenotype expressed on cell surfaces is the result of codominant Mendelian inheritance. For example, if the maternal HLA type is ab and the paternal type is cd, the offspring can end up ac, ad, bc, or bd. The inheritance of HLA is complicated by genetic crossovers that, as expected, occur in proportion to the distance between the alleles on the sixth chromosome.

The D allele of the HLA system, also designated class II, is different from the others, because its definition is based on a more complex biological phenomenon, the mixed lymphocyte response (MLR). In other words, the cell surface configuration expressed by this allele is too subtle to be recognized by specific complement-fixing antibodies. Rather, its detection requires the active participation of lymphocytes. The HLA-D antigen appears to be expressed uniquely on the surface of B lymphocytes. If B lymphocytes of one person are genetically different at the D determinant from those of another person and are mixed with the nonidentical person's T lymphocytes, several days' cultivation of the mixture of lymphocytes will cause the T lymphocytes to undergo a blastogenic response. This response is detected by means of a stimulation of incorporation of radioactive thymidine into the lymphocyte DNA.

The MLR is especially important for bone marrow transplantation, because HLA compatibility is required both for the complement-fixation-determined antigens and the MLR-related antigens in order for an acceptable probability of engraftment to occur. This strict compatibility is not so necessary in kidney allografting. However, even "perfect" matching of nonidentical twins with respect to the HLA and MLR antigens does not invariably ensure engraftment or prevent graft-versus-host disease. Clearly, as yet undefined antigens must evoke immunological recognition, therefore, except for identical twins, some degree of immunosuppression is necessary to ensure successful transplantation. Nevertheless, improvements in immunosuppressive therapy have permitted the transplantation of marrow from increasingly less well-matched donors. Indeed, a national registry has been established to permit transplant centers to identify potential donors for recipients lacking sufficiently histocompatible siblings or other relatives.

Technology of Marrow Grafting

Insofar as most candidates for marrow transplantation suffer from immunodeficiency or decreased numbers or function of phagocytes (i.e., impaired phagocyte activity), they are susceptible to infection. Therefore, an initial supportive effort is often required to eradicate existing infection and to place the patient in a protected environment in which further infection can be avoided. If thrombocytopenia and bleeding are occurring as part of the underlying disease, appropriate transfusions are given, although only if absolutely necessary in order to minimize immunization against antigens that could compromise the graft.

Hematopoietic stem cells can "home" from the blood to the bone marrow. For reconstitution of lymphoid stem cells, as few as a half-million to 1 million nucleated bone marrow cells will suffice. To establish an entire hematopoietic stem, 10 times more cells are needed. These numbers of cells can be obtained from 50 to 500 ml of bone marrow. This quantity of marrow cells is easily derived from multiple aspirates of the pelvic bone marrow. This procedure must be performed with the subject under general anesthesia. The anticoagulated samples procured are strained through steel mesh to remove bone spicules and fat aggregates; they are then infused into the histocompatible recipient.

The preparation required of the recipient for this infusion depends on the disease being treated and on the degree of immunological compatibility between donor and recipient. For the ideal case of a transplant between identical twins for the treatment of severe combined immune deficiency, no preparation is required. For the much more common setting of transplants between HLA-identical and MLR-non-reactive siblings for immune deficiency, bone marrow aplasia, or leukemia, varying degrees of immunosuppression and sometimes total marrow irradiation of the recipient are required. In establishing immunological competency in the patient with severe combined immune deficiency, the major problem in the immunodeficient recipient is graft-versus-host disease, rather than graft rejection. Therefore, the strategy is to administer immunosuppressive drugs after the beginning of engraftment, giving enough treatment to try to prevent graft-versus-host disease without compromising the growth and differentiation of the lymphoid graft.

In the case of replacement of narrow hematopoietic stem cells to a failed bone marrow, more vigorous immunosuppression is necessary to inhibit graft rejection and graft-versus-host disease. The potent immunosuppressive drug *cyclosporine* (which acts on T cells), methotrexate, and alkylating agents are commonly used. A technique used to gain initial immunosuppression without compromising the viability of the graft is to give a transfusion of "buffy coat" cells from the donor before the marrow infusion, followed by an immunosuppressive drug. The buffy coat is the leukocyte- and platelet-rich interface between the red cells and plasma of a unit of whole blood after centrifugation. The goal is to expose the recipient's immune system to any antigens in donor blood cells that might be foreign. The lymphoid cells responding to the antigens begin to undergo "blast" transformation, a state in which they have an increased susceptibility to toxic therapy. This flushing out of potentially reactive lymphocytes permits them to be exposed to a vigorous dose of immunosuppressive therapy at a time when this treatment does not compromise the graft. Even after infusion of the marrow, at some point immunosuppressive treatment in more moderate amounts is given to suppress rejection and graft-versus-host disease. Another strategy is

to deplete cytotoxic T-cells from a donor's bone marrow aspirated for reconstitution of a recipient.

The most recent use of total marrow reconstitution has been as therapy for genetic diseases and leukemia. Genetic bone marrow disorders treated by means of this approach have included the Wiskott-Aldrich syndrome, severe congenital neutropenia, and severe neutrophil functional disorders. Bone marrow transplantation was initially attempted in patients with acute leukemia after several relapses, but more recently it is being evaluated as earlier therapy for acute nonlymphocytic leukemia for young adult patients with acute lymphatic leukemia in remission and, most recently, chronic granulocytic leukemia. In this setting, an additional requirement is the need to destroy completely the malignant or genetically abnormal stem cells from the recipient's bone marrow. This sterilization of the bone marrow is often accomplished by means of total-body irradiation.

After conditioning and infusion of the donor's marrow, a period of waiting and supportive care follows. In the case of severe combined immune deficiency, donor T lymphocytes appear in the blood within 2 weeks of transplantation. By 1 to 2 months, the recipient demonstrates the capacity to mount specific immune responses, and immunoglobulins are synthesized.

In the setting of transplantation for marrow failure, genetic disease, or leukemia, the appearance of reticulocytes and nucleated erythrocytes at about the sixth to tenth day heralds the beginning of expression of a successful graft. Phagocytes appear later, and platelets appear last, by about 4 weeks. Hematopoietic hormones (Ch. 1) accelerate the emergence of mature blood cells from an engrafted marrow. The failure of a graft to "take" usually means that immunological rejection has occurred. In this circumstance, a second attempt at transplantation with more vigorous immunosuppression may then be tried.

The increase in peripheral blood counts that

occurs after a transplantation attempt may not necessarily indicate engraftment. Rarely, the bone marrow recovers in idiopathic aplastic anemia after immunosuppressive therapy, possibly because the cause of such cases is an autoimmune reaction against the patient's own hematopoietic stem cells. In acute leukemia and for genetic disorders there is the possibility that the recovery of peripheral blood cells is actually a result of insufficient sterilization of the host marrow and reflects a return of the recipient's own blood cells. To document engraftment, it is possible to use a number of genetic markers of peripheral blood cells. If the transplant is from male to female or vice versa, the appearance or disappearance of the Y chromosome is useful. Most other tests for engraftment involve detecting changes in cell surface antigens such as blood groups by immunological procedures.

The overriding factor currently determining the success of a transplant is the availability of a histocompatible donor. A second consideration is the recipient's age. The older the recipient, the higher the incidence of graft-versus-host disease; the ability of the patient to withstand the complications of bone marrow failure declines with age as well. At present about half of patients with aplastic anemia who have received marrow transplants survive 2 to 3 years, whereas about 20 percent of untransplanted patients with this disease are alive after these intervals. These figures are mainly applicable to relatively young persons, because engraftment is rare (and therefore rarely attempted) in patients over 40 years of age. The survival data are best for patients under 20 years of age.

Future Possibilities of Bone Marrow Allotransplantation

If progress continues in surmounting immunological and other problems besetting bone marrow allografting, the uses of the treatment will expand. Marrow transplantation may be useful in restoring metabolic pathways to patients with certain inborn errors of metabolism and with storage diseases. As the knowledge of the immune system increases, more sophisticated immunological engineering may permit engraftment of marrow across histocompatibility barriers without immunosuppression. This achievement would dramatically increase the number of patients able to benefit from the procedure.

Autologous Marrow Therapy

Destruction of hematopoietic stem cells with resulting bone marrow failure is often a consequence of intensive therapy of hematologic and nonhematologic malignancy. This complication can limit the amount of antitumor treatment. In theory, if bone marrow stem cells could be removed before administration of chemotherapy or irradiation and returned to the patient afterward for engraftment, this limitation could be circumvented. The fact that it is now possible to preserve bone marrow stem cells indefinitely in a frozen state and the lack of immunological barriers to autotransplantation are attractive features of this therapeutic approach. However, two problems limit the success of this technology. First, the toxicity of anticancer therapy in high doses is such that organs other than the blood can be irreversibly damaged. Therefore, even if very high doses of treatment are given and the patient is hematologically reconstituted with autologous marrow, the treatment causes unacceptable damage to other organs. Second, there is often the possibility that the patient's bone marrow contains tumor stem cells as well as normal hematopoietic stem cells. Studies are being directed at eradicating such tumor cells from bone marrow samples by means of ex vivo chemotherapy or monoclonal antibody techniques. An exciting future direction for autologous bone marrow treatment will be the insertion of genes into bone marrow stem cells. This genetic engineering may be applicable to patients with congenital hemolytic disorders and other genetic diseases.

SUGGESTED READINGS

O'Reilly, R.J. (1986) New promise for autologous marrow transplants in leukemia. N. Engl. J. Med. *315*:186.

Thomas, E.D. (1987) Bone marrow transplantation. CA *37*:291.

Thomas, E.D. (1987) Bone marrow transplantation in hematologic malignancies. Hosp. Pract. Feb 15:77.

Index

Page numbers followed by t denote tables; those followed by f denote figures.